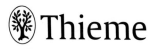

Dedication

To our parents, teachers, patients, students, and children, all of whom have given us so much.

Pocket Atlas of Chinese Medicine

Edited by

Marnae C. Ergil, MA, MS, LAc, Dipl. OM (NCCAOM)
Professor
Finger Lakes School of Acupuncture
and Oriental Medicine
New York Chiropractic College
Seneca Falls, NY, USA

Kevin V. Ergil, MA, MS, LAc, Dipl. OM (NCCAOM)
Associate Professor
Finger Lakes School of Acupuncture
and Oriental Medicine
New York Chiropractic College
Seneca Falls, NY, USA

With contributions by

Simon Becker, Dipl. Ac and CH
(SBO-TCM, NCCAOM)
President
Swiss Professional Organization for TCM
Waedenswil, Switzerland

Stephen Birch, PhD
The Stichting (Foundation) for the
Study of Traditional East Asian Medicine
(STEAM)
Amsterdam, the Netherlands

Mary Garvey, BA, PracDipAc, MHlthSci,
MLitt
College of Traditional Chinese Medicine
University of Technology Sydney
Sydney, Australia

Michael McCarthy, MA(ThB), LAc,
DipCHM, D-Tuina, MIRCHM, MTCMCI
Institute of East West Medical Sciences
Dublin, Ireland

Anne Reinard, BA
Luxembourg, Luxembourg

Yves Réquéna, MD
Private Practice
Aix-en-Provence, France

Professor Douglas Wile, PhD
Alverno College
Milwaukee, WI, USA

172 color plates

Thieme
Stuttgart · New York

Library of Congress Cataloging-in-Publication Data is available from the publisher.

Important note: Medicine is an ever-changing science undergoing continual development. Research and clinical experience are continually expanding our knowledge, in particular our knowledge of proper treatment and drug therapy. Insofar as this book mentions any dosage or application, readers may rest assured that the authors, editors, and publishers have made every effort to ensure that such references are in accordance with **the state of knowledge at the time of production of the book.**

Nevertheless, this does not involve, imply, or express any guarantee or responsibility on the part of the publishers in respect to any dosage instructions and forms of applications stated in the book. **Every user is requested to examine carefully** the manufacturers' leaflets accompanying each drug and to check, if necessary in consultation with a physician or specialist, whether the dosage schedules mentioned therein or the contraindications stated by the manufacturers differ from the statements made in the present book. Such examination is particularly important with drugs that are either rarely used or have been newly released on the market. Every dosage schedule or every form of application used is entirely at the user's own risk and responsibility. The authors and publishers request every user to report to the publishers any discrepancies or inaccuracies noticed. If errors in this work are found after publication, errata will be posted at www.thieme.com on the product description page.

© 2009 Georg Thieme Verlag,
Rüdigerstrasse 14, 70469 Stuttgart, Germany
http://www.thieme.de
Thieme New York, 333 Seventh Avenue,
New York, NY 10001, USA
http://www.thieme.com

Cover design: Thieme Publishing Group
Illustrator: Karin Baum, Paphos, Cyprus
Typesetting by Sommer Druck, Feuchtwangen, Germany
Printed in Germany by Offizin Andersen Nexö, Zwenkau

ISBN 978-3-13-141611-7

1   2   3   4   5   6

Acknowledgements

We would like to acknowledge the editorial and production team at Thieme Publishers, particularly Angelika Findgott and Anne Lamparter, for their patient and persistent commitment to the production of the *Pocket Atlas of Chinese Medicine*. We are also very grateful to Bob Felt of Paradigm Publications for supporting our involvement in this project. Given the history of its production, the fact that when we were invited on as editors and authors, it had already been in the works for some time, and that our initial contribution was to make its production take longer than originally intended, Angelika Findgott's determination to see this project emerge in print was fundamental to its publication and is a tribute to her vision and dedication.

We are grateful to the authors who have contributed their scholarship to this text. Simon Becker, Stephen Birch, Mary Garvey, Anne Reinard, and Yves Réquéna came to the project well before we did, and were good natured and generous with their time as the editorial and design characteristics of the book became clearer (especially to the editors) and revisions of already submitted chapters became necessary. Simon Becker kindly allowed his extensive and well-written contribution, in which he shares his comprehensive knowledge of Chinese medicine, to be substantially edited. We are also grateful to Doug Wile and Michael McCarthy, who joined the project later and contributed their substantial expertise to it.

We are indebted to the Finger Lakes School of Acupuncture and Oriental Medicine of the New York Chiropractic College, and to our colleagues for providing an environment that supports scholarship and the time-consuming endeavor of writing and editing. We thank Ai Zhong Li, PhD, LAc, who provided her expertise in guiding, and posed for many of the illustrations for the *tui na* chapter. We thank our students who contributed to the content of numerous photos.

Finally, we must recognize the extent to which this work as a whole, and particularly our work as authors, depends on the generosity of scholars, our teachers, patients, and students, who have kindly provided us with any actual knowledge or understanding that we might have about the tradition of Chinese medicine. We are particularly indebted to the profound and generous scholarship of Nigel Wiseman and Feng Ye. As editors we have endeavored to use Wiseman and Ye's standard glossary throughout the text, thereby making Chinese medicine terms transparent to the reader. As authors we relied heavily on Wiseman and Ye's *Fundamentals of Traditional Chinese Medicine*, and the *Practical Dictionary of Chinese Medicine.* In addition, we could not have proceeded without the works of Paul Unschuld, Tie Tao Deng, Yi Tian Ni, as well as others too numerous to mention here.

If, as is likely, there are any errors in this text, we, as editors and authors are entirely responsible for them.

Foreword

Chinese medicine belongs to all of us. People in all cultures value its perspectives. It is a distinctive treasure because its 2000 years of continuous—if often contrasting—commentary represent the best example of the subtlety and power emerging from the examination of human experience. Chinese herbalism is more sophisticated than other herbal traditions because the Chinese were persistent in observing and recording their experiences.

As Western society became familiar with Chinese medicine in the late 20th century, acupuncture was emphasized because it was an easy fit with the licensed, private practice professionalism characteristic of health care in the West. Related methods of acupressure, *qi gong*, and *tui na* were largely ignored. Acupuncture was progressively revised to emphasize the idea that mechanical action in a precise location creates a specific effect, a recasting of traditional acupuncture concepts into a linearity that felt comfortable to Westerners.

In actuality, acupuncture grows out of the profound nature of human touch and the relationship of vital energy between people. Locating points by touch is more effective than using purely anatomical guides, since the therapist feels the movement of *qi* just as a *qi gong* practitioner does, and is guided by the dynamic of sensation between patient and therapist.

Chinese medicine begins with an appreciation of life and vital energy (*qi*). When *qi* flows smoothly it provides balance and protection. Treatment enhances and facilitates the flow of *qi*. In an acupuncture treatment we help patients help themselves, by inviting *qi* to move as it needs to. From this perspective, the location of stimulus and the timing of sensations are considered valid according to the perceptions of patient and practitioner, rather than according to a static chart.

I was born with a bilateral cleft palate. Consequently, I owe my life to Western technological medicine. Most aspects of technological medicine involve surgery, prostheses, and testing, all of which have clear practical value and are easily integrated into different cultural paradigms. However, a cultural contrast is revealed when we compare Chinese medicine and Western pharmaceutical medicine.

In medical school we learned that disease is an alien process that needs to be attacked. We learned that the body itself is frequently the source of disease. As a consequence of this philosophy, most pharmaceuticals are designed to suppress one or another of the functions of components of our body. Significantly, pharmaceuticals which are not suppressive of physiological function, such as penicillin and digoxin, are derived from herbal traditions and incorporated into Western medicine.

As a clinician, I have observed that pharmaceutical medicine and its implicitly adversarial model can drain its practitioners. In contrast, Chinese medicine seems to have an invigorating effect on practitioners, perhaps because it recognizes, and uses, the experiences of the patient and the intuition of the therapist in each treatment. The clinician partners with the patient. Increased self awareness of the therapist can have a clear and beneficial impact on treatment outcome.

Western medical research seeks information about life by testing linear models of cause and effect. Greater accuracy depends on a lack of confounding variables, and a simple model: one action leads to one outcome. Only a limited number of variables can be traced statistically. While these analytical methods provide statistical power, they underestimate our body's complexity. The heart or lungs, which behave more like machines, are widely studied and well understood using this model. Parts of the body that have more layered functions, such as the liver and the flora of the intestinal lumen, are less well understood.

The Austrian philosopher Karl R. Popper asked us to focus on assertions that are specific enough so that it is possible to prove them false given the right kind of evidence. While this is appropriate in many settings, it does not apply to most biological situations, where the issues posed by high degrees of complexity challenge its reductive orientation. The evolution of life includes complexity and redundancy at every level and every moment of existence, posing real challenges to reductionistic models.

No survival traits could be more important than homeostasis, tissue repair, and the removal of toxins. We need to appreciate the body's healing intelligence as a product of evolution. Let me refer to my own clinical experience: I was asked to help a pregnant woman during an unproductive labor. I chose SP-6, a point on the lower leg commonly used to assist labor. I needled it, hoping for stronger labor. Instead, the patient fell asleep for 4 hours, woke up and delivered the baby in 2 hours. I made a suggestion; the body adapted and prioritized its processes according to its needs.

To summarize, there are three significant contrasts between Chinese medicine and Western medicine:

1) Chinese medicine builds upon active homeostatic bodily function. Western pharmaceutical medicine seeks balance by suppressing certain components of physiological systems.
2) Western research focuses on linear models, while Chinese medicine accepts the challenge of our complex biological world.
3) Chinese medicine is a welcoming context for long-term change and self development.

The editors, authors, and publisher of this beautiful book felt it was important to present a full, well-rounded picture of Chinese medicine and its engagement with health and disease. In today's world, we need a health care model that focuses on more complex bodily needs. I believe that this book offers a unique window on the ways in which Chinese medicine understands the world and the body. Thank you, Thieme, Marnae, and Kevin Ergil for helping us find a more open path to the future.

Michael Smith, MD
Director, Lincoln Recovery Center
Associate Professor of Psychiatry,
Cornell University
Founding Chairperson, National
Acupuncture Detoxification Association
Bronx, New York, USA

Preface

The *Pocket Atlas of Chinese Medicine* is a unique book and one that, we hope, will offer a rich overview of the history, theory, and practice of Traditional Chinese Medicine. The unique character of the book emerges out of two characteristics. The first is the distinct concept of the pocket atlas, which, by using very informative text pages coupled with related illustrations, provides an exceptionally vibrant and rich source of information that is also convenient to skim and sample as required by the reader. The second is that this book has been produced by experts in Chinese medicine who teach, study, and practice on three continents, signaling both the internal consistency of modern professional Chinese medicine and its distribution throughout the world.

What this book is and who it is for

This book is a comprehensive exposition of the history, theory, and practice of Chinese medicine as it is practiced today in China and throughout the world. It offers a concise and accurate discussion of Chinese medicine history, fundamental theory, diagnosis, acupuncture, traditional pharmacotherapy, *tui na*, *qi gong*, *tai ji quan*, Chinese dietetics, and acupuncture research. In writing and editing this book we sought to provide information that is fundamental to understanding the way in which Traditional Chinese Medicine is practiced with a degree of detail that is unusual in introductory texts. Each chapter offers a substantial amount of information in a format designed to support the reader with no knowledge of the subject, but with a depth from which we believe even the experienced practitioner will glean insights and information that are new to them.

While no chapter exhausts its subject, or can stand in place of the numerous standard references or texts that must be assimilated to cover each topic treated here, each chapter encompasses the core principles and complete structure of these theoretical and clinical domains providing the reader with a complete and faithful description of the topic.

Written to be accessible to any reasonably educated person who is interested in acquiring or deepening an understanding of Chinese medicine, the book is designed to be a resource for anyone who is unsatisfied with limited and limiting 'popular' books on the subject and who needs a broader and deeper understanding of Chinese medicine. We think that it will be of great value to students or professionals in any discipline who need a comprehensive overview of the field of Chinese medicine.

We wrote and edited with two particular audiences firmly in mind: students training to join our profession and professionals across a range of disciplines who desire a stronger understanding of Chinese medicine.

Students of Chinese medicine who need to lay a firm and broad foundation on which to build their future knowledge will benefit enormously from this book. The early stages of Chinese medicine studies involve engagement with huge amounts of information. Often this detail can obscure the structure that informs it. Those beginning their studies in Chinese medicine need to be able to understand the structure of the medicine and its therapeutic domains so that they can engage in systematic study from a more informed perspective. This book offers detailed discussions of key principles in an organized and efficient way.

The *Pocket Atlas of Chinese Medicine* supplies the physician, the pharmacist, the nurse, the chiropractor, and other traditional and non-traditional providers of health care with the level of information that professionals require for understanding without the extensive technical detail that is required for clinical practice. It is our hope that being able to engage the richness and complexity of this medicine more fully will help increase understanding, improve collaboration, and possibly improve the quality of research design where Chinese medicine is investigated in the West.

How to get the most from this book

This book is written as a series of distinct chapters and each chapter can be read in isolation. In fact some pages and groups of pages can be read as concise primers on specific ideas and topics. However, the book is intended to serve the reader best if it is read from beginning to end as, especially in the first three chapters, concepts are developed and linked to each other. An impatient reader can read the first three chapters on history, theory, and diagnosis, and then proceed to read about any of the therapeutic domains: acupuncture, herbal medicine, Chinese dietetics, *tui na*, *tai ji quan*, or *qi gong*.

As we wrote our chapters and worked with other authors, we incorporated the histories of three patients from Marnae's clinical practice (no accurate identifying information has been provided). These three patients—*Jeremy*, *John*, and *Alice*—are introduced in the chapter on diagnosis and are encountered in the chapters on acupuncture, *tui na*, and Chinese pharmacotherapy. We chose three patients who represented three important aspects of Chinese medicine and used them throughout the chapters to show how diagnostic and therapeutic thinking works in Chinese medicine. *John* has a chronic condition associated with aging and ill health, *Jeremy* is typical of many patients with an acute respiratory ailment, and *Alice* illustrates some perspectives on gynecological conditions. These patients do not represent the complete range of patients encountered in clinics or cared for with Chinese medicine, their conditions are not complex, but they do provide a sample of a typical outpatient population and offer the reader a window into the application of the clinical reasoning process in Chinese medicine.

Marnae C. Ergil and Kevin V. Ergil

Geneva, New York, USA

Table of Contents

1

History

Marnae C. Ergil

Introduction

The history of Chinese medicine is a history of China (**A**). Statements concerning the antiquity of Chinese medicine vary. Mythological histories assert a 5000-year-old tradition, while more scholarly works suggest a 2000-year-old tradition. The earliest written records are just over 2000 years old. It is not the actual age of Chinese medicine that is important, so much as the sense of history that is embodied in it. As political, social, and religious trends rose and fell, aspects were incorporated into a constantly changing and continually developing medical system. From early ancestor worship, to the systematization of Confucian thought and the Daoist search for immortality, from the reinterpretation of ancient classics to the introduction of the medical thought of the West; all of these, and more, influenced the traditional medicine of China and impacted the medicine that we now call Chinese medicine.

Today, a medicine that retains many aspects of these historical developments is practiced in China, Taiwan, Hong Kong, Japan, Singapore, Korea, Vietnam, and, more recently, in Europe, the United States, and Australia. As this medicine has traveled across the world, it has absorbed new ideas and continued its development. Medicine is not a static entity that comes into being and then never changes, and practitioners of traditional medical systems, just like those in biomedicine, will respond to new ideas and new theories. What is distinctive about Chinese medicine is that over its long development it has been able to incorporate the new ideas while also retaining older therapeutic and diagnostic perspectives.

The Creation of the World

As is true of any culture, there is a creation myth to explain the origins of the Chinese people. In China, the legend is the story of Pan Gu. One of the many legends of Pan Gu relates the story thus. In the beginning, the cosmos was a gas that solidified into a colossal stone. Out of a cosmic egg was born a creature named Pan Gu, who lived 18 000 years, growing 3 m (10 ft) a day, and spending his time chopping the stone into two parts, one of which became the heavens (*yang*) and the other the earth (*yin*). When Pan Gu completed his work and died, his head became the mountains, his breath the wind and clouds, his voice thunder, his left eye the sun, and his right eye the moon. His muscles and veins became the matrix of the earth and his flesh the soil. His hair and beard became the constellations and his skin and body hair became plants and trees. His teeth and bones became metals and his marrow became pearls and precious stones. His body became the rain and the lice upon him were impregnated by ether and became humans (Wong and Wu 1936).

Dynasty	Period
Xia	Ca. 2100–ca. 1600 BCE
Shang	Ca. 1600–ca. 1100 BCE

Zhou
  Western Zhou
  Eastern Zhou, including Spring and Autumn Period
	Ca. 1100–ca. 771 BCE
	770–475 BCE

Warring States	475–221 BCE
Qin	221–206 BCE
Han	206 BCE–220 CE
Three Kingdoms	220–265 CE
Western and Eastern Jin	265–420 CE
Northern and Southern Jin	420–581 CE
Sui	581–618 CE
Tang	618–907 CE
Five	907–960 CE
Northern and Southern Song	960–1270 CE
Jin	1115–1234 CE
Yuan	1271–1368 CE
Ming	1368–1644 CE
Qing	1644–1911 CE

Republic of China
  Mainland
  Taiwan
	1912–1949 CE
	1949 CE–present

People's Republic of China	1949 CE–present

Note: For a detailed outline of major medical events in the dynasties see pp. 50–51.

A Chinese dynasties. Note that many of the periods overlap. Dynasties were often established before the overthrow of an existing regime, or co-existed in different areas of China.

This myth is interesting because of the idea of Pan Gu's body furnishing the environment for life. One of the fundamental aspects of Chinese medicine is the recognition of a very close relationship between human physiology and the outer environment. As we explore Chinese history, we shall see that the health of the emperor's body was closely related to the health of the world (China), and if natural disasters occurred, then the emperor's relationship with the heavens was thought to be out of balance, causing illness in the world. This relationship between the earth and the body is an important element of the philosophy of Chinese medicine, and one that appears not only in medical theory but also in political theory and Chinese statecraft.

The Legendary Origins of Chinese Medicine

From approximately 2900 BCE, three legendary rulers were said to have governed China in succession. Each is closely associated with the creation of Chinese culture and Chinese medicine. They are Fu Xi (the Ox-tamer—**A**), Shen Nong (the Divine Husbandman—**B**) and Huang Di (the Yellow Emperor).

Fu Xi, said to have lived in 2953 BCE, was miraculously conceived and was born after a 12-year gestation period. He is said to have invented the first pic-ture symbols as a form of written communication, to have established rules of marriage, and to have taught fishing and the rearing of domestic animals. His contribution to medicine was the construction of the eight trigrams (*ba gua*—**C**) on which were based the *Book of Changes (Yi Jing* or *I Ching)*, and many of the principles of medical philosophy.

Shen Nong is said to have reigned from 2838–2698 BCE. He was the inventor of the plow and hoe, the inaugurator of settled agriculture, the founder of public markets, and most importantly, the purported author of the first materia medica, *The Divine Husbandman's Materia Medica (Shen Nong Ben Cao)*. He is said to have tasted 70 different kinds of plants, animals, or minerals in a single day, thereby establishing the art of herbal medicine (see p.224). In addition, Shen Nong expanded the usage of the eight trigrams developed by Fu Xi into the 64 hexagrams currently in use. Shen Nong is the patron god of herbalists and considered to be the father of herbal medicine. Traditionally, on the first and 15th day of each month, incense and offerings are put before his shrine and, in some places, a discount on all herbs is given on these days. Evidence indicates that the first materia medica was not actually written until the first century BCE, despite its attribution to Shen Nong.

A One of the three legendary rulers, Fu Xi (born 2953 BCE), is famous for establishing rules of conduct and how to live as a settled people, rather than as nomadic tribes. He is thought to have created the eight trigrams *(ba gua)* upon which many later philosophical and medical ideas were based.

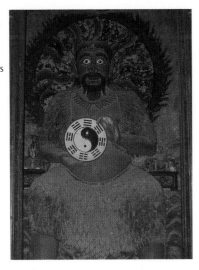

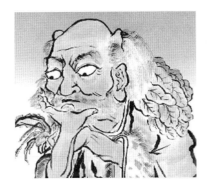

B Shen Nong. Shen Nong is said to have reigned from 2838–2698 BCE. As the mythical author of the *Divine Husbandman's Materia Medica,* he is the patron god of herbalists. He has been incorporated as a deity in the Daoist pantheon of gods.

C Ba gua. This version of the *ba gua* is referred to as the Sequence of Pre-Heaven. The trigrams are correlated with the four cardinal directions, with south at the top and north at the bottom. The trigram associated with south and summer is the trigram for heaven and the one for north and winter is the trigram for earth. The trigrams found opposite each other are meant to balance one other. This is the sequence that is said to have been arranged by Fu Xi. Other versions are commonly seen; however, this is the one that is considered to be the oldest version.

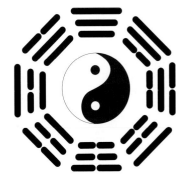

Huang Di (**A**) is perhaps the most widely recognized figure of Chinese medicine. Said to have lived from 2698 to 2598 BCE, he, along with his minister Qi Bo, is the mythical author of *The Yellow Emperor's Classic of Medicine (Huang Di Nei Jing)*—sometimes also called *The Yellow Emperor's Inner Classic*—the text to which future generations linked their ideas and theories and that continues to be cited today to support the practice of Chinese medicine. The first compilation is more correctly dated to ca. 200 BCE. The text is, in fact, a compilation of writings by many different people, and it has been edited and revised many times. However, it is in this book that the traditional medicine of China is first expressed in a form that is familiar to us today.

The text is divided into two books: the *Simple Questions (Su Wen)* (**B**) and the *Spiritual Pivot (Ling Shu)*, sometimes also known as the *Spiritual Axis*. The *Simple Questions* deals with medical theory such as the principles of *yin* and *yang* and the five phases and the *Spiritual Pivot* focuses on acupuncture and moxibustion. The two texts are written as a series of questions and answers between Huang Di and his advisor, Qi Bo. Qi Bo, like Shen Nong, is said to have tested the actions of drugs, cured people's sickness, and written books on medicine and medicinal therapeutics. Huang Di is also thought to have developed the art of silk-making, to have built the first boats, made the first carts, designed the bow and arrow, and created the written language. He is often called the "Father of the Chinese Nation."

The text that is attributed to the Yellow Emperor includes essays on such topics as:

- the *yin yang* doctrine
- the five-phase doctrine
- the body and its organs
- blood and *qi*
- the vessels
- pathogenic agents
- diseases
- examination
- invasive therapies
- substance therapies
- heat therapies

Credit for being the inventor of the traditional medicine of China is variously ascribed to any one of these three legendary rulers (see p. 4). In fact, probably none of the three actually existed but they serve the important function of explaining the origin of Chinese medicine. Shen Nong and Huang Di, and the texts that bear their names, continue to be important to the basic theory of Chinese medicine and are constantly referred to as the support for the theory and practice of Chinese medicine.

These essays show the diversity of material covered and, as many of these remain the major topics of discussion in Chinese medicine, also point to the continuity of the tradition.

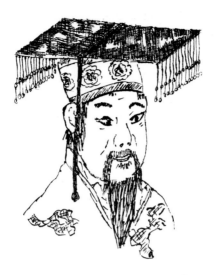

A Huang Di. Huang Di (the Yellow Emperor) is the mythical being who is said to have authored the text *The Yellow Emperor's Classic of Medicine (Huang Di Nei Jing)*. Actually, this text is a compilation of disjointed essays that have been edited and re-edited many times over the past 2000 years. However, this is still the text that modern practitioners cite to support the theory and practice of Chinese medicine.

"In former times there was Huang Di.
When he came to life, he had spirituality and magic power.
While he was [still] weak, he could speak.
While he was [still] young, he was quick of apprehension.
While he grew up, he was sincere and diligent.
When he had matured, he ascended to heaven."

(Cited in Unschuld 2003, p. 9)

B Quote from *Huang Di Nei Jing Su Wen*.

Early Archaeological Evidence— the Shang Dynasty

The Shang dynasty (ca. 1600–1100 BCE) is the first Chinese dynasty of which there is clear archaeological evidence. Of earlier peoples, there are stories, but no evidence to support them. Most likely, prior to the Shang, stone-age nomadic cultures were scattered around Northern China, with no central ruler. The Shang dynasty developed out of interaction between tribes, who then created a powerful and far-reaching authority. Among the archaeological evidence of the Shang are many artifacts, including what are called oracle bones, indicating that there were therapeutic activities occurring during this time.

Important to understanding these therapeutic activities is knowledge of some of the basic structures of Shang society. The first Chinese scripts were developed during this time, allowing information to be passed on. The Shang had clearly delineated social relationships. There was a king and nobility, and the society had become sedentary. Most importantly, there was a definite understanding that the living and the dead existed in an interdependent relationship. The dead required food from the living and the living were dependent upon the dead for health and well-being, for success or failure, and for a stable and beneficial climate. This relationship developed into the beginnings of ancestor worship, an idea that, in differing forms, has remained with the Chinese to the present. The relationship between the living and their ancestors was important to therapeutic

activity because this relationship mediated all events in life, including health and illness.

Evidence of actual therapeutic activity exists only in relation to the kings, indicating that the king mediated between the ancestors and the living. As long as the ancestors were content and cared for, the condition of the country was harmonious, and the people were generally healthy.

Shang Diagnosis of Disease

The king consulted the ancestors through oracle bones and the interpreters of the oracle bones, the *wu* (shamans). The oracle bones were usually either the scapula of oxen or tortoise carapaces. Holes were drilled into the bones or carapaces (**A**), the king (**B**) would pose a question and the bone or carapace would be heated to very high temperatures and quickly cooled, creating cracking between the drilled holes. The cracks could be read and interpreted by the king in order to know the will of the ancestors. Queries posed to the ancestors ranged from questions about the weather, hunting, dreams, illness, war, and the future. For the most part, the cause of any disease or trouble, including social, physical, or natural problems, was the curse of an ancestor who had been offended in some way.

There is also some evidence that disease was understood to have environmental causes such as snow and wind. These concepts were to become much more developed within the practice of medicine and remain important today.

A A tortoise carapace oracle bone with characters inscribed on it.

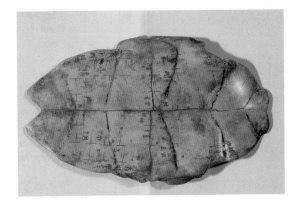

B Character for "king." The character *wang* depicts the relationship of the ruler to the heavens or ancestors and to the earth or people. The top line represents the heavens or the ancestors, the bottom line represents earth or humans, and the middle line represents the ruler. The perpendicular line connecting the three shows how the ruler is the intermediary between heaven or the ancestors and earth or humans, communicating with the ancestors to keep the earth and humankind healthy and harmonious.

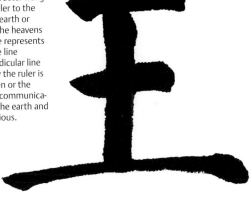

Shang Treatment of Disease

When disease is caused by giving offense to the ancestors, then treatment is relatively straightforward: appease the offended ancestor. This might in clude making offerings, changing the way the ancestor was buried, or revising the conduct of political affairs. Although the king was solely responsible for communication with the ancestors, he would only intervene in the illnesses of individuals who were members of his family or the nobility. Individuals outside of the king's immediate circle needed to find other ways to address their diseases. Only if the sickness posed a severe threat to the people (an epidemic) and only when failure to act might erode his authority would the king engage the ancestors on behalf of the people. It was the king's ability to communicate with the ancestors that gave him authority, and upon which his continued leadership depended. If he lost this ability to communicate, or if individuals felt that the relationship was no longer effective, he would lose his power. Interestingly, the idea of the king/emperor communicating with and receiving the approval of the ancestors or heaven became the guiding principle by which dynasties were created and overturned up until the final imperial dynasty fell in 1911.

If the ruler lost his ability to communicate with the ancestors and to heal the people of social and natural disasters, he could be legitimately replaced by someone who had that power. Here we can see the close relationship between the ruler, the ancestors, the health of the nation and emerging medical therapeutics. Over time, a medical system developed that was more directed at preventing disease or treating the individual, but that system was still informed by its political roots.

As time passed, ancestor worship led to the development of many complex philosophical systems, including the system of *feng shui* (wind and water), which began as a method of divining the winds and waters so that the graves of ancestors were placed in propitious places. Many of the ideas of Confucius were based on the concept of ancestor worship, most especially his emphasis on filial piety and the veneration of one's ancestors.

To this day, ancestor worship continues to be practical in places such as Taiwan and Singapore. Temples are erected to the ancestors and tablets for each are placed within them. Qing Ming Day (literally clear and bright festival), commonly known as "Tomb Sweeping Day," is a national holiday in Taiwan and mainland China. It is the day that people return to the graves of ancestors, bringing food and money for the afterlife (see also **A, B, C**).

A Qing dynasty ancestral shrine. This picture shows the entrance to an ancestral shrine. Inside the shrine are found the ancestral tablets that represent all of a given family's ancestors. Often there will be hundreds of tablets within a single shrine.

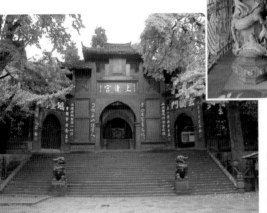

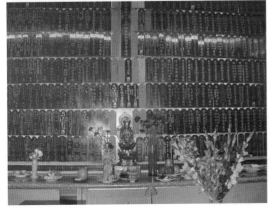

B Family temple. In front of this ancestral shrine one can see the traditional fu dogs (one male and one female) guarding the entrance.

C Ancestral tablets inside an ancestral shrine. Traditionally, these would have been made of stone.

The Zhou Dynasty and Demonological Medicine (1100–475 BCE)

When the Shang originally consolidated power, many tribes developed relationships with them, while remaining independent of their authority. One such group, the Zhou, in addition to allying themselves with the Shang, allied themselves with early Tibetan tribes, for whom the Shang people had a great animosity. Ultimately, the Zhou, with the help of the Tibetan tribes, overthrew the Shang and established their own dynasty (see p. 3 and 50). One of the longest dynasties, the Zhou did not establish a completely unified state, rather a system of allied city-states, similar to European feudal society (Hucker 1975).

For much of the Zhou dynasty, the consultation of oracle bones continued as it had in the Shang dynasty. The *wu* (**A, B**, see also p. 8 and 14) of the Shang period are also found during the Zhou dynasty, but, toward the end of the dynasty, the *wu*, who had been principally members of the royal family, lost much of their political power. As a result, they established themselves as healers and diviners among the ordinary people. Their role amongst the nobility was, in part, taken over by priests who were able to communicate with the heavens to understand the future (a very different function from communicating with ancestors to determine if they were angry).

With the decentralization of power produced by the city-state system, there was little clarity about the ultimate source of political authority. Allegiances were focused on regional leaders at the expense of the king. Additionally, natural disasters were prevalent. Both conditions—environmental calamities and the lack of strong central leadership—provoked confusion an anxiety among the commoners. Distant dwellers in other city-states might not share their beliefs and loyalties. Which leader guided the rituals of the people?

Out of this pervasive sense of anxiety grew the notion that the uncared for ancestors of peoples who failed to observe the correct rites could come to roam the land as demons, visiting illness and disaster upon others. Unlike ancestors, demons were not connected to populations by posthumous family ties and obligation, but struck where they wished. From these concerns the practice of "demonic medicine" was born. Because it was no longer clear if the king had direct contact with the beings of the other world, the *wu* took on the role of interpreting the demon's desires for the people and of exorcising the demons and evil winds from the sick, a position with less rank, but ultimately longer-lasting.

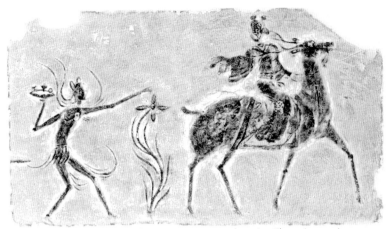

A *Wu* with wings. Rubbing taken from a Han Dynasty tomb carving. The *wu* is preparing an herbal medication.

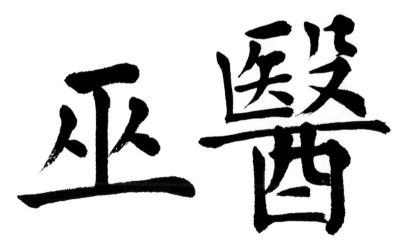

B Characters for *wu* and *yi*. The character for medicine and physician or healer *(yi)* may have been created during the Zhou dynasty. It originally had the character for *wu* on the bottom with the upper half depicting a quiver with an arrow on the left and a spear on the right. Later, the bottom half of the character was changed to depict the character for alcohol, an important component of medicinal wines.

It is possible that the concept of untended spirits as demons unassociated with individuals sprang from the development during the Zhou dynasty of the concept of human souls. The Zhou conceived of humankind as having two souls: the ethereal soul (*hun*), and the corporeal soul (*po*). The corporeal soul exists in the body from birth and dies at death. The ethereal soul enters the body some time after birth and can leave the body during sleep to wander through the world. After death, the ethereal soul continues to travel the world until it finds another body that it wishes to enter. The precept of demonic medicine, especially as it developed toward the end of the Zhou dynasty is that this ethereal soul is inherently evil and wishes to hurt humankind. The *wu* have the power to exorcise these homeless souls and banish them from the world of the living; however, in this model, adherence to proper social norms no longer protects the individual from illness or danger, as it did when the ancestors prevailed

Treatment of Disease Caused by Demons

Although the belief that demons could cause disease is clearly documented in archaeological artifacts of the late Zhou and Warring States period, the actual treatment of demonological disease is less clear. There is some evidence that the *wu* attempted to treat demons in the same way in which warriors attempted to expel invaders, by attacking them with spears. *The Book of Rites (Liji)* of the Zhou dynasty states that

"several times a year, and also during certain special occasions, such as the funeral of a prince, hordes of exorcists would race shrieking through the city streets, enter the courtyards and homes, thrusting their spears into the air, in an attempt to expel the evil creatures" (Unschuld 1985, p. 37). In addition to using spears and fear, the *wu* used medicinal drugs to expel or destroy demons. Some of the drugs used included "aromatics, prepared animals or parts of animals, herbs, a woman's menstrual cloth, and others" (ibid., p. 41).

Warring States: Creating Order from Chaos

The decline of the Zhou dynasty was long and dramatic. The final years were filled with wars and battles until finally any semblance of unity fell apart and the period known as the Warring States began (**A, B**). The Warring States period (see also pp. 3 and 50) officially began in ca. 475 BCE and lasted until 221 BCE, however, from around 771 BCE the Zhou nation was in disintegration and there was no order of any sort. Out of this chaos many attempts to bring order emerged, including Confucian thought and Daoism.

Kong Fu Zi (Confucius), perhaps the most influential man in Chinese history, lived during the Warring States period, and created the philosophical doctrine that was to substantially influence Chinese culture for the rest of time.

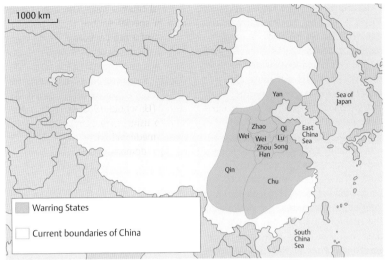

A Map of China during the Warring States period (ca. 475 BCE–221 BCE).

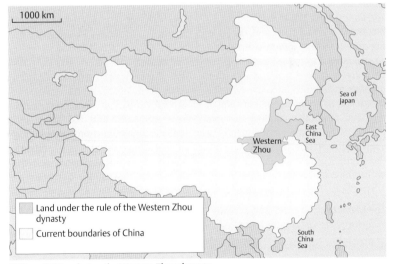

B Map of China during the Western Zhou dynasty.
A and B These two maps show how the territory that is China has changed. Over time, the territory covered by the Chinese empire has grown and shrunk several times. The area depicted on modern maps includes several contested regions, called Autonomous Regions, including the area comprising Tibet.

Confucius lived from 551 to 479 BCE. Although he was a scholar and a teacher, he wanted to be involved in politics, however, without passing the imperial examinations (which he failed to do) there was no route into the imperial bureaucracy. Ironically, many years after his death, he was to have immense influence on every aspect of Chinese life, including medicine.

Confucius believed in a natural order to things, which was also a moral order. The decay and chaos of the nation was due to the leadership of inferior men who were not performing the rites of feudal society correctly. If men were virtuous and strictly observed the rites of the ancients then the country would be orderly and all would be well in society and nature. The Confucian doctrine was based on a hierarchy of social roles and the practice of associated virtues, which must be maintained in order for the roles to be correct (**A, B, C**). If the roles are properly maintained, then there will be health and harmony in one's life and in the land. Improper conduct disrupts the social order. The maintenance of appropriate relationships will maintain the strength and vitality of China and of the Chinese.

The Medicine of Systematic Correspondence

Although the moral order of Confucian thought was not directed at medicine, it had a great effect on the development of medicine. What is today called the "Medicine of Systematic Correspondence" (Unschuld 1985) emerged, along with the Confucian moral code, out of the chaos of the Warring States. This system of medicine was not designed to appease ancestors or demons, but rather was a rationally based system that managed observed somatic and environmental relationships to bring order to chaos.

As it developed, the Medicine of Systematic Correspondence incorporated several major ideas, all of which developed as separate philosophical notions during the Warring States period. Although aspects of these ideas have entered into the realm of religious or cultural practices, what has been retained in the traditional medicine of China, hearkens back to the practices of the Warring States. Today, Chinese medicine includes Warring States' ideas, such as: a belief in the unity of humankind and nature, *yin yang* and five-phase theory, and the concept of *qi* as the basis of life. While not explicitly a part of contemporary Chinese medical theory, the image of a united, harmonious, smoothly functioning empire transposed onto the healthy body versus a nation out of balance, with stagnation and disunity transposed onto the sick body, continues to be a pervasive, if implicit, theme, both in Chinese medicine and in society. Other ideas, such as ancestor worship and the *wu*, while no longer strictly a part of the medical system, continue to manifest in Chinese culture and in folk shamanic practices.

Five Key Relationships	Appropriate Virtues
Father to son	Filial piety
Ruler to subject	Loyalty
Brother to brother	Brotherliness
Husband to wife	Love and obedience
Friend to friend	Faithfulness

A The Confucian hierarchy of social roles. This table depicts the five relationships that were key to understanding Confucian philosophy and the virtues that were incumbent upon the subordinate in each relationship.

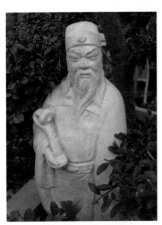

B Statue of a Confucian scholar.

"If we were to characterize in one word the Chinese way of life for the last two thousand years, the word would be Confucian. No other individual in Chinese history has so deeply influenced the life and thought of his people, as a transmitter, teacher and creative interpreter of the ancient culture and literature, and as a molder of the Chinese mind and character. The other ancient philosophies, the religious systems of Taoism and Buddhism, all have known their days of glory and neglect; but the doctrines of Confucianism, since their general recognition in the first century before Christ have never ceased to exert a vital influence on the nation down to our own century. Many Chinese have professed themselves to be Taoists, Buddhists, even Christians, but seldom have they ceased at the same time to be Confucianists. For Confucianism since the time of its general acceptance has been more than a creed to be professed or rejected; it has become an inseparable part of the society and thought of the nation as a whole, of what it means to be a Chinese, as the Confucian Classics are not the canon of a particular sect but the literary heritage of a whole people."

(DeBary, Chan & Watson 1960, p. 15)

C Quote from *Sources of Chinese Tradition*.

Unity of Humankind and Nature

The first element of the Medicine of Systematic Correspondence, the belief in the unity of humankind and the natural world, is perhaps the aspect of Chinese medicine that is most appealing to us today. Essentially, this belief implies that there is a relationship between the greater environment (the macrocosm) and the environment of the body (the microcosm). This is most commonly and clearly expressed in terms of the natural environment and its effect on the body. For example, exposing oneself to wind can result in being "struck by wind," which can manifest as a common cold or as facial paralysis. The other aspect of humankind's relationship to the natural environment is expressed within the body, where internal wind can be stirred up if there is an insufficiency of fluids causing dryness or if there is internal heat. This may result in spasms, seizures, or even paralysis. This is analogous to the state of the natural world where drought causes great winds that create sandstorms and destroy crops, causing famine.

This unity however, does not apply only to the natural environment, but also to the social environment. If one's social relationships are inappropriately maintained, then one's emotions are affected, that is, anger rather than love between husband and wife, which is then reflected in one's body, manifesting as headaches, palpitations, and so on. Thus, maintaining the appropriate relationship to the natural environment and maintaining appropriate social relationships are equally important to the maintenance of health.

Yin Yang Theory

The next element of the Medicine of Systematic Correspondence, which emerged as a response to the chaos of the Warring States period, is the understanding of *yin* and *yang* and the five phases (*wu xing*). These two theories of correspondence developed as separate philosophical and political schools, which were not specifically concerned with medicine, but which later became the basis for medical thought.

The theory of *yin* and *yang* is the most fundamental concept in the philosophy of Chinese medicine. Originally, the two characters signified no more than the sunny side of a hill (*yang*) and the shady side of a hill (*yin*) (Wilhelm and Byrnes 1967, p. 297; Unschuld 1985, p. 55) (**A**). The very different environments that exist on either side of a hill, the brightly lit, warm, active side and the shaded, cool and quiescent side, came to represent a set of opposites, which must always be present simultaneously, which contain elements of the other and that can transform into each other. The *yin yang* school grew up as a school of philosophy that attempted to explain the world in terms of these paired oppositions. Later, these ideas were also applied to the body to express ideas about both normal physiological and pathological processes (**B, C**).

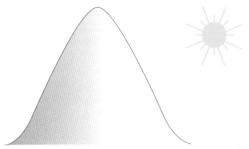

A *Yin* **and** *yang* can be thought of as the shady and sunny side of a hill. *Yin:* the shady side of the hill. *Yang:* the sunny side of the hill.

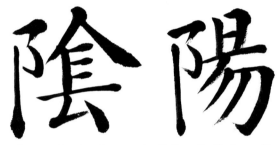

B Characters for *yin* **and** *yang,* **each with the radical for "mound" on the left.**

"Heaven is *yang,* earth is *yin.*
Spring is *yang,* fall *yin.*
Summer *yang,* winter *yin.*
Daytime is *yang,* nighttime *yin.*
The larger state is *yang,* the smaller *yin.*
The ruler is *yang,* the minister *yin.*
The superior is *yang,* the inferior *yin.*
The male is *yang,* the female *yin.*
The father is *yang,* the son *yin.*
The elder brother is *yang,* the younger brother *yin.*
All of the *yang* categories emulate heaven. Heaven exalts proper order.
Overstepping proper order is dissemblance.
All of the *yin* categories emulate the earth.
The virtue of the earth is being placid and quiet, properly ordered and tranquil."

(Cited in Unschuld 2003, p. 87)

C Quote from *Huang Di Nei Jing Su Wen.*

One of the most important aspects of *yin yang* philosophy is that every phenomenon must be identified as *yin* or *yang* in relation to specific surroundings. In terms of the body, the outside of the body, the skin and hair are *yang* in relation to the inside of the body and the organs, the upper part of the body is *yang* in relation to the lower part of the body, and the back of the body is *yang* in relation to the front of the body. *Yin* and *yang* can be defined only in relation to each other, not as individual entities existing without each other. For example, spring is *yin* in relation to summer because it is cooler and is a time of development toward the *yang* of summer, but spring is *yang* in relation to winter because it is warmer and indicates that the seasons are moving toward warmth. Thus, the *yin* or *yang* nature of any phenomenon is not definite, but ever-changing in relation to the environment (see also p. 56ff).

One of the discussions of the *yin yang* school is the debate over the physical existence of *yin* and *yang*. Are *yin* and *yang* merely concepts used to organize phenomena in relation to each other or are they actual, tangible phenomena or substances that can rise and decline both in nature and in the human body, causing imbalance between *yin* and *yang* and thus creating disharmony or illness in the body (Farquhar 1987)? When considering the body in Chinese medicine, it is important to understand *yin* and *yang* as both concept and substance so as to be able to organize the body in terms of *yin* and *yang*, and also to be able to systematically observe and treat imbalances and insufficiency of *yin* and *yang* substances.

Five-phase Theory

Five-phase theory, which is based upon definite lines of correspondence (**A**) into which all things in the universe can be placed, is quite Confucian (see also p. 60ff). If the proper relationships between these lines of correspondence are maintained, then there is harmony in the body and in the universe, just as there is harmony if the proper virtues are practiced in relationships. The phases are not static but constantly changing in relation to each other and to the environment. Included in the theory of the movement of the five phases is an engendering cycle in which one phase is responsible for producing the next (that is, wood engenders fire) and also a restraining phase in which one phase is responsible for restraining another (that is, wood restrains earth) (**B**). When the phases are out of balance then there is an effect on the actions of the other phases. Because each phase is correlated with an organ system, imbalances in the body reflect in the associated organ systems.

Phase	Wood	Fire	Earth	Metal	Water
Tone/note	Jue	Zhi	Gong	Shang	Yü
Colors	Cyan	Red	Yellow	White	Black
Seasons	Spring	Summer	Long summer	Autumn	Winter
Numbers	Eight	Seven	Five	Nine	Six
Emperors	Fu Xi	Yan Di	Huang Di	Shao Hao	Zhuan Xu
Spirits	Spirit of trees	Spirit of fire	Spirit of soil	Spirit of the West	Spirit of water
Creatures	Shelled	Feathered	Naked	Hairy	Armored
Gods	God of household	God of oven	God of soil	God of door	God of roads
Animals	Cock	Sheep	Ox	Horse	Pig
Climate	Wind	Heat	Damp	Dryness	Cold
Directions	East	South	Center	West	North

A Five-phase correspondences. This table of five-phase correspondences shows some of the correspondences as they relate to the world, to government, and to culture, but does not depict the relationships of the body. This more historical chart shows how the five phases group phenomena or concepts. They can also be used to represent the body as a system of interrelated systems that are linked to the environment. These linkages will be made more clearly in Chapter 2.

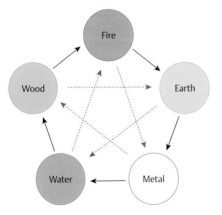

B The engendering and restraining cycles of the five phases.

These explicitly defined relationships of engendering and restraining are easily incorporated into the Confucian model of maintaining order. Essentially, the Confucian moral order, the theory of *yin* and *yang* and the order of the five phases all imply that both the tangible and the intangible elements of life are mutually dependent upon each other through lines of correspondence, through maintaining appropriate relationships, and through appropriate coexistence.

It is from these theories, which were philosophical responses to political strife, that many of the fundamental ideas of the Chinese medicine we practice today emerged. It is important to remember, however, that these ideas did not emerge first as theories of medicine, but rather as ideas that could be applied to the political chaos existing in China in order to unify the nation. The five phases had wide-ranging applications. We see them in the five-note musical scale of China, in traditional calendrics, which assigned a phase to every year, and even to the governmental regulation of water, fire, metal, wood, and soil, which had to be harmoniously attended to (Unschuld 1985, p. 60).

Qi

The classical character for *qi* (**A**) embodies that which creates and nourishes the human body: air and food. The upper part of the character represents the rising of vapors or breath, while the lower part of the character represents cooked rice, both of which are essential for the continued survival of the human body. The character thus represents "vapors rising from food" (Unschuld 1985, p. 72). During the Warring States period, *qi* seems to have had the meaning of vapors, breath, and even life, as well as that which makes up all tangible matter. Thus, *qi* was both that from which we were formed and also that which kept us alive. Over time, the idea of *qi* has become extremely broad, encompassing almost every aspect of natural phenomena (**B, C**). During the Warring States period, however, *qi* became important as it was related both to environmental influences on the body, and to vacuity or repletion of *qi* in the body causing disease.

In the Han dynasty (206 BCE to 220 CE, see also p. 50) the philosophical ideas, *yin* and *yang*, the five phases, and Confucian morality, came together with the ideas of the relationship between the body and the environment, ideas such as the invasion of evil spirits, and the notion of *qi* as the essence of life, to form the Medicine of Systematic Correspondences, a medicine that incorporated the language of government and politics and superimposed it onto the body.

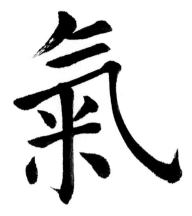

A The classical character for *qi*.

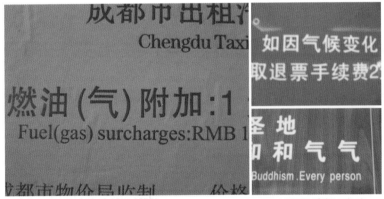

B Photos of *qi* on billboards in China. The complex character for *qi* is made up of the radical (root) for rising vapors above with the character for cooked rice below, representing "vapors rising from food," or life. The characters depicted here are the simplified form, in which the radical for rice is removed.

毒氣	*du qi*	poisonous gas
氣泵	*qi beng*	air pump
氣氛	*qi fen*	atmosphere
氣憤	*qi fen*	indignant, furious
氣性	*qi xing*	temperament, disposition

C There is a wide range of usages for the character *qi*.

Daoism as a Response to Chaos and its Influence on Medicine

Lao Zi (**A**) and Chuang Zi, two important characters in the Daoist movement probably lived at about the same time as Confucius. The development of Daoist and Confucian philosophy (**B**) was a response to the chaos of the late Zhou/early Warring States period. Like Confucius (**C**), Lao Zi, Chuang Zi, and the Daoists were exploring ways of creating a viable political system. While the systems ultimately were at variance with each other, it was not unusual to find the Confucian scholar who, in his later years, retreated into an individual search for the Dao (the path).

Daoism is not a homogeneous system of thought. It has been influenced by many people over hundreds of years. In fact, the term Daoism often groups together differing, sometimes opposing intellectual schools that have nothing more in common than that they are based on a concept of Dao.

While Confucian thought was concerned with how humankind should behave in society, Daoism emphasized how humans could conform to the laws of nature. After Confucian thought, Daoism has probably been the most influential native philosophy. Early Daoist writings were about a return to a simpler life where humankind was in harmony with nature, and death was a natural event. However, that humans had lived longer in "ancient" times and that humans living during the Warring States period were not living their lives to the fullest was a prevalent idea. As

Daoism developed, it became a doctrine of individualism in unity with nature. For some Daoists, unity with nature evolved into a search for immortality, which led to involvement with medicine and therapeutics.

The Daoists influenced the development of herbal medicine as they searched for an herb of immortality. It is likely that Shen Nong was made divine by the Daoists and that the organization of *The Divine Husbandman's Materia Medica* was created by the Daoists. The book was divided into three sections: superior herbs, which could be taken long term without harm and had rejuvenating properties; medium herbs, which had tonic effects but could be toxic if taken long term; and inferior herbs, which were used for curing disease, were considered poisonous and could not be taken for a long time. Drug therapy was also of interest to the Daoists because herbs were not controlled by any social order, but worked independent of human relationships. For this reason, herbal medicine did not hold great interest for Confucian medical scholars because it operated outside the context of constructed social relations (see also p. 224).

In addition to herbal therapeutics, the Daoists developed many breathing exercises to keep the circulation of *qi* smooth and they emphasized the idea of humankind's unity with nature, with the environment, with the seasons, and so on (see also chapters 2, 8, and 9).

A Statue of Lao Zi. Lao Zi, often considered the father of Daoism, is the purported author of the *Dao De Jing/Tao Te Ching or The Book of the Way* (amongst many translations of the title). At various times in Chinese history, Daoism had great political influence. Its influence on Chinese medicine is seen primarily in the development of the various materia medica.

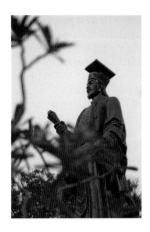

Confucian Thought	Daoism
A burden of social responsibility	Flight from conventional duties of society
Concern for things human	Vision of "other" world of the spirit
Moralism/common sense	Paradoxical, mystical, poetic
Scholar-gentleman, good family man, good bureaucrat, good citizen	Scholar-gentleman, recluse, interested in the beauty of nature and the spirit world

B Differences between the Confucian scholar-gentleman and the Daoist scholar-gentleman. Not always so clearly demarcated, in reality, the two were often intertwined and it was not unusual for the Confucian scholar to also be a Daoist. The Daoist leanings often came out more as the gentleman-scholar retired from public life.

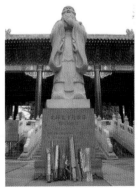

C Statue of Confucius. Confucius and Lao Zi both lived during the Warring States period. Confucius (551–479 BCE) was a scholar who wanted to become a governmental bureaucrat but instead was a teacher and librarian. After his death, his writings were compiled by his students and his thought became the dominant political doctrine that was to influence Chinese culture for the next 2000 years.

Although none of the major texts that were to influence medicine through the next 2000 years were written during the Warring States period, the major ideas and philosophies that would inform medicine evolved during this period as responses to the chaos, unrest and lack of order.

The Reunification of China and the Emergence of the Traditional Medicine of China

For a brief period (221 to 206 BCE) China was reunified under the Qin dynasty (see pp. 3 and 50). The Qin leadership have been classified as "legalists" who were primarily interested in law and not in philosophy or medicine. Although there were no great advances in medicine during this time, the emperor, Qin Shi Huang Di, created China's first truly centralized government. He created a non-feudal, non-hereditary bureaucratic system with administrative districts and counties that were responsible to the central government. To work, this system required complete obedience to the central government and, consequently a strong, even dictatorial leader. Qin Shi Huang Di therefore prohibited philosophical discussion and forbade both criticism of the current government and praise of earlier governments. In 213 BCE, all writings other than official Qin historical documents and treatises on divination, agriculture, or medicine were collected and burnt. Copies were maintained only in the imperial library.

The strict adherence to law and to the central government did not last long, but it was during this period that major unification projects, such as roads connecting the empire, waterways, irrigation systems, canals and the Great Wall, were begun, with the help of forced labor (**A, B**). The dynasty fell apart under the second emperor, the son of Qin Shi Huang Di, who was too weak to maintain the central government.

In 206 BCE, China was unified under the Han dynasty (see pp. 3 and 50). During this dynasty, a stable aristocratic order was established and China expanded geographically, economically, and politically, influencing regions that are now Vietnam and Korea. This dynasty is considered by many as the beginning of civil society in China and even today, the Chinese call themselves *Han ren* or people of the Han. The Han dynasty was a period of great advancement for China. The Confucian doctrine was deeply integrated into political life. It was also during this period that the Medicine of Systematic Correspondence, the medicine that bears a relationship to the medicine with which we are familiar today, fully emerged. As described earlier, this medicine developed from the inclusion of diverse ideas from diverse schools of thought. The Medicine of Systematic Correspondence began as and remained a heterogeneous set of theories, each of which may be appropriate in any given circumstance, but which may also contradict each other.

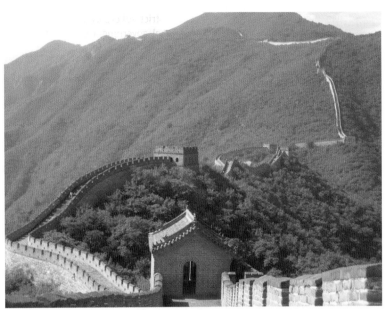

A The Great Wall of China. Although seemingly a huge project, the wall was actually built in stages. The great accomplishment of Qin Shi Huang Di was to connect the walls protecting many of the Northern cities, thereby beginning the creation of the Great Wall. His thought was to build a wall to keep the barbarians of the North out of China. Unfortunately, this did not work, as much later, the Mongols (1271 under Kubla Khan) were able to overcome China from the North and establish the Yuan dynasty. The building of the Great Wall was manageable only through massive conscriptions of workers, a feat that was accomplished because of the immense control exercised by Qin Shi Huang Di.

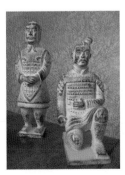

B Figures of the Terracotta Army. The Terracotta Army of the first emperor Qin Shi Huang Di was unearthed in 1974, near Xi'an in Shanxi Province. The life-size figures vary in height according to their army ranking and include generals, warriors, horses, chariots, and more. Although they have not all been unearthed, it is estimated that there are about 7000 soldiers, 130 chariots, and nearly 700 horses.

The Textual Basis of Chinese Medicine

During the Han dynasty the major texts (**A**) that form the corpus of medical theory were written or compiled. Two of these, *The Yellow Emperor's Classic of Medicine* and the *Divine Husbandman's Materia Medica*, are traditionally attributed to the legendary emperors, Huang Di and Shen Nong.

The Yellow Emperor's Classic of Medicine is the most well known and often referred-to medical classic. However, it is not a text from which a homogeneous system of ideas can be understood. It is a compilation of essays describing the ideas and teachings of various schools and teachers. It includes ideas popularized through demonic medicine, it discusses *qi*, the circulation of *qi* in the channels, and about 300 acupuncture points. There is discussion of *yin* and *yang* and the five phases, the functions and the relationships of the viscera and bowels, acupuncture and moxibustion, and diagnostics. *The Yellow Emperor's Classic of Medicine* mentions some herbal formulas, but it is primarily a theoretical and philosophical text that attempts to link varied ideas within a conceptual structure, rather than a book about treatment. This text uses the language of goverscribe the body. Just as a well-managed nation runs well because the necessary ministers are functioning as they ought and the waterways and passages are free or a nation is disrupted because the functions of some bureaucratic official are impaired, causing stagnation or a breakdown in communication and movement, so too do the administrative centers of the body (the viscera and bowels) affect the function of the body. Finally, it should be remembered that *The Yellow Emperor's Classic of Medicine* to which we have access today is a greatly altered text from the text of 100 BCE. Over time, the text has been adapted, edited, and commented upon so that today there are many versions based upon different interpretations.

Besides *The Yellow Emperor's Classic of Medicine* and the *Divine Husbandman's Materia Medica*, several more texts are important to the development of Chinese medicine. Though not well known, medical texts considered to be older than *The Yellow Emperor's Classic of Medicine* were unearthed from three tombs in Hunan Province called the Ma Wang tombs. They discuss magical and demonic concepts of medicine and some less well-developed ideas about the Medicine of Systematic Correspondence. The texts identify 11 vessels (six originating on the feet and five originating on the hands) through which vapor (it is not called *qi* in these texts) flows, and which are described as being either *yin* or *yang* vessels. The Ma Wang texts mention moxibustion and the use of heated stones, but not acupuncture or acupuncture points, an omission that has led to the hypothesis that the channels of the body were described prior to the recognition of acupuncture points (see also p. 222).

Text	Probable Original Dates and Authorship	Significance in the History of Chinese Medicine
Various texts from the Ma Wang tombs	Ca. 200 BCE Author unknown	Buried in 168 BCE and found in 1973, these medical texts are related to, but older than *The Yellow Emperor's Classic of Medicine*. They provide the support for the theories of physiology and pathology and the acupuncture treatments found in the *Classic*
Huang Di Nei Jing Su Wen and *Ling Shu (Yellow Emperor's Classic of Medicine: Plain Questions and Spiritual Pivot)*	Ca. 100 BCE–100 CE Attributed to Huang Di (the mythical Yellow Emperor) Actually by various unknown authors and compilers	Perhaps the most important texts of Chinese medical history. The ideas and treatments found in these texts have continued up to the present to be a valuable source of theoretical and practical information. Evidence indicates that these texts were a series of essays that were first compiled in about 100 CE
Nan Jing (The Classic of Difficulties)	Ca. 100 CE Attributed to Bian Que of the Zhou dynasty Actual author is unknown	Compiled during the first century, this text was thought to be merely a commentary or explication of *The Yellow Emperor's Classic of Medicine*, but it is now more aptly regarded as a stand-alone text that makes theories presented in the *Classic* accessible to the medical practitioner
Shen Nong Ben Cao (Divine Husbandman's Materia Medica)	Ca. 100–200 CE Attributed to Shen Nong Actual author unknown	Substances were divided into three classes: upper, middle, and lower. The upper substances are the sovereigns, the middle substances are the ministers, and the lower substances are the assistants and envoys. The text clarifies the roles of each class and how to combine classes to create an effective formula
Shang Han Za Bing Lun (Treatise On Cold Damage and Miscellaneous Diseases)	Ca. 150–219 CE Compiled by Wang Shu He (210–285 CE) from the no longer available text written by Zhang Zhong Jing *(Zhang Ji)*	This is the first known text to attempt to apply the Medicine of Systematic Correspondence, a system primarily used for the practice of acupuncture, to medicinal therapeutics. It discusses the many different manifestations of externally contracted disease, especially cold. It addresses the nature of the invading evil, and the constitution of the body and how the constitution affects the outcome of the illness. Originally written as one text, Wang Shu He divided the text into two, the *Shang Han Lun (On Cold Damage)* and the *Jin Gui Yao Lue (Essential Prescriptions of the Golden Coffer)*

A The major medical texts through the Han dynasty.

The *Nan Jing (The Classic of Difficulties)* (**A**), although attributed to a physician of the Zhou dynasty named Bian Que, was probably compiled some time during the first or second century CE. It is an extremely systematic book, which covers "all aspects of theoretical and practical health care perceivable within the confines of the *yin yang* and five-phases doctrines, as defined by the 'original' Medicine of Systematic Correspondences" (Unschuld 1986, p. 4). It is important because it marks a shift in medical thinking from purely theoretical to practical. This is the first text to systematically apply the theory of disease as expressed in *The Yellow Emperor's Classic of Medicine* to the practice of medicine. It is also important because the magical and demonological aspects of medicine have, for the most part, been discarded as unsystematic. The focus is on the concepts of systematic correspondence. The body is presented as a coherent, functional whole and, the practice of acupuncture is directly discussed. Although not as culturally important to the story of the traditional medicine of China as *The Yellow Emperor's Classic of Medicine*, the *Classic of Difficulties* is considered by many to be a more complete, useful, and mature text.

Around the same time, Zhang Zhong Jing (142–220 CE; aka Zhang Ji) (**B**) wrote *Shang Han Za Bing Lun (Treatise On Cold Damage and Miscellaneous Diseases)*, a herbal medicine text that was based on Zhang Zhong Jing's clinical experiences and observations (see p. 226). Like the *Classic of Difficulties*, this was a clinical text. Most importantly, it is the earliest text to emphasize physical signs and symptoms and the course of disease, as well as the method of treatment. Unfortunately, Zhang's work was not well received at the time he wrote it and it was not until much later (960 CE) that his ideas were recognized as clinically important. Like *The Yellow Emperor's Classic of Medicine*, this text has gone through numerous changes over time, and today appears in two volumes, *Shang Han Lun (On Cold Damage)* and the *Jin Gui Yao Lue* (*Essential Prescriptions of the Golden Coffer*, see also p. 226).

Hua Tuo (110–207 CE) (**C**), a legendary culture hero of Chinese medicine also lived during the Han dynasty. He is said to have discovered the first anesthetic and used it in surgical practices. He supposedly had a secret powder that would produce numbness, thus allowing him to open the abdomen and remove any diseased organs. He was also an acupuncturist and herbalist and he developed some of the early forms of *qi gong* based on animal postures (see Chapter 8). Unfortunately, Hua Tuo seems to have failed to pass his surgical knowledge on to anyone else, as the art of surgery in the Chinese tradition remained confined to minor procedures (see also pp. 320 and 356).

"The scripture states: there are five palaces (bowels) and six depots (viscera). What does that mean?
It is like this: [Usually one speaks of] six palaces, but actually there are five palaces. Although [one commonly speaks of] five depots, there are also [arguments pointing out an existence of] six depots. They state that the kidneys consist of two depots. The one on the left is the kidney; the one of the right is the gate of life. The gate of life is the place where the essence and the spirit are harbored. In males it stores the essence; in females it holds the womb. The influences of the gate of life are identical with [those of] the kidney. That is why [some] speak of an existence of six depots.
There are five palaces. What does that mean?
It is like this. Each of the body's five depots has one palace associated with it. The Triple Burner is a palace, too, but even so it is not related to any of the five depots. Hence [some] speak of an existence of [only] five palaces."

(Cited in Unschuld 1986, p. 399)

A Quote from the *Nan Jing* *(The Classic of Difficulties:* The Thirty-ninth Difficult Issue).

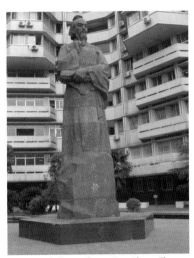

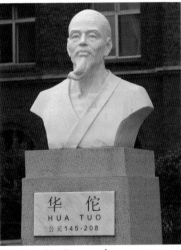

B Statue of Zhang Zhong Jing. Zhang Zhong Jing is the author of the *Shang Han Za Bing Lun (Treatise On Cold Damage and Miscellaneous Diseases).* Today his image is found on the campus of nearly every school or hospital of Chinese medicine in China.

C Hua Tuo. Hua Tuo was a famous surgeon, acupuncturist, and herbalist. His diagnostic skills were said to be so great that he could predict the outcome of any condition. He is said to have developed the *qi gong* exercise entitled "The Frolics of the Five Animals"(see p. 322), which would remove disease, strengthen the body, and ensure health. His fame lies in his purported discovery of an anesthetic drug that allowed him to perform surgery wherever it might be necessary.

Another influence on medicine during the Han dynasty was the introduction of Buddhism from India. Buddhism was introduced to China sometime around 100 CE, by monks traveling across the Silk Road (**A, B**), an important trade route that ran from China all the way to modern-day Turkey. Unlike Daoism and Confucian thought, Buddhism did not initially have a strong following in China, although around 400 CE it made some inroads into popular Chinese culture.

In terms of medicine, while the theories of Indian or Buddhist medicine never became important, some aspects of the Indian pharmacopeia were integrated into the Daoist pharmacopeia, especially in relation to the search for an herb of immortality. Perhaps most importantly, the Buddhists introduced to China the concept of hospitals and medical care for the peasant population. Buddhist monasteries were also hospitals, and the monks were willing to treat anyone who needed their services. In order to prevent the Buddhists and Buddhism from becoming too influential, other medical practitioners eventually had to follow their path and treat the peasants as well as the elite.

The Han dynasty is the time period to which most of the ancient traditions of Chinese medicine can be traced. During this time, the groundwork was laid for the rest of the development of medical practice in China. This does not mean that the medicine of China remained static from 220 CE to the present, but rather that the foundation for further examination and development was established. The first mention of acupuncture as a therapeutic modality and the first herbal prescriptions were written during this dynasty. However, the actual practice of Chinese medicine was limited to a few scholar-officials who found the topic interesting. Throughout the next 1800 years, new theories would continue to be presented and old ideas re-examined, but the texts of the Han dynasty, most especially *The Yellow Emperor's Classic of Medicine*, *The Divine Husbandman's Materia Medica*, the *Classic of Difficulties*, and *Treatise On Cold Damage and Miscellaneous Diseases* were to remain the foundation texts of the traditional medicine of China.

It is important to remember that the Medicine of Systematic Correspondence was the medicine of the elite, of the gentry, not the medicine of the general population. Eighty percent of the total population of China consisted of farmers and peasants living at subsistence level and dependent upon the soil for their life. These people developed their own traditions, primarily based in eclectic religious beliefs and herbal lore, but they did not participate in the development of the traditional medicine of China. The medicine of the elite was a text-based tradition that was available only to the literate segments of society.

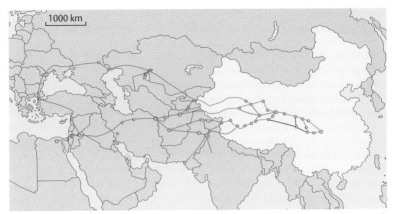

A The Silk Road. The Silk Road is a series of ancient trade routes that, when connected, traversed over 8000 km from Chang'an (modern-day Xi'an) all the way to what is today Istanbul in Turkey. Over this route, trade and knowledge passed into and out of China to and from India, Greece, Egypt, and Rome. Buddhist monks first entered China from India over this route, bringing with them both a new religion and new information about health and disease.

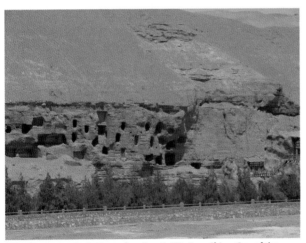

B Dunhuang grotto in Gansu Province in Western China. One of the places that many Buddhist texts have been found is in the Dunhuang grotto in Gansu Province, an area on the Silk Road. The first cave was established around 366 CE. At one time there were over 1000 caves, although only about 490 currently remain. Within the Buddhist scriptures found here are also several medical texts that include information about diagnosis, medical remedies, acupuncture and moxibustion, and materia medica.

The Maturation of Chinese Medicine

To this point, we have explored the oldest roots of Chinese medicine and pinpointed ancient theories that have, in one form or another, continued to develop within the tradition. The Han dynasty fell in 220 CE, and was followed by another period of strife and unrest. During this time, the Medicine of Systematic Correspondence continued to develop, as seen by the publication of Huang Fu Mi's (215–286 CE) *Systematic Classic of Acupuncture and Moxibustion (Zhen Jiu Jia Yi Jing)* and Wang Shu He's (210–285 CE) *Pulse Classic (Mai Jing)*. In 581, the Sui dynasty (see pp. 3 and 50) reunified China and again began the outward expansion of the empire. By this time, all of the elements that were going to inform the development of medicine in China until the introduction of Western medicine had appeared, including: Confucian thought, Daoist philosophies and exercises, Buddhist philosophies and exercises, as well as fundamental theories such as *yin* and *yang*, the five phases, the concept of *qi*, and the notion of the unity of the body with the environment. Chinese medicine did not become stagnant, however. Rather, the next stage of development revolved around a reexamination of the classics and the creation of treatment principles or strategies based on new interpretations of the fundamental concepts that had evolved during the Han dynasty.

Short-lived as it was, the Sui dynasty did not see a large contribution to the development of medicine. However, there are records indicating government support for farms for the cultivation of herbs.

In 618, the Sui dynasty was succeeded by the Tang dynasty (**A**, see also pp. 3 and 50), which continued to spread the influence of China through Central Asia and Vietnam and into Korea and Japan. During this period, considered by some to be the apex of China's cultural development, both Buddhism and Daoism strongly influenced medical thought.

Several important steps in the development of medicine occurred during the Tang dynasty, especially in the realm of education. For the first time, educational ranks were developed for imperial physicians. While most Confucian, Daoist, and Buddhist scholars (**B**) had a certain amount of medical knowledge, in the seventh century an imperial school of medicine was founded and medical institutions developed, further highlighting the difference between the classically trained literate elite and the folk traditions and regional practitioners. Classical medicine, which had been a pastime for scholar-officials now became a path toward advancement in the imperial bureaucracy. The students in the imperial school were all classically trained in Confucian doctrine prior to entering the medical academy. In the medical academy, they would study *The Yellow Emperor's Classic of Medicine*, the *Divine Husbandman's Materia Medica*, the *Pulse Classic*, the *Systematic Classic of Acupuncture and Moxibustion*, and other fundamental texts, after which time they could specialize in any given course of study.

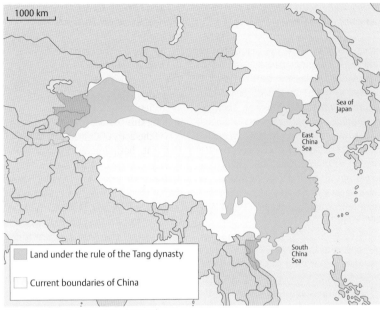

A Map of Tang dynasty China (700 CE).

Land under the rule of the Tang dynasty

Current boundaries of China

1000 km

Sea of Japan

East China Sea

South China Sea

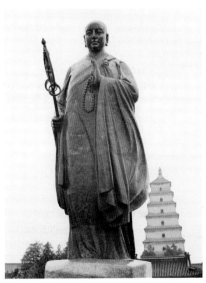

B Xuan Zang. Xuan Zang (603–664 CE) was a Tang dynasty Buddhist monk who, frustrated with the lack of information available in Chinese, traveled to India to study Buddhism. He learned Sanskrit and later returned to China, bringing with him over 600 Buddhist texts. Upon his return to China, he established a large translation bureau in Chang'an. He translated texts from Sanskrit to Chinese, making over 1000 fascicles of scriptures available.

By the Tang dynasty, several branches of medicine were recognized. They included: internal medicine, pediatrics, diseases of the eyes, ears, mouth and teeth, cupping, massage, and exorcism. Additionally, four kinds of practitioners were differentiated: physicians, acupuncturists (**A**), manual therapy practitioners, and exorcists. Unfortunately, while the profession of medicine was considered a benevolent practice, practitioners were relegated to a lower social position, being placed in the category of artisans, along with fortune-tellers, and astrologers (Wong and Wu 1985, p.76). The imperial schools were founded solely for the training of physicians to the emperor and his retinue. It was not until the Song dynasty (960–1270 CE) (see pp.3 and 50) that schools were established to train physicians for the average citizen.

Another important development of the Tang dynasty was the field of medical ethics. Sun Si Miao (581–682 CE), was a famous physician and literary scholar of the period who was well versed in Daoist and Buddhist practices. One of his texts, the *Thousand Ducat Prescriptions (Qian Jin Yao Fang)* contains a section entitled "On the Absolute Sincerity of Physicians," which established him as China's first medical ethicist (**B**). His essay sparked discussion of appropriate behavior for physicians in relation to who they treated and the fees that they could accept. He also addressed the need for continued scholarship among physicians and for compassion and high moral standards. Despite the scholarly achievements of men like Sun Si Miao, because of their practice of medicine, they were still relegated to the class of artisans and considered to have wasted their talents.

The Systematization of Medicine and Medical Education

In the Song dynasty a major change occurred in the bureaucracy of China. The hereditary aristocracy was replaced by the scholar-official whose position was based on merit. Merit, rather than rank or position became the criterion for advancement, and civil servants became the elite of China. One effect of this shift was a return to the precepts of Confucian morality as the guiding political force and the sweeping of Buddhism and Daoism into the status of popular religions. This neo-Confucianism emphasized Confucian morality, principles of education, and the proper order of relationships. The Song also saw an increase in literacy due to the spread of printing, the establishment of systematic educational institutions and the use of civil service examinations as the method of entry into the bureaucratic system. This increase in literacy led to a profusion of new texts in all areas, including medicine, and to huge enterprises in the reinterpretation of the classics.

During the Song dynasty medicine became very specialized. Texts on specific diseases and their treatment were published, and the first practical handbook on acupuncture and moxibustion was compiled. Overall, focus was on treatment of disease and specialization led to in-depth discussion of treatment strategies.

A A bronze acupuncture model.
In 1027 CE, the emperor had two bronze figures made to illustrate the location of acupuncture points. The models had holes drilled at the location of the points. For study purposes these would be covered with wax and filled with water. When a point was correctly located, water would drip out of the holes.

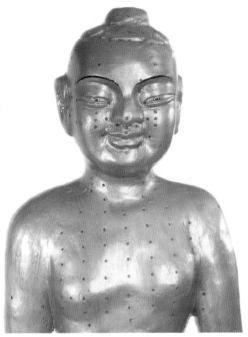

"Whenever a Great Physician treats diseases, he has to be mentally calm and his disposition firm. He should not give way to wishes and desires, but has to develop first of all a marked attitude of compassion. He should commit himself firmly to the willingness to take the effort to save every living creature.

If someone seeks help because of illness or on the ground of another difficulty, [a Great Physician] should not pay attention to status, wealth or age, neither should he question whether the particular person is attractive or unattractive, whether he is an enemy or a friend, whether he is Chinese or a foreigner, or finally, whether he is uneducated or educated. He should meet everyone on equal ground... Finally, it is inappropriate to emphasize one's reputation, to belittle the rest of the physicians and to praise only one's own virtue. Indeed, in actual life someone who has accidentally healed a disease, then stalks around with his head raised, shows conceit and announces that no one in the entire world could measure up to him. In this respect, all physicians are evidently incurable."

(Unschuld 1979, pp. 30–31)

B Quote from the section "On the Absolute Sincerity of Physicians" from the Thousand Ducat Prescriptions *(Qian Jin Yao Fang)* by Sun Si Miao.

One of the most important medical movements of the Song dynasty was the incorporation of herbal therapeutics into the Medicine of Systematic Correspondence. Previously, herbal medicine had remained a field separate from the more systematic medicine of the imperial academy, generally practiced by Daoists, family lineage practitioners, and folk practitioners. During the Song however, several extensive herbal pharmacopeias were published under imperial decree and herbal medicine became a part of the classical training of a physician. Because of the emphasis on Confucian relationships there was also an emphasis on the validation and compilation of correspondences. As a result, the Medicine of Systematic Correspondence was extended to the herbal pharmacopeia. This is when tastes and temperatures were assigned to herbs according to their *yin* or *yang* nature and specific functions were assigned to individual herbs. Herbal medicine, which had once been the property of the Buddhists and Daoists, was integrated into the Confucian system. This was the first attempt to apply the theory of one system to the practice of another therapeutic system and it transformed the practice of herbal medicine into an orderly and hierarchical system.

As a part of the revision of herbal medicine, the theories of Zhang Zhong Jing, the author of *Treatise On Cold Damage and Miscellaneous Diseases*, were revived (see p.226). This revival had a huge influence on the theory of herbal medicine, and several hundred years later was to precipitate the formation of a new theoretical school, the School of Warm Diseases (*Wen Bing Xue*). While the theoretical underpinnings of Chinese medicine lie in the Han dynasty, the form that we recognize today was established during the Song dynasty with its emphasis on classification and order. Thus, the five phases were further developed, as were the functions of the organs. The emphasis on systematic correspondence stems from the Song dynasty, as well as all attempts at reconciliation of opposing theories.

During the Song dynasty, the imperially trained medical practitioner began to use both acupuncture and herbal therapies to treat the sick. Herbal therapies were incorporated into the Medicine of Systematic Correspondence and attempts were made to reconcile the discrepancies in theory and practice that had emerged over time. Still, however, the well-trained practitioner of Chinese medicine remained primarily a scholar. The practice of Chinese medicine was taken up as an avocation, not as a primary profession.

Despite the advances of the Song, there also were struggles, most notably in the realm of education. A large number of schools of medicine opened during the Song dynasty. Who would be permitted to attend these schools and whether attendance at these schools was mandatory in order to practice medicine was at issue.

Plates **A, B, C** trace the developmental progress of important medical events, medical bureaucracy, and medical education over the preceding dynasties, which resulted in their systematization during the Song dynasty.

One of eight administrations under Court of Imperial Sacrifices:

- Two directors (junior and senior)
- Two deputy directors
- Four chief medical directors
- Eight assistant medical directors (clinical)
- X physicians (clinical)

- X practitioners (clinical)
- Eight pharmacists
- 24 apprentices in materia medica
- Two curators of medicinal gardens
- Eight apprentices of medicinal gardens

A Tang dynasty medical bureaucracy. Also under this bureau were four teaching departments, which consisted of the departments and personnel shown in **C** (adapted from Wang and Wu 1985).

491 CE	First permanent hospice with a dispensary established (Buddhist)
493 CE	Examinations for qualification to practice and teach medicine first appear
510 CE	First charitable government hospital established
620 CE	Hospital and clinic established inside the Imperial Compound
620–630 CE	Imperial Medical College founded
653 CE	Buddhist and Daoist monks and nuns forbidden to practice medicine
734 CE	Government supported orphanages and infirmaries for the poor
845 CE	Buddhist Hospitals (Compassion Pastures) transferred to lay control and called *Bing Fang* (Patients' Compounds)

B Important medical events of the Sui and Tang dynasties.

Department	Faculty, Staff, and Students	Texts	Lectures/Courses
General medicine (physicians)	One professor, one lecturer, 20 physicians, 100 practitioners, 40 students, two dispensers	Various materia medica *Pulse Classic (Mai Jing)* *Yellow Emperor's Classic of Medicine*	General medicine Sores and ulcers Pediatrics Eyes, ears, nose, and mouth Cupping
Acupuncture	One professor, one lecturer, 10 physicians of acupuncture, 20 acupuncture practitioners, 20 students	Specialized in sphygmology and acupuncture, learning the system of points on the surface of the body where needling should take place in accordance with the signs indicated by the pulse and other diagnostic aids	
Massage	One professor, four physicians of massage, 16 massage practitioners, 15 students	Medical exercise (for example *qi gong*), massage, trauma, and bone-setting	
Exorcism and incantation	One professor, two physicians of exorcism and incantation, eight practitioners of exorcism and incantation, 10 students	Exorcism and incantation	

C Tang dynasty medical education (adapted from Needham 1970, pp. 387–88).

Much of the conflict over education stemmed from the differing views of imperially trained physicians and independent physicians on the practice of medicine as a livelihood or as a natural outgrowth of scholarly pursuits. By the 12th century, given the emphasis on neo-Confucian thought and order and the growing importance of the examination system for entrance into the official class, the imperially trained physicians won the argument. Attendance at medical schools was limited to the classically trained Confucian scholar and the practice of medicine was limited to those trained in the medical academies. This limited the resources and abilities of the lay physician and jeopardized their ability to continue to practice medicine. This decision also institutionalized disdain for anyone who chose to practice medicine as a vocation rather than an avocation. The result was that Buddhist and Daoist monks continued to practice medicine for the people and to include the use of incantations and exorcisms in their practice, while the neo-Confucians rejected these elements of medicine and focused on the physical rather than the spiritual or psychological aspects of medicine. Of course, the Medicine of Systematic Correspondence continued to and continues to recognize the influence of the emotions on the health of the body, but the influence of nominally "spiritual" aspects of medicine such as the role of the spirits in health and disease was diminished. Thus, when we hear that Chinese medicine lost its "spiritual" aspect with the advent of the Communist Party, this is simply not true. In fact, the clear separation of naturalistic medicine from magical practices began in the 11th century, long before Communism.

Medicine in the Late Imperial Period: 1368–1911 CE

The academic medicine and systematic therapeutics of the Song dynasty continued through the next two dynasties, the Jin and the Yuan (see pp. 3 and 50), with such scholars as Liu Wan Su, founder of the School of Cooling, Zhang Zi He, founder of the School of Purgation, Li Dong Yuan, author of the *Discussion of the Spleen and Stomach (Pi Wei Lun)*, and Zhu Dan Xi, founder of the school of *Yin* Nourishment. These four are considered the classic scholars of the Jin/Yuan period and their theories continue to be evaluated, discussed, and used.

During the Ming dynasty, Li Shi Zhen (**A**) wrote his *Comprehensive Herbal Foundation (Ben Cao Gang Mu)* (**B**), which included discussion of 1892 substances, including substances such as ginseng and kelp (see p. 226). This book continued the incorporation of medicinal drugs into the framework of systematic correspondence. In addition to his materia medica, Li Shi Zhen authored the text that was to become the basis for pulse diagnosis in modern Chinese medicine, the *Lakeside Master's Study of the Pulse (Bin Hu Mai Xue)*.

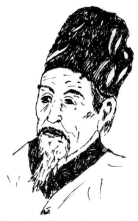

A Li Shi Zhen. Li Shi Zhen was the author of two major texts that have remained important to the practice of Chinese medicine to this day: the *Comprehensive Herbal Foundation (Ben Cao Gang Mu)* and the *Lakeside Master's Study of the Pulse (Bin Hu Mai Xue)*.

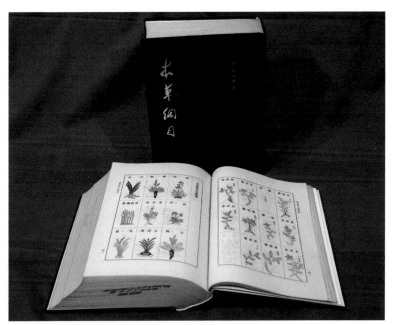

B Page from the *Comprehensive Herbal Foundation (Ben Cao Gang Mu)*.

The exploration of linkages between disease causation and therapeutics continued and several new medical sects emerged. In response to an epidemic in 1641, Wu You Ke (1592–1672 CE) used a treatment method that was based on the idea of "pestilential *qi*" causing epidemics and that treated with the use of cold substances. His text, *Discussion of Warm Epidemics (Wen Yi Lun)* explored the basis for his treatment. This discussion continued into the Qing dynasty as the School of Warm Diseases developed. The *Discussion of Warm Disease (Wen Re Lun)* by Ye Tian Shi complemented Zhang Zhong Jing's method of diagnosing and treating diseases caused by cold with an equally systematic method of diagnosing and treating those caused by heat (see also p. 226).

The most important occurrence of the Qing dynasty was the introduction of Western influence, technology, and medicine into China. Initially, the influence of the West was limited by the emperor, but as missionaries moved deeper into China, they brought new medical ideas, including missionary hospitals, and they used medicine to influence converts. To many, the old, "non-scientific" theories began to seem implausible, and there was disharmony in the medical community. In 1822, the Imperial Medical College declared that "the discipline of acupuncture … will henceforth be discontinued indefinitely" (Taylor 2005, p.44). With this statement, acupuncture became the medicine of the lower classes.

Medicine in Modern China

With the collapse of the Qing, and the formation of the Republic, the groundwork was laid for the elimination of Chinese medicine from the landscape. Sun Yat Sen (**A**), the founder of the Chinese Republic, was trained in Western medicine in Japan, and a series of clashes over the regulation, establishment, or elimination of practitioners of Chinese medicine occurred under the national government in an attempt to save the profession, practitioners from a variety of schools and traditions came together, and despite their differences, worked to create a unified medical system, using the term "Chinese medicine" or *zhong yi*. The theories and practices of Chinese medicine that had traveled through history to be incorporated into *zhong yi* included the theories of *yin* and *yang* and the five phases, the concept of *qi* as the basis for life, the understanding of the unity of the body with nature and the body as a microcosm of nature and, though somewhat obscure, some of the demonological concepts such as the idea of disease evils remained in the corpus of the literature.

However, the Nationalists disdained the medicine because of its lack of scientific proof and the early Communists, under Mao Zi Dong (**B**), disdained the medicine because it referred back to the feudal period in China to support its theories. The period from 1911 to 1950 was a difficult time for practitioners of Chinese medicine and extinction seemed imminent, no matter which political party prevailed.

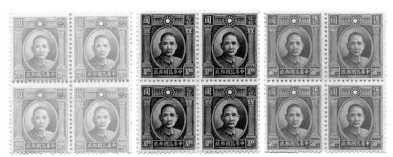

A Stamps showing the image of Sun Yat Sen, the founder of the Chinese Republic.

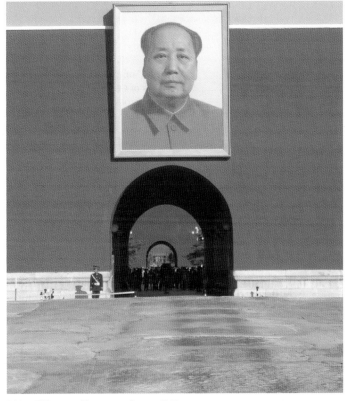

B Mao Zi Dong on Tiananmen Square, Beijng.

After the Communist takeover of 1949, Mao Zi Dong softened his view of Chinese medicine slightly. In 1954, a group of older doctors from Nanjing were convened to discuss the future of Chinese medicine. From this meeting came the first modern attempts at state-run schools of Chinese medicine. The first school opened in Nanjing in 1954, to be followed in 1956 by the opening of four academies of Chinese medicine in Beijing, Shanghai, Guangzhou, and Chengdu. Mao had wanted the students to be physicians choosing to study Chinese medicine, but early experiments with this were not successful and so the schools opened to others in order to increase the number of available physicians in China. These schools were not ranked as high as medical schools, but they were at the level of most colleges, and attendance was state-sponsored. From 1956–1959, the first set of standardized textbooks for a five-year curriculum were created by physicians from all five of the academies. These textbooks would continue to be revised and updated over the next 50 years, and are currently in their seventh edition.

When, in 1958, Mao declared "China's medicine and pharmacology is a great treasure house" (Taylor 2005, p.120), he was envisioning a single medicine in which physicians would be trained in biomedicine, and also study Chinese medicine. Rather than one medicine, however, two medicines developed, and today, the medicine, marketed by the Chinese to the West as Traditional Chinese Medicine, continues to be taught and practiced throughout China and the West.

In general, colleges and universities of Chinese medicine (see **A** for an example of a typical curriculum) in China today are divided into three main departments: the Department of Chinese Medicine (focused on the practice of herbs), the Department of Acupuncture, and the Department of Pharmacy (focused on the harvesting, preparing, and dispensing of herbs). These institutions are attended by students who have completed high school, indicated that they were interested in studying medicine, and tested sufficiently high on the college entrance examination. Many see the study of Chinese medicine as a path to the practice of biomedicine. Others have chosen the field because their parents were physicians of Chinese medicine and dictated their choice, and a small minority chose these colleges because of a desire to study Chinese medicine (Ergil 1994).

After graduation, most practitioners work in one of the large hospitals of Chinese medicine found throughout China. These hospitals, many of which are also equipped with high-tech biomedical diagnostic tools such as CAT and MRI scanners, have both in-patient and outpatient wards where the primary treatment is Chinese medicine. Other routes to employment include opening a private practice (a somewhat complex endeavor in modern China) or for a small number, continuing with one's education and completing a Master's Degree or PhD in Chinese medicine. Advanced degrees are usually focused on either animal research or research on the classics. Additionally, much emphasis is placed on the integration of Chinese and Western medicine.

Year	Semester	Course	Hours	Credits
First year	First semester	Foreign Language	72	2.5
		Physical Education	54	2
		Classical Medical Chinese	72	3
		Fundamental Theory of Chinese Medicine	90	5
		Human Anatomy	108	5
		Medical Biology	36	2
		History of Chinese Medicine	36	2
	Second semester	Foreign Language	72	2.5
		Physical Education	54	2
		Classical Medical Chinese	72	3
		Materia Medica	90	5
		Chinese Medicine Diagnostics	108	5
		Embryology	54	2
Second year	First semester	Foreign Language	72	2.5
		Physical Education	36	2
		Materia Medica	72	3
		Formulas	108	5
		Chinese Medicine Internal Medicine I	90	5
		Biochemistry	72	4
	Second semester	Foreign Language	72	2.5
		Physical Education	36	2
		Biology	90	5
		Chinese Medicine Internal Medicine II	90	5
		Shang Han Lun (On Cold Damage)	90	5
		Public Health and Emergency Medicine	72	3
Third year	First semester	Foreign Language	72	2.5
		Traditional Health Protection Physical Education	36	1
		Pathology	90	4
		Chinese Medicine Gynecology	72	4
		Warm Disease Theory	72	4
		Acupuncture	108	5
		Chinese Medicine Ophthalmology	40	2
	Second semester	Chinese Medicine Pediatrics	70	4
		Pharmacology	50	3
		Foreign Language	40	1.5
		Chinese Medicine Ears, Nose, and Throat	40	2
Fourth year	First semester	Traditional Health Protection Physical Education	36	1
		Fundamentals of Western Diagnostics	108	5
		Jin Gui Yao Lue (Essential Prescriptions of the Golden Coffer)	90	4
		The Yellow Emperor's Classic of Medicine I	90	4
		Chinese Medicine Traumatology	72	4
		Western External Medicine	54	3
	Second semester	Traditional Health Protection Physical Education	36	1
		Heterodox Schools of Chinese Medicine	90	5
		The Yellow Emperor's Classic of Medicine II	36	2
		Western Medicine Internal Medicine	72	4
		Computers and Medicine	90	3
		Chinese Medicine External Medicine	72	4
		Emergency Care	54	2
Fifth year	First and second semester	Graduation Practice		

A Department of Chinese Medicine Curriculum of a modern college of Chinese medicine in China.

As the medicine that has its roots in China has spread through the world, it has evolved and adapted to its adopted cultures. So the medicine that is practiced in Japan, for example, continues to look to the Chinese classics for its roots, but has privileged different texts or different theoretical paradigms. As a result there are several, extremely varied, schools of thought in Japan, ranging from practitioners who practice much as practitioners in China do, to those who do not even insert a needle. In Korea and Vietnam, distinct systems and theories that rely on the basic theory of Chinese medicine have developed. Many scholars from these countries also choose to study in China to gain greater insight into the medicine by studying at its source. In some Asian countries, the practice of Chinese medicine is limited to those trained as biomedical physicians. In Japan, one can be trained as an acupuncture practitioner or a moxibustion practitioner, but only physicians are permitted to practice the herbal tradition, *kampo* (meaning Chinese method).

The ideas of Chinese medicine were introduced to the West through many different avenues. In France, men such as George Soulié de Morant were highly influential, while in Britain, individuals like Royston Low and Jack Worsley played very important roles. The styles of acupuncture that were developed by these individuals diverge greatly in some respects from the medicine that is practiced in China today, but at their root, they are all based on the same fundamental theories.

When the ideas of Chinese medicine were eventually introduced to the West, it was the theory of the acupuncture channels and the corresponding therapeutic technique of acupuncture that was popularized and first taught. The practice of herbal therapeutics, despite being the primary internal medicine therapy in China, took much longer to gain momentum.

Although the practice of Chinese medicine first came to the United States with Chinese immigrants, it was focused in the Chinatowns (**A**) and did not gain any popularity amongst the larger society. In the United States, acupuncture gained visibility after James Reston, a *New York Times* reporter visiting China just prior to Richard Nixon's visit developed appendicitis. After having his appendix removed surgically, with standard surgical procedures, he received acupuncture for the treatment of post-surgical pain. The article about his experience appeared on the front page of the *New York Times* and captured the imagination of many US citizens (**B**). Today, in Europe, Japan, and North America, most practitioners of Chinese medicine are allowed to practice acupuncture, and many also practice herbal medicine. Laws and educational standards vary greatly from one country to another and even within countries such as the United States and Canada where each state or province has its own regulation.

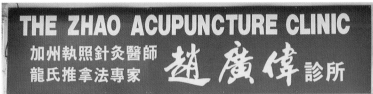

A Chinese clinic in Chinatown, San Francisco.

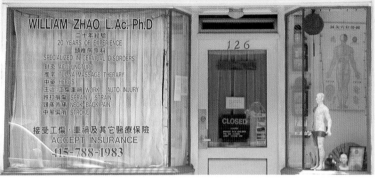

"Now, let me tell you about my appendectomy in Peking.
In brief summary, the facts are that with the assistance of 11 of the leading medial specialists in Peking, who were asked by Premier Chou En-lai to cooperate on the case, Prof. Wu Wei-jan of the Anti-Imperialist Hospital's surgical staff removed my appendix on July 17 after a normal injection of Xylocain and Bensocain, which anesthetized the middle of my body.
There were no complications, nausea or vomiting. I was conscious throughout, followed the instructions of Professor Wu as translated to me by Ma Yu-chen of the Chinese Foreign Ministry during the operation, and was back in my bedroom in the hospital in two-and-a-half hours.

However, I was in considerable discomfort if not pain during the second night after the operation, and Li Chang-yuan, doctor of acupuncture at the hospital, with my approval, inserted three long thin needles into the outer part of my right elbow and below my knees and manipulated them in order to stimulate the intestine and relieve the pressure and distension of the stomach.
That sent ripples of pain racing through my limbs and, at least, had the effect of diverting my attention from the distress in my stomach. Meanwhile, Doctor Li lit two pieces of an herb called *ai*, which looked like the burning stumps of a broken cheap cigar, and held them close to my abdomen while occasionally twirling the needles into action."

(Reston 1971)

B Quote from James Reston (*New York Times*, Monday July 26, 1971).

Translation and Terminology

One of the more challenging aspects of the West's engagement with Chinese medicine was that books were available only in Asian languages, languages that were typically inaccessible to the Westerner. Early translations of the texts fell into one of three categories:

1. Translations done by the Chinese of very simplified acupuncture texts that were translated into primarily biomedical terminology. These were often very poor translations and the use of biomedical terminology caused a great deal of confusion and loss of important concepts.
2. Translations done by native English speakers that offered a great deal to the field, but, neglected to follow some of the simple rules of translation, such as the creation of a glossary to allow the reader to return to the terms of the original text. These texts also suffered from over-simplification for the English reader.
3. Original books based on the author's own study of Chinese medicine, which while useful, were colored by the author's interpretation.

As schools of Chinese medicine developed outside of China, the demand for textbooks increased along with a recognition of the need for quality translations that were true to the Chinese ideas, did not conflate Chinese medical terms with biomedical terms, and provided a glossary that allowed the reader to fluently return to the actual terms or characters of the original (Ergil and Ergil 2008) (see **A, B, C** for examples of translation issues).

Since the publication of *Fundamentals of Chinese Medicine* (Wiseman and Ellis 1985), and the subsequent publication of the *Glossary of Chinese Medical Terms* (Wiseman 1989), the translation debate has centered around the use of a standardized, glossed terminology with a dictionary to support its use and a non-standardized terminology that was dependent upon translator interpretation of usage. The debate, centered aroun source-oriented vs. target-oriented translations (Wiseman 2007) has gone on for many years with no clear resolution, but as more practitioners learn Chinese and the amount of translated material increases, more and more use is being made of standardized terminology and source-oriented translation.

It is the belief of the editors that standardized terminology frees the translation from unnecessary interpretation and allows the reader to interpret what they believe the author of the original text was saying. It also allows the non-native English speaker who is familiar with Chinese characters to return to the original Chinese and to know that throughout the text, the terminology will be consistent. Although this text is not a translation, the terminology used sticks as closely as possible to the terminology of Wiseman and Ye, and the source-oriented approach, as published in the *Practical Dictionary of Chinese Medicine* (Wiseman and Ye 1998). The question of language in Chinese medicine is just one more aspect of the history of the movement and evolution of Chinese medicine.

Chinese	Source-oriented Translation	Biomedical-/Target-oriented Translation
风火眼 *feng huo yan*	Wind fire eye	Acute conjunctivitis
痹 *bi*	Impediment	Arthralgia

A Examples of term translation problems. In the upper line, wind fire eye as a Chinese medicine concept has a much broader meaning than acute conjunctivitis. Acute conjunctivitis has nothing to do with wind or fire, nor was it a concept that historic figures knew anything about when they saw a red, teary eye. In the lower line, impediment refers to musculoskeletal pain conditions due to wind–cold-damp or other combinations of evil and it does not occur only in the joints (adopted from Wiseman 2007).

Chinese	Source-oriented Translation	Biomedical-/Target-oriented Translation
痿 *wei*	Wilting	Flaccidity syndrome
痰核 *tan he*	Phlegm node	Subcutaneous nodule
喉蛾 *hou e*	Throat moth	Tonsillitis
疝 *shan*	Mounting	Hernia

B Further examples of the use of biomedical terms (adapted from Wiseman 2007).

Chinese	Source-oriented Translation	Biomedical-/Target-oriented Translation
活血 *huo xue*	Quicken the blood	Promote blood circulation
神 *shen*	Spirit	Consciousness
邪 *xie*	Evil	Pathogenic factor
泻 *xie*	Drain	Sedate

C Simplifying the meaning or using a term with an already understood (connotative) definition that obscures the original meaning but the chosen term is "easier to understand."

Chinese	Source-oriented Translation	Biomedical-/Target-oriented Translation
哮 *xiao*	Wheezing (a sound that often accompanies panting)	Asthma
喘 *chuan*	Panting (severe breathing difficulty, with discontinuity of breathing	Asthma
哮喘 *xiao chuan*	Wheezing and panting	Asthma
心悸 *xin ji*	Heart palpitations	Palpitations
惊悸 *jing ji*	Fright palpitations	Palpitations
怔忡 *zheng chong*	Fearful throbbing	Palpitations

D Using one term to translate many different terms in Chinese conflates ideas, may cause clinical confusion or errors, and results in the loss of meaning and concepts.

Table of Dynasties

Dynasty	Period	Major Medical Events
Xia	Ca. 2100–ca. 1600 BCE	No archeological proof of its existence
Shang	Ca. 1600–ca. 1100 BCE	True archaeological evidence of its existence
		Ancestor worship and oracle bone divination by the king are the main forms of medicine
		Disease is equated with the curse of an ancestor
		Oracle bones are interpreted by the king and the *wu* (shamans)
Zhou Western Zhou Eastern Zhou, including Spring and Autumn Period	Ca. 1100–ca. 771 BCE 770–475 BCE	Ancestor worship continues, the *wu* are more prevalent and begin to play a role in the healing of sick individuals, not just the king
		As the dynasty declines, there is a time of chaos and unrest, which results in demonological therapy, magical correspondence, and ancestor worship. Disease may now be caused by a demon or by magic, not just by an ancestor
		Confucius lives (551–479 BCE)
Warring States	475–221 BCE	Continued chaos and unrest allows demonological therapy to thrive
		A time of great philosophical thinking: – development of *yin yang* school – development of five-phase school – Confucius dies (479 BCE) and development of Confucian doctrine by his students Lao Zi and Zhuang Zi live – development of Daoism
Qin	221–206 BC	Reunification of China under a legalist regime that requires strict adherence to the emperor
		Major works such as the Great Wall are completed
		Philosophy is banned and all books that are not supportive of the regime are burned
Han	206 BCE–220 CE	China is reunified after the fall of the Qin. The Confucian doctrine takes its place as the political school of thought that will continue to influence China for the next 2000 years
		Yin yang and five-phase schools are integrated into the Confucian doctrine
		The Medicine of Systematic Correspondence, which is based in Confucian thought, develops
		The major medical classics are written or compiled, including The Yellow Emperor's Classic of Medicine, Classic of Difficulties, On Cold Damage, and The Divine Husbandman's Materia Medica
		Buddhism comes to China from India
Three Kingdoms	220–265 CE	
Western and Eastern Jin	265–420 CE	
Northern and Southern dynasties	420–581 CE	
Sui	581–618 CE	Focus on unifying China
		Farms for the cultivation of herbs established by government
		All of the elements that informed the development of medicine in China are present: Confucian thought, Daoist philosophy, search for immortality, Buddhist exercises, treatment of the masses, *qi*, Medicine of Systematic Correspondence and so on. From this point on, changes in the medicine of China were variations on a theme

Dynasty	Period	Major Medical Events
Tang	618–907 CE	Chinese culture closely tied to Buddhist philosophy
		In medicine, there is interest in examining that which already existed, not furthering philosophical thought
		Educational ranks are established for imperial physicians
		Imperial school of medicine is founded
		Medicine is broken into four specialties: acupuncture, massage, internal medicine, incantations
Five dynasties	907–960 CE	
Northern and Southern Song	960–1270 CE	Scholar-officials replace aristocracy as dominant class
		Medicine becomes more specialized
		1027: bronze acupuncture men created for use in the Imperial Academy
		System of correspondences expanded to include herbs
		Revival of theories of Zhang Zhong Jing *(Shang Han Lun)*
		Struggle over education of physicians: imperial vs. apprenticeship
		Attempts to explain away contradictions within medicine and a shift away from the spiritual aspects of medicine
Jin and Yuan	1115–1234 CE 1271–1368 CE	Four masters: Liu Wan Su (School of Cooling), Zhang Zi He (School of Purgation), Li Dong Yuan (Spleen Stomach School), Zhu Dan Xi (School of *Yin* Nourishment)
		Foreign (Mongol) dynasty, China completely taken over by Mongols
Ming	1368–1644 CE	Considered one of the high points of the late imperial era
		Medicinal drugs fully incorporated into the Medicine of Systematic Correspondence
		Li Shi Zhen lives (1518–1593)
		Development of *Wen Bing* (Warm Diseases) theory
		Interest in empirical evidence (what actually works)
Qing	1644–1911 CE	Foreign dynasty (Manchu) and the last imperial dynasty
		Early Qing: economic, political, and cultural stability
		Influx of Westerners into China
		Return to classics as protection against foreigners
		Medical unrest: lack of satisfaction with old theories
		Introduction of Western medicine has a huge influence: modernization vs. tradition
Republic of China Mainland Taiwan	1912–1949 CE 1949 CE–present	Encouraged the move toward modernization
		Modernization = scientization
		Chinese medicine nearly lost. Saved by the creation of *zhong yi* (Chinese medicine)
People's Republic of China	1949 CE–present	Traditional Chinese medicine used on the Long March
		Schools with standardized curriculum and texts established (1954–1959)
		Move toward integration of Western and Chinese medicine

A Chinese dynastic chart with major medical events.

2

Fundamental Theory of Chinese Medicine

Kevin V. Ergil

Introduction

When students in colleges of Traditional Chinese Medicine begin their studies, one of their first courses addresses what is called "Fundamental Theory" (中医基础). This course presents the core theoretical models that underlie every aspect of Traditional Chinese Medicine practice. It is intriguing to note that, while these courses are taught in modern classrooms to students who graduate to practice in hospital settings furnished with conventional biomedical diagnostic and therapeutic resources, every element of the course can be directly mapped onto the 2000 years of Chinese medical practice and scholarship that precedes this modern age.

The reorganization of traditional medical education by the Marxist-Maoist educators of the 1950s made it possible to systematically educate thousands of young men and women as TCM physicians. However, the basis for this educational program was and is the classic texts of Chinese medicine, such as *The Yellow Emperor's Classic of Medicine, On Cold Damage*, and others.

This chapter presents the core ideas of Chinese medicine: *yin* and *yang*, the five phases, the bodily substances (*qi*, blood, essence, and fluids), spirit, the channels, the viscera and bowels, the extraordinary organs, the triple burner, and the causes of disease. The Chinese medicine understanding of an embodied mind is discussed as well. These ideas are essential to understanding all aspects of Chinese medicine diagnosis and treatment. In some cases these ideas will seem easy enough to grasp at once; in other cases these ideas will re-emerge with greater clarity in later chapters.

Fundamental Theory (see **A** for an outline) is just that, fundamental. As we begin our discussion of *yin* and *yang*, and as the ideas strike us as at once simple and profound we may confuse the ease with which we understand these ideas with mastery. I have frequently experienced lectures presented by senior teachers of Chinese medicine who, in teaching their colleagues, begin with a recapitulation of such fundamental ideas: *yin* and *yang*, the natural rhythm of sun and shade, or hot and cold. Chinese members of the audience listen carefully; others often listen carelessly, wondering why such basic ideas are being recapitulated to an audience that must already know them well. What the scholars and senior clinicians know, and the neophytes do not, is that the deeper truths of the core theory of Chinese medicine reveal themselves only through years of application and experience.

As a former student once said to me as we sat on a park bench together and admired the spring weather: "When I began my studies, *yin* and *yang* were simply words to understand, now everywhere I look I see that the interplay of *yin* and *yang* and the five phases surround me on every side."

Fundamental Theory Outline	Topics Discussed
Yin and *yang*	• *Yin* and *yang* in medicine
The five phases	• The four cycles of the five phases
Qi, blood, fluids, essence, and spirit	• *Qi* • Blood and fluids • Essence and spirit • The pathology of *qi*, blood, and body fluids
The channels	• The eight extraordinary vessels
Viscera and bowels	• The heart and pericardium • The lung • The spleen, stomach, and intestines • The liver and gallbladder • The kidney and urinary bladder • The triple burner • The extraordinary organs • Development, reproduction, and aging
The three causes of disease	• External causes: the six evils • Internal causes: the seven affects • Neither internal nor external causes
The healthy body as an orderly landscape	

A Fundamental Theory outline: topics discussed in this chapter.

Yin *and* Yang

Yin and *yang* express the idea that any given phenomenon can be understood to exist in balance in relation to a given complementary phenomenon. These phenomena then exist in a state of dynamic equilibrium. From alterations in that dynamic relationship, different conditions arise. As was discussed in Chapter 1, the idea of *yin* and *yang* was first expressed with the image of the contrasting climates of sunny and shady hillsides. Imagine, for a moment, the different environments that exist on either side of that hill: on the bright, sunny side, plants and animals that enjoy light are more prevalent, the air is drier, and the rocks are warm; on the dim, shaded side, the air is moist and cool, animals take refuge from the heat of the day. *Yin* and *yang* exist in relationship (**A**, see also p. 20).

Yin phenomena are characterized as moist, cool, passive, nurturing, interior, dark, and deep, while *yang* phenomena are warm, active, consuming, exterior, light, and superficial. *Yin* and *yang* are used to describe the cycle of the seasons, the cycle of a day as it moves from dawn to dusk and then to dawn again, the viscera and bowels, and the acupuncture channels.

This type of analysis depends on the continuously divisible nature of *yin* and *yang*. The cycle of the seasons can be analyzed in this way (**B**). Summer is *yang* within *yang*, fall is *yin* within *yang*, winter is *yin* within *yin*, and spring is *yang* within *yin*. Thus, the coldest, darkest, and most *yin* period is *yin* within *yin*, whereas spring, when the *yang* begins to emerge from the *yin*, is *yang* within *yin*.

A world that is seen through the lens of *yin* and *yang* is seen in ecological perspective: each phenomenon is seen in relation to its surroundings, and it is expected that each phenomenon will exert upon, and receive from its surroundings, influences that can be understood in *yin* and *yang* terms. "Just as the language of ecology is the language of interrelation and interdependence, the language of Chinese medicine is a language of interrelation and interdependence. The external landscape, or human environment, is understood to be in profound and dynamic relationship with the internal landscape, or human organism" (Ergil 2006, p. 384).

Human beings have a nature and structure inseparable from *yin* and *yang* and as such are inseparable from the world around them. Every aspect of life partakes of a *yin* or a *yang* aspect. Understanding of this fact and living life in accord with *yin* and *yang* supports life itself. According to the ancient physician-sages, "To follow (the laws of) *yin* and *yang* means life; to act contrary (to the laws of *yin* and *yang*) means death" (*Huang Di Nei Jing Su Wen* Chapter 2 in Unschuld 1988, p. 13).

Yang	Yin
South side of a hill	North side of a hill
North side of a river	South side of a river
3, 7, 9	2, 6, 8
Bright	Dark
Heaven	Earth
Sun	Moon
Day	Night
Spring	Autumn
Summer	Winter
Hot	Cold
Sunshine	Cloudy
Dry	Damp
Male	Female
Fast	Slow
Movement	Stasis
Light	Heavy
Front	Back
Up	Down
Outside	Inside
Fire	Water
Wood	Metal
Left side	Right side

A *Yin* and *yang* correspondences.

B *Tai ji di tu* with seasons. The familiar "*yin yang* symbol" is the *tai ji di tu* or the map of the supreme ultimate conveying the idea of the profound meaning implied in this simple image. Here it is shown surrounded by shaded areas indicating the division of the primary duality of *yin* and *yang* into the four seasons.

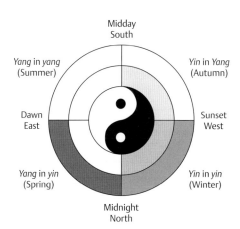

Midday
South

Yang in *yang*
(Summer)

Yin in *Yang*
(Autumn)

Dawn
East

Sunset
West

Yang in *yin*
(Spring)

Yin in *yin*
(Winter)

Midnight
North

Yin and *Yang* in Medicine

While it is probably easiest to think about *yin* and *yang* as qualitative descriptive terms that help the Chinese physician organize information, it should be remembered (especially in traditional pharmaceutics) that the *yin* and *yang* constituents of the body are actual things that can be reinforced by specific substances or actions.

This relationship between *yin* and *yang* is often represented by a lit candle. If one considers the *yin* aspect of the candle to be the wax and the *yang* aspect to be the flame, one can see how the *yin* nourishes and supports the *yang* and how the *yang* consumes the *yin* and thus burns brightly. When the wax is gone, so is the flame. *Yin* and *yang* exist in dependence on each other.

The dynamic physiology of *yin* and *yang* is a recurring theme as we examine narrower concepts such as the *qi* and blood or the viscera and bowels. Movement within the body can be analyzed in terms of *yin* and *yang*. Light and mobile, and hence *yang*, substances move up and out, while dense and viscous *yin* substances move down and in to produce an interior dynamic that is fundamental to Chinese medicine physiology.

A describes the five sets of relationships between *yin* and *yang* that obtain when *yin* and *yang* are viewed as actively counterbalanced qualities or substances; the analysis is the same in either context. This approach is used to understand pathological processes and is summed up in the following funda-mental principle, "When *yin* prevails, there is cold; when *yang* prevails, there is heat. When *yang* is vacuous there is cold; when *yin* is vacuous there is heat"[*].

For instance, repeated exposure to cold combined with a diet replete with cold foods, raw vegetables, and cold beverages produces a repletion of *yin*, which comes to dominate the *yang* factors of the body, producing signs of cold in the body. This is what is meant by *yin* prevailing. It is quite common to encounter individuals whose body's *yin* substances have become depleted. This can occur through illness, taxation, or the chronic use of some drugs. It can also occur through the aging process (a form of taxation) and is often seen in peri-menopausal women where signs such as night sweats, flushing, hot flashes, etc., are seen as a sign of insufficient *yin*, In this case "where *yin* is vacuous there is heat," is the interpretation.

While simple, these concepts are fundamental to organizing concepts of physiology, pathology, diagnosis and treatment and sections of this text will return to them often.

---

[*]   Statements such as this are classically derived aphorisms that are core axioms in Chinese medicine reasoning. This text refers to them as "critical principles" and they appear in quotes when presented. While these expressions can be found in many texts most of those presented here can be found in Wiseman (1996 and 1998).

Yin and *Yang* Balanced

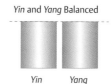

Yin   Yang

Balanced *yin* and *yang* is considered
physiologically normal.

Replete *Yin*

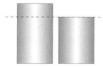

Yin   Yang

Abnormal abundance of *yin*, presents signs
of cold and abundant *yin*.

Vacuous *Yin*

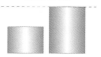

Yin   Yang

Normal *yang* unrestrained, presents
signs of heat and *yang* overactivity.

Replete *Yang*

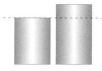

Yin   Yang

Abnormal abundance of *yang*, presents signs
of heat and overactivity of *yang*.

A Balance of *yin* and *yang.*

Vacuous *Yang*

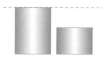

Yin   Yang

Normal *yin* is not warmed and balanced
when *yang* is insufficient, presents signs
of cold and abundant *yin*.

The Five Phases

The five phases are earth, metal, water, wood, and fire. In Chinese, *wu* (五) means "five" and *xing* (行) expresses the idea of movement, "to go." Sometimes *wu xing* is translated as "the five elements," but this translation fails to convey the dynamism of the Chinese concept, instead focusing on the apparent similarities between the *wu xing* and the elements of ancient and medieval Greco-Roman medicine. While the *wu xing* may, and has historically, included the implication of material elements, the five phases are used to describe a set of dynamic relations occurring among phenomena (see also p. 20).

The relationships, which are described in detail below, are based on the idea that every phenomenon has qualities or characteristics in common with one of the phases. Thus, wood with its quality of flexible, forceful growth is seen in relation to the season of spring, the wind, and the affect of anger, all of which partake of suddenness and force. The heart, summertime, the heat of the noon day, the tongue, unbridled joy, and the surging pulse that rises forcefully to the surface all conjure the redness, outward movement, and heat of fire. All of these associations can be seen in **A**. These associations convey diagnostic and therapeutic meaning in their own right. A patient with unresolved grief may present with a history of lung

conditions. A patient with a predilection for moist sweet foods may burden the spleen, which responds with the production of superfluous flesh.

The five phases have many functions in Chinese medicine. Their correspondences and relationships are used to understand the roles and relationships of the viscera and bowels. Emotional experiences, foods, seasons, and sounds can all be linked to the activities of the organs, their function, and physical expression. All theory concerning the viscera and bowels is deeply informed by five-phase thinking. The five phases are also applied in traditions of diagnosis and treatment that employ very strict constructions of classical thought. This can be seen in systems of acupuncture therapy that are based in the tradition of the *Classic of Difficulties (Nan Jing)* and use five-phase theory extensively to integrate ideas about organ function, pulse signs, and acupuncture point selection (this is discussed in greater detail in the Chapters 3 and 4).

The five-phase correspondences outlined in **A** provide a clear sense of how we might think with the five phases. Laughter is the sound of the heart and red is its color. Unrestrained laughter, a red face, a pulse that is felt more forcefully in the heart position suggests some disturbance in the heart. **B** and **C** show the directional associations of the five phases and the relationships between the five phases and *yin* and *yang* respectively.

Category	▽ Wood	△ Fire	☐ Earth	◇ Metal	○ Water
Season	Spring	Summer	Late summer	Autumn	Winter
Time of day	Before sunrise	Forenoon	Afternoon	Late afternoon	Midnight
Climate	Wind	Heat	Damp	Dryness	Cold
Direction	East	South	Center	West	North
Development	Birth	Growth	Maturity	Withdrawal	Dormancy
Color	Cyan	Red	Yellow	White	Black
Taste	Sour	Bitter	Sweet	Acrid	Salty
Viscus	Liver	Heart	Spleen	Lungs	Kidney
Bowel	Gall-bladder	Small intestine	Stomach	Large intestine	Urinary bladder
Sense organ	Eyes	Tongue	Mouth	Nose	Ears
Tissue	Sinews	Vessels	Flesh	Skin/body hair	Bones
Mind	Anger	Joy	Thought	Sorrow	Fear
Odor	Goatish	Scorched	Fragrant	Raw fish	Putrid
Vocalization	Shouting	Laughing	Singing	Weeping	Sighing
Spirits	Ethereal soul	Spirit	Reflection	Corporeal soul	Will
Body fluid	Tears	Sweat	Saliva	Mucus	Urine
Manifestation area	Nails	Complexion	Lips	Body hair	Head hair

A Five phase correspondences.

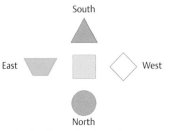

B The directions of the five phases.

Phase	Yin Yang Relationships	
▽ Wood	*Yang* in *yin*	*Shao yang*
△ Fire	*Yang* in *yang*	*Tai yang*
☐ Earth	Balanced *yin* and *yang*	
◇ Metal	*Yin* in *yang*	*Shao yin*
○ Water	*Yin* in *yin*	*Tai yin*

C Five phases and *yin* and *yang*.

The Four Cycles of the Five Phases

The four cycles portray the dynamic relationship between the phases. The first two cycles are "physiological" indicating normal relations in the body's viscera and bowels, homeostasis, or balance in the system (**A**).

The engendering cycle is the cycle of growth and development. It expresses the mother–child relationship, the mother conveying her *qi* or vital substance to the child in the act of nurturance. This is the cycle of seasonal change as spring (wood) gives rise to summer (fire), which produces long summer (earth) (mid-July to mid-August) and then autumn (metal), which is followed by winter (water) and so on with the return of spring.

Wood is the image of vigorous forceful growth, of a sapling bursting forth in the spring. Wood fuels fire and the heat of summer is captured in the image of fire. Just as fire consumes wood leaving earth-like ash behind, so the ripening grains of long summer emerge from the fire of summer. Metal is observed to be derived from metallic oxides in the earth and so is seen as the child of earth. The essence of earth: fruits, nuts, and grains are collected during the fall harvest, as plants are cut with metal tools. Fall gives way to winter as metal produces water. Moist breath exhaled by the lungs, or the use of metal mirrors to condense water from the atmosphere in arid environments, is the basis for this analogy.

The restraining cycle depicts the healthy control of one phase by another. The engendering cycle is a positive feedback system, without restraint it will become unbalanced. The restraining cycle shows the "grandmother" phase controlling its "grandchild." Fire, earth's mother, is the grandmother of metal, and controls its grandchild. Wood controls earth as wooden spades and bulwarks were used to shape and control earth. In turn, earthen dams and ditches guide and restrain water to productive purpose. Water can dampen the ardor of fire and fire can be used to melt and shape metal.

The negative feedback of the restraining cycle balances the positive feedback of the engendering cycle.

The next two cycles are "pathological" and manifest in a body out of balance (**B**). They are produced when a phase becomes weak or exuberant. The overwhelming cycle occurs when one phase becomes weak or exuberant and disturbs the restraining cycle. If the spleen (earth), associated with normal digestion, becomes weakened then the liver (wood) overwhelms it, causing digestive disturbances. This can also occur where the liver (wood) becomes replete and overwhelms the spleen (earth).

The rebellion cycle occurs when the grandchild phase either becomes exuberant or when the grandmother weakens and the restraining cycle is counteracted. The heart (fire), instead of being restrained by the kidney (water), rebels and flaring of heart fire with *yin* vacuity occurs.

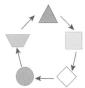

The engendering cycle *(xiang sheng)*
Engendering: each phase relates
to the next as mother to child.
Earth engenders metal.

The restraining cycle *(xiang ke)*
Restraining: the grandmother restrains
the grandchild. Earth restrains water.

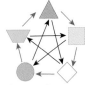

Engendering and restrainig shown together

A Two "Physiological Cycles".

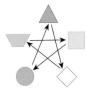

The overwhelming cycle *(xiang cheng)*
reflects a pathological situation in which
the restraining cycle is over expressed
and the restraining phase over powers the
restrained phase. Earth overwhelms water.

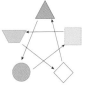

The rebellion cycle *(xiang wu)* is a
pathological situation that occurs when
the restrained phase rebels against the
restraining phase. Water rebels against
earth.

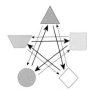

Overwhelming and rebellion shown together

B Two "Pathological Cycles".

Qi, *Blood, Fluids, Essence, and Spirit*

Qi

After *yin* and *yang*, no concept is more crucial to Chinese medicine than that of *qi*, the idea that the body is pervaded by a subtle material and mobile influence that produces most physiological functions and maintains the body's health and vitality. *Qi* and blood are closely linked, in fact they are virtually inseparable since *qi* and blood are said to flow together through the channels and nourish the organs. Blood and *qi* have a *yin* and *yang* relationship: *qi* is the active, *yang* substance; it warms and gives the body vitality. Blood is the *yin* substance moistening and nourishing the organs. The close relationship between *qi* and blood is expressed by the critical principle that states, "*Qi* is the commander of blood and blood is the mother of *qi*." This expresses the *yang* aspect of *qi* in its role of actively conducting blood through the body and the *yin* role of blood, which nourishes *qi* and smoothes its way through the body.

Sometimes *qi* is translated as *energy*, but this conceals the distinctly material attributes of *qi* and its close relationship with the tangible and substantive aspects of our embodied experience. While *qi* has an energetic character (in the sense that energy is defined as the capacity of a system to do work) it is important to remember the physicality of *qi*. The analogy of wind filling the sails of a boat is used to convey the idea of invisible but forceful *qi* moving throughout the body (see also pp. 22 and 324).

The Yellow Emperor suggests that *qi*, blood, fluid (liquid and humor), essence, and the vessels are all different forms of *qi*. There are many different types of *qi* in the body and each type is distinguished by its source, location, and function. Thus, the *qi* that causes the lungs to respire and to remain clear is the lung *qi*. The *qi* that defends the body from heat, cold, and infection is the defense *qi* and so on. Generally, all the *qi* of the body is characterized as source *qi* or original *qi* and is produced through the combination of the "great *qi*" or the air we breathe, the "essence of grain and water" or the food we eat, and the "essential *qi* of kidney" or the metabolic factors and capability of the body. When source *qi* is actively engaged in maintaining the health of the body and counteracting disease processes it is referred to as "right" or "correct" (*zheng*) *qi*. Here the idea of the right, the physiological and healthy is opposed to the idea of a disease evil. **A** depicts the production of *qi*.

Once source *qi*, the undifferentiated *qi* of the body, is produced, it is stored and distributed. Source *qi* is considered to have five major divisions. All *qi*, regardless of its location has five functions: activation, warming, defense, transformation, and containment, and a distinctive dynamic: moving inwards and outwards, up and down as it moves through the channels, organs, and around the body (**B**, **C**, **D**).

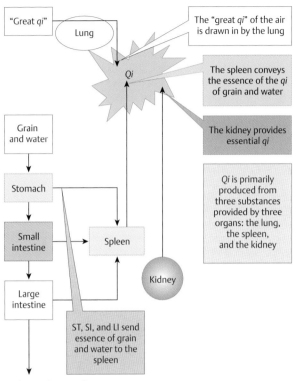

A The production of *qi*.

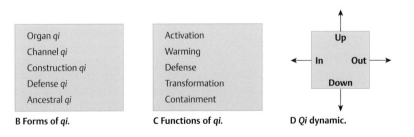

B Forms of *qi*.

Organ *qi*
Channel *qi*
Construction *qi*
Defense *qi*
Ancestral *qi*

C Functions of *qi*.

Activation
Warming
Defense
Transformation
Containment

D *Qi* dynamic.

Blood and Fluids

In relation to *qi*, blood and fluids constitute the *yin* aspects of the body. Blood is produced when the essence of food and water is raised by the spleen to the lungs (**A**). Blood and construction *qi* are closely linked and travel together in the vessels. Blood nourishes the body.

Fluids are a general term for thin (liquid, *jin* 津) and viscous (humor, *ye* 液) substances that moisten and lubricate the body. Like *qi* and blood, they are produced from food and drink and the transformative process of the body. Humor is thick, pertains to the organs, and lubricates the joints. Liquid is thin and is responsible for moistening the skin, eyes, and mouth.

Essence and Spirit

Qi, essence, and spirit make up the "three treasures" (*san bao* 三包). Essence is the gift of one's parents, and spirit the gift of heaven. Essence is the substance of the kidney, and spirit dwells in the heart.

Essence is "that which is essential to life," the fundamental support of physiological processes, which must be replenished by food and rest. Essence is also understood in a very narrow sense as "reproductive essence," the reproductive substances (sperm and ova). Essence is divided into "earlier heaven" (congenital, "prenatal") essence that is the genetic endowment combined with the nourishment received during gestation. At the moment of the first breath, the production of "earlier heaven" ceases and the production of "later heaven" (acquired, "post-natal") begins. This is the essence formed using one's congenital essence to transform the essence of grain and water. Both congenital and acquired essence are stored in the kidney and support the development and function of the body.

Insufficiency of essence can manifest in developmental disorders in early life, problems with growth and maturation. In later life, damage to essence can hasten the aging process or reduce the body's ability to fend off disease and to heal quickly. It is generally understood that congenital essence is a finite resource, the loss of which is inevitable and leads to decline and death. The rate of decline, and the quality of life is controlled by how quickly congenital essence is lost and how effectively the acquired essence is developed. The management and preservation of essence is an object of specific practices in *qi gong, tai ji quan,* dietetics, and herbal medicine.

Spirit (*shen* 神) is the amalgam of vitality and consciousness suggesting healthy mental and physical function. It is the alert and appropriate engagement of a human being with the world around them. We encounter spirit in the luster of the eyes and face in healthy people, as well as in their ability to think and respond to the world around them.

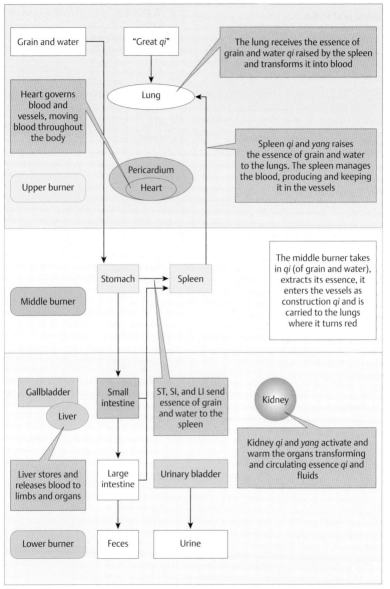

A The production and distribution of blood in relation to *qi* fluid, and the triple burner.

The Pathology of *Qi*, Blood, and Body Fluids

The pathological processes associated with *qi*, blood, and body fluids illustrate very fundamental ideas about these three closely related substances (**A**). All three depend on nourishment and movement. The vital substances are healthiest when produced abundantly and traveling freely through their established pathways. Poor nutrition, illness, overuse, and aging can deplete *qi*, blood, and fluids. *Qi* can become stagnant, blood static, and fluids congested through impaired organ function inhibiting their movement, or through the blockage of channels by disease and trauma.

Qi, blood, and fluids are produced from the *qi* of grain and water. If the organs that produce and distribute them fail to function properly, the substances become insufficient. Chronic illness can damage organs, impairing the production of *qi*, and aging, overwork, or placing demands on the body beyond its normal capacity can lead to taxation fatigue. In all cases, *qi* vacuity can occur; in this case insufficiency of the source *qi* leads to generalized fatigue and, typically, *qi* vacuity associated with specific organs. For example, spleen *qi* vacuity could lead to digestive upset, bloating, fatigue after eating, and loose stools. *Qi* fall is a special case of *qi* vacuity where the containing function of the spleen *qi* is weakened and rectal or uterine prolapse occurs.

Blood vacuity arises with blood loss from either profuse bleeding or chronic loss of small amounts of blood. Failure of the spleen to produce blood, or of the liver to store blood can lead to general signs of blood vacuity.

Damage to liquid and humor desertion occur with substantial loss of fluids due to diarrhea, sweating, and vomiting. Both blood and fluid are *yin* substances and can be damaged by fever.

Qi becomes stagnant in the channels or organs when its normal movement is impeded. This can occur with the early onset of illness, emotional upset, or trauma. While any obstruction of *qi* can cause pain, *qi* stagnation can produce a diffuse pain as the movement of *qi* is not completely blocked. *Qi* counterflow is a special case of *qi* stagnation; here obstruction causes reversal of the normal movement of *qi*. Coughing caused by obstruction of the lungs is counterflow lung *qi*.

Blood stasis is caused by many factors. It is a frequent consequence of trauma, including sprains and strains. It is often seen in gynecological conditions where prolonged *qi* stagnation or blood vacuity has given rise to static blood leading to menstrual pain. Sharp stabbing pain is often associated with blood stasis.

Water swelling and phlegm-rheum both occur where the ability of the visceral *qi* to transport and transform fluids is impaired.

As we shall see later in this chapter, static blood and phlegm–rheum can behave as pathological agents in their own right (see p. 93).

Pathology	Possible Causes	Signs and Symptoms
Qi vacuity	Chronic illness, feeble constitution, aging, taxation fatigue, poor diet	Weak and easily fatigued Lung *qi* vacuity: shortness of breath, a low voice Spleen *qi* vacuity: reduced appetite, indigestion, loose stools Kidney *qi* vacuity: frequent urination, low back pain
Qi stagnation	*Qi* dynamic is disturbed in a channel or organ by emotional disturbance, poor diet, illness, or trauma	Often seen in early stages of many diseases. Localized pain, distension, sensations of pain that are not fixed
Qi counterflow	*Qi* dynamic is disturbed in a channel or organ by dysfunction or illness and *qi* moves abnormally	Cough is an example of lung *qi* counterflow Nausea, vomiting, and hiccough are examples of counterflow stomach *qi*
Qi fall	*Qi* dynamic is disturbed, typically by insufficiency of the spleen *qi* and the *qi* fails to contain and support	Diarrhea, uterine prolapse, rectal prolapse
Blood vacuity	Blood loss, taxation, poor diet, or failure of the spleen to produce blood	Dizziness, pallid complexion, palpitations, pale lips, insomnia, dry skin
Blood stasis	*Qi* stagnation, *qi* vacuity, blood vacuity, heat, cold, and trauma interrupt the ability of blood to move freely in the vessels	Dark or dull complexion, cyanotic lips, local stasis produces a fixed stabbing pain, bleeding may occur in gynecological disorders
Blood heat	Produced by heat toxin entering the blood, typically in febrile disease	Coughing or vomiting bright red blood, deep red macules or papules; if severe, delirium, coma
Qi stagnation and blood stasis	Where *qi* and blood are simultaneously obstructed, typically after trauma or following *qi* stagnation	Fixed stabbing pain and areas of distended pain. Typically seen in gynecological presentations, trauma, and organ damage such as nephritis or ulcers
Qi and blood vacuity	The production of *qi* and blood are closely linked, or failure of *qi* to contain blood can lead to chronic bleeding and anemia	Pallid complexion, shortness of breath, fatigue, dizziness, palpitations
Damage to liquid and humor desertion	Fever, sweating, profuse urination, vomiting, diarrhea, hot environments, lack of fluids	Thirst, dry throat and tongue, dry skin, dry hard stools, scanty concentrated urine
Water swelling and phlegm-rheum	Illness or insufficiency causes transformative function of the lung, spleen or kidney *qi* to be impaired leading to poor movement and transformation of fluids	Various signs of fluid accumulation including edema, inhibited urination, abdominal fullness, cough and panting with expectoration of phlegm, and pulmonary edema with cardiac failure

A Pathology of qi, blood, and body fluids.

The Channels

The typical acupuncture figurine (**A**) suggests the complexity of acupuncture channels and points. However, the image of a human figure traversed with lines punctuated with dots presents only the very basic structure of the surface course of the 12 regular channels and two of the extraordinary channels. The architecture of the channels and networks is a complex inferential anatomy describing interior relationships that permit communication between the viscera and bowels, and the surface of the body and the interior. This topic is discussed extensively in Chapter 4. For our purposes it is important to understand the channels and networks as producing a system of communication between all the areas of the body so that the observed movement of *qi*, blood, fluids, and essence, as well as the effects of acupuncture can be understood.

There are two major groups of channels. The first are the 12 regular channels (*shi er jing luo* 十二经络). The regular channels have several associated subsidiary channels: the 12 sinew channels, 12 cutaneous regions, and 12 divergent channels (see Chapter 4 and **A**).

The regular channels are divided into six *yang* and six *yin* channels, which are distributed bilaterally on the body. The *yin* channels run along the inner surface of the limbs (three on the arms and three on the legs) and across the chest and abdomen (**B**). Each *yin* channel is associated with a viscus. The *yang* channels run along the outer sur-

faces of the limbs (three on the arms and three on the legs) and along the buttocks, flanks, and back (with the exception of the stomach channel, which traverses the sides of the abdomen). Each *yang* channel is associated with a bowel.

Each of the six *yin* channels is paired with its interiorly-/exteriorly-related *yang* channel. This pairing expresses an important physiological connection between the associated viscera and bowel.

The Eight Extraordinary Vessels

The second major group of channels are the eight extraordinary vessels. They are extraordinary for two reasons. They do not have a continuous, interlinking pattern of circulation. While they have connections with each other and with the 12 regular channels, they do not link, one to the next, as the 12 regular channels do.

Second, the eight extraordinary vessels are not associated with a specific organ system. Instead, they function as reservoirs of *qi* and blood and furnish connections between different organ and channel systems. They fill and empty as required by the changing physiology of the regular channels and organs. Surplus *qi* or blood from the regular channels may be stored in the eight extraordinary vessels and released when required. The eight extraordinary vessels are closely related to the functions of the liver and kidney systems and also to the functioning of the uterus and the brain.

A The surface pathways of the channels and the acupuncture points are displayed on this model.

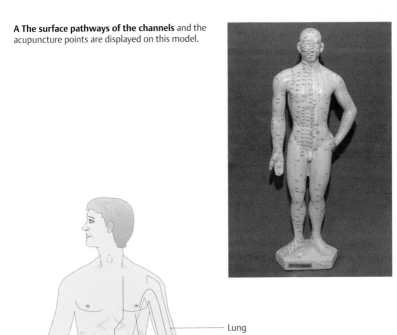

- Lung
- Pericardium
- Heart

- Spleen

- Liver

- Kidney

Tai yin	(lung + spleen)
Jue yin	(pericardium + liver)
Shao yin	(heart + kidney)

B Channel pairings: The three great *yin* channels. See p. 167 for all 12 regular channels.

Viscera and Bowels
(Zang and Fu 脏腑)

Through the 16th century, the Chinese view of human anatomical structures was similar to that of their European contemporaries. Human dissection occurred in China but never reached the level of organized extensive exploration into the structure of the body that was occurring in Europe by that time. Instead, Chinese medicine, though rooted in an understanding of familiar anatomical structures, produced a system in which organs serve as markers of associated, but wide-ranging physiological functions rather than being collections of well-described tissue whose functions remained restricted by their location and histology.

There are 12 organs, divided into the "viscera," which are also called six *zang* or solid organs, and the "bowels," which are also called six *fu* or hollow organs. These organs are understood to be the physical structures that we associate with conventional anatomy (with one exception, the triple burner). The six *yin* viscera are the heart, lungs, liver, spleen, kidneys, and pericardium. The six *yang* bowels are the small intestine, large intestine, gallbladder, stomach, urinary bladder, and the triple burner (*san jiao* 三焦). These organs are linked to physiological functions that are often similar to those associated with them in biomedicine, but which also might be very different. The liver is said to store blood and to distribute it to the extremities as needed. The spleen is understood as an organ of digestion. The Chinese understood the physical structure and loca-

tion of the organs, but because systematic dissection was not pursued, the observation of physiological function formed the basis of medical thought.

The circulation and elimination of fluids was observed and attributed to an organ that was said to have a name, but no form, the "triple burner." This organ (see p. 85) has come to be considered as the combined activity of other organs (lung, spleen, and kidney) in fluid metabolism, illustrating the importance that physiological function, rather than structure and histology, plays in the role of an organ in Chinese medicine.

The organs of viscera and bowel are paired in the *yin* and *yang*, or interior–exterior relationship. The heart is linked with the small intestine, the spleen with the stomach, and so on. Each viscus and each bowel has an associated channel that runs through the organ, through the paired organ, within the body, and across the body's surface, then connects with the channel of the related organ. The complex ramifications of the channels describe the connections that allow the organs to interact and influence each other. Ancient understandings of physiology described the organs as a harmoniously functioning team of imperial officials loyally serving the monarch (heart) and furthering the aims of its embodied consciousness (spirit). Each official is given a title that reflects its role (**A**).

The following sections present the viscera and their related organs and their functions through the "critical principles," or traditional aphorisms that function as axioms in the physiology of Chinese medicine (**A**).

"The heart holds the office of the monarch."

"The pericardium holds the office of the courier."

"The lung holds the office of the minister."

"The spleen and stomach are the officials of the granaries."

"The small intestine is the official of receiving bounties."

"The large intestine is the official of conveyance."

"The liver holds the office of general whence strategies emanate."

"The gallbladder is the official of justice."

"The kidney is the official of labor from whence agility emanates."

"The bladder is the official of the municipal waterworks."

"The triple burner is the official who controls irrigation."

A Critical principles: the viscera and bowels as imperial officials (adapted from thue *Huang Di Nei Jing Su Wen*).

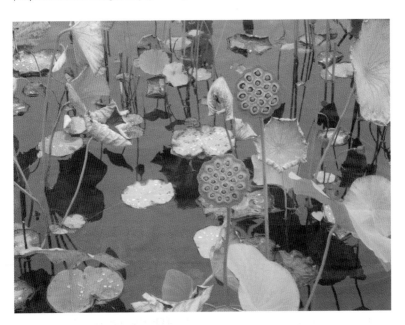

The Heart and Pericardium

The heart and pericardium (**A**) are two distinct, but closely related organs. The heart is the emperor, governing the movement of blood and the conduct of the organs, and housing consciousness or spirit. The pericardium is the heart's intermediary, acting as the portal through which the spirit engages the world.

Two critical principles stated in *The Yellow Emperor's Classic of Medicine* present the fundamental role of the heart: "The heart is the great governor of the five viscera and the six bowels and is the abode of the spirit." "The heart governs the blood and vessels of the body." The heart ensures that the body is nourished and all organs are supplied with blood.

In its role of storing spirit, the heart is the seat of consciousness. It "governs the spirit light" and is the place from which consciousness encounters the world. Spirit refers to clarity of consciousness and the strength of the mental faculties. The role of the pericardium is that of a minister or courier who permits the transmission of information between the heart/spirit and the greater world. "The pericardium holds the office of minister and courier; from it joy and pleasure emanate." The pericardium is not generally a subject of direct clinical interest unless there are severe alterations of consciousness produced by an obstruction of the pericardium. Clinically these conditions can involve patterns such as phlegm clouding the pericardium or heat entering the pericardium. The channel pathways and acupuncture points associated with the pericardium are frequently used in treating a variety of conditions.

The function of the heart is dependent on the vital substances of the body. Abundant *qi* and blood ensure a regular heartbeat and a moderate and forceful pulse. Insufficiency of heart *qi* and blood can produce an irregular beat, lusterless complexion, palpitations, even clinical signs of blood stagnation such as green-blue complexion, especially where heart *yang* is insufficient. Where heart blood or *yin* becomes insufficient the ability of the heart to store the spirit properly can be affected, producing insomnia and dream-disturbed sleep.

The *yin* heart is paired with the *yang* organ, the small intestine. This relationship is diagnostically and therapeutically relevant since close channel relationships allow heat to flow out of the heart via the small intestine.

The tongue is the sprout of the heart and while clinical signs of the heart's status are found primarily on the tip of the tongue, the color and quality of the tongue, and the ability to speak clearly all point to the health of the heart. Because the heart governs the other organs and manifests in the tongue, the tongue can be used to investigate the status of all the organs.

Yin viscus:	heart
Yang bowel:	small intestine
Yin viscus:	pericardium
Yang bowel:	triple warmer

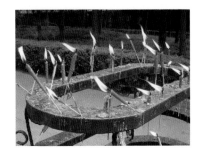

Critical Principles

"The heart governs the blood and vessels of the body."

"All blood is subordinate to the heart."

"The heart stores the spirit."

"The heart governs the spirit light."

"The tongue is the sprout of the heart."

"The bloom of the heart is in the face."

"The heart governs speech."

A The heart and the pericardium.

Fire Phase Correspondences	
Season	Summer
Climate	Heat
Direction	South
Development	Growth
Color	Red
Taste	Bitter
Viscus	Heart
Bowel	Small intestine
Sense organ	Tongue
Tissue	Vessels
Mind	Joy
Odor	Scorched
Vocalization	Laughing
Body fluid	Sweat
Manifestation area	Complexion

The Lung

While the heart conveys blood to the organs, the lung (**A**) gathers in the "great *qi*," creating and replenishing source *qi* in conjunction with the spleen and kidney. Thus, the lung "governs *qi*." "The lung holds the office of assistant, whence management and regulation emanate." In addition to its role in regulating the waterways, the lung functions as an assistant to the heart, furnishing the *qi* that assists in propelling the blood through the body. The lung is also critical in the final transformation of the essence of grain and water into blood.

Lung *qi* "faces the hundred channels, governs the regulation of the waterways, conveys essence to the skin and [body] hair, and governs the defensive exterior of the whole body." The lung controls *qi* and fluids, supports the movement of *qi* and blood, and the ability of the skin and the interstices to repel evils. This depends on the lung's diffusion, and depurative downbearing. Diffusion refers to the movement of *qi* and fluids to the surface of the body, thus providing for the defense of the body, and ensuring that the skin and body hair is moist and nourished. Depurative downbearing is the free flow of air in and out of the lungs, the transmission of inhaled *qi* to the kidneys, and the descent of water to the kidneys and bladder for excretion. The impor-

tant role of the lung in the movement of water is expressed in the principle that "the lung is the upper source of water," since the lung is responsible for the smooth movement of water out to the surface of the body and down to the kidneys.

The lung is depicted as a tender and moist canopy protecting and covering the other organs, and, when healthy, infusing them with *qi* and moisture. Like the metal condensing mirrors of ancient China, the lung focuses and distributes the body's moisture. If lung *qi* is obstructed or insufficient, the free flow of *qi* and fluids becomes impeded causing conditions such as non-diffusion of lung *qi*, or congestion with phlegm due to the failure of depurative downbearing. The lung is easily susceptible to damage from external evils. The lung is responsible for the strength of the body's first line of protection, the defense *qi*. Thus, the lung is critical to the overall health of the body.

The lung is related to the large intestine through the channels and a particular affinity due to their shared relationship to fluids. Where "the lung governs the regulation of the waterways," "the large intestine governs liquid." Both have critical roles in the distribution and excretion of water. Where these are impaired by illness, it is often possible to use the relationship between the two organs for their mutual benefit.

Yin visceris:	lung
Yang bowel:	large intestine

Critical Principles

"The lung is the tender organ."

"The lung is adverse to cold."

"The lung is the canopy of the viscera."

"The lung governs *qi*."

"The lung regulates the waterways."

"The lung governs diffusion and depurative downbearing."

"The lung governs the skin and body hair."

"The lung governs the exterior of the entire body."

"The lung opens at the nose."

"When the lungs are harmonious the nose is able to distinguish smells."

A The lung.

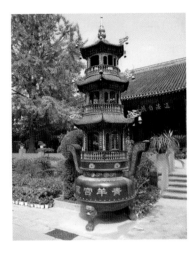

Metal Phase Correspondences	
Season	Autumn
Climate	Dryness
Direction	West
Development	Withdrawal
Color	White
Taste	Acrid
Viscus	Lungs
Bowel	Large intestine
Sense organ	Nose
Tissue	Skin/body hair
Mind	Sorrow
Odor	Raw fish
Vocalization	Weeping
Body fluid	Mucus
Manifestation area	Body hair

The Spleen, Stomach, and Intestines

The spleen and stomach (**A**) are the officials of the granaries. They transform and distribute the essence of grain and water and are the root of acquired essence. Although the small intestine is the heart's bowel and the large intestine is the lung's, both are important in digestion. *The Yellow Emperor's Classic of Medicine* states, "The spleen, stomach, small and large intestines ... manage the granaries and are the seat of construction; they are called receptacles, having the ability to transform the five flavors entering and the waste leaving the body."

The spleen and stomach form a *yin yang* pair and their digestive roles reflect the relationship. The *yang* stomach "governs the intake and decomposition of grain and water," conveying food to the small intestine and so "governs downbearing of the turbid." The small intestine is the official of receiving bounties and governs humor; it "governs separation of the clear and the turbid." The turbid is waste and the clear is essence, and this refers to the extraction of the thick nourishing aspects of fluid, the humor, from the chyle. The large intestine is the official of conveyance and governs liquid; it governs the transformation and conveyance of waste. The small and large intestines strain off fluid and nutrients from waste returning them to the spleen for distribution. The *yin*-spleen in turn, "governs the movement and transformation of grain and water and distribution of its essence." After food is digested under the spleen's influence, it is responsible for transformation and the transportation of its essence, whether to the lungs to create blood or as *qi* throughout the body. The spleen's *qi* moves essence upwards, thus "the spleen governs upbearing."

"The spleen manages the blood," refers both to the part the spleen plays in the production of blood and its role in containing blood in the vessels. This is an extension of the role of containment that we saw linked to *qi* earlier. The spleen *qi* is essential to the containment of blood.

"The spleen governs the flesh and limbs, and opens into the mouth." A healthy form as opposed to emaciation and weakness or obesity and constitutional dampness are the product of a well-regulated spleen. The ability to distinguish and savor tastes is under the influence of the spleen.

Clinical issues of the spleen involve digestion, weight problems, anemia, bleeding disorders, and the accumulation of dampness and phlegm. Insufficiency of the upbearing spleen *qi* can cause center *qi* fall, causing prolapsed organs or hemorrhoids. In contrast, disturbance of normally descending stomach *qi* can lead to counterflow ascent of stomach *qi* with vomiting. The small and large intestines are susceptible to heat and dryness. Blood or fluid insufficiency affecting the large intestine can cause dryness and constipation.

Yin viscus:	spleen
Yang bowel:	stomach

Critical Principles

"The spleen governs the movement and transformation of grain and water and distribution of its essence."

"The spleen governs upbearing."

"The spleen dislikes damp and likes dryness."

"The spleen manages the blood."

"The spleen stores reflection."

"The spleen governs the flesh and limbs, and opens into the mouth."

"If the spleen is functioning harmoniously, then the mouth can taste the five flavors."

"The stomach governs intake and the spleen governs the grinding down."

"The stomach governs intake and decomposition of grain and water."

"The stomach governs downbearing of the turbid."

"The stomach is the sea of water and grains."

"The stomach dislikes dryness and likes damp."

Yin viscus:	heart
Yang bowel:	small intestine

"The small intestine governs separation of the clear and the turbid."

"The small intestine governs humor."

Yin viscus:	lung
Yang bowel:	large intestine

"The large intestine governs the transformation and conveyance of waste."

"The large intestine governs liquid."

A The spleen, stomach, and intestines.

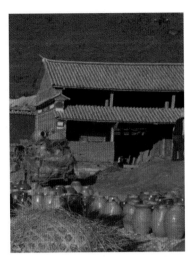

Earth Phase Correspondences	
Season	Late summer
Climate	Damp
Direction	Center
Development	Maturity
Color	Yellow
Taste	Sweet
Viscus	Spleen
Bowel	Stomach
Sense organ	Mouth
Tissue	Flesh
Mind	Thought
Odor	Fragrant
Vocalization	Singing
Body fluid	Saliva
Manifestation area	Lips

The Liver and Gallbladder

The liver (**A**) is critical to the orderly distribution of *qi* and blood within the body and, next to the heart, is the organ most closely related to emotion and judgment. While the heart governs blood and the lungs govern *qi*, the liver governs "free coursing," which refers to its role in maintaining an orderly *qi* dynamic. It is said that "the liver governs upbearing and the lung governs downbearing," describing the predominant directionality of each in the *qi* dynamic. At the same time the "liver governs blood," which describes its role of storing and releas- ing blood as needed. Thus, the liver harmonizes the movement of *qi* and blood, facilitating the free movement of *qi* through the organs and channels, and releasing blood to the limbs as required for activity. Because of the liver's important role in nourishing the limbs and supporting muscular activity it is said that "the liver governs the sinews."

The liver's role in facilitating the free movement of *qi* and releasing blood reflects its desire for unimpeded action. The liver is compared to a general in charge of strategy and tactics, exercising judgment and taking action. The liver, like a shoot in the spring, pushes firmly in its determined direction, and reacts forcefully to constraint and obstruction. Known as the "unyielding viscus" because of its preference for unobstructed "orderly reaching" the liver reacts to impediments to smooth movement with force. Thus, disturbances of the liver's free coursing can manifest as pain in its channel pathway, especially along the sides of the rib cage, headache from the upward movement of its obstructed *qi*, and anger.

The liver's channel pathway is important to understanding the liver's role. The channel reaches from the crown of the head to the feet, reaches the eyes, and connects closely with the genitals. While the kidney is considered to primarily govern reproduction, the liver has an important role in sexuality and its blood supports female reproductive capacity. As the kidney stores essence, the liver stores blood; liver blood and kidney essence are mutually dependent and so are said to be "of the same source." Visual acuity depends on liver blood and so "the liver opens at the eyes."

The liver has a *yin* and *yang* relationship with the gallbladder. The surplus liver *qi* is channeled into the gallbladder where it accumulates and forms into bile, which is then controlled by the gallbladder. The gallbladder is said to be "responsible for what is just and exact." The gallbladder is particularly associated with decision-making. Stagnation or repletion of liver or gallbladder *qi* can produce anger or ill-considered decisions, while fright suggests insufficient liver *qi*, and indecision and timidity signify insufficient gallbladder *qi*.

Yin viscus: liver

Yang bowel: gallbladder

Critical Principles

"The liver is *yang* within *yin*."

"The liver governs free coursing."

"The liver stores blood."

"Liver *qi* and liver yang tend toward superabundance while liver blood and liver *yin* tend toward insufficiency."

"The liver governs fright."

"The liver governs the sinews; its bloom is in the nails."

"The liver opens at the eyes."

A The liver and gallbladder.

Wood Phase Correspondences	
Season	Spring
Climate	Wind
Direction	East
Development	Birth
Color	Cyan
Taste	Sour
Viscus	Liver
Bowel	Gallbladder
Sense organ	Eyes
Tissue	Sinews
Mind	Anger
Odor	Goatish
Vocalization	Shouting
Body fluid	Tears
Manifestation area	Nails

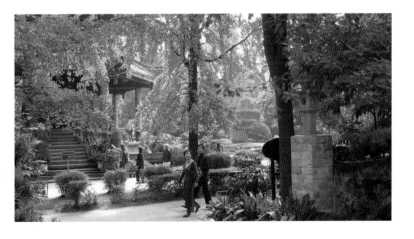

The Kidney and Urinary Bladder

The "kidney is on the left and the life gate is on the right," expresses what is known as the "double nature" of the kidney and why the Chinese classics carefully assign plurality to them. Traditionally the left kidney has the *yin*-supportive functions of the kidney viscus, while the right has the *yang* functions, which are attributed to the *ming men huo* or "life gate fire." This anatomical localization, which becomes quite relevant in pulse diagnosis, for instance, reminds us that the kidney has both *yin* and *yang* attributes. Each of the body's viscera depend on the kidney to support their functions and so it is said, "Kidney *yin* and kidney *yang* are the root of the *yin* and *yang* of all the organs" (**A**).

We have already encountered the kidney as fundamental to the production of *qi* and as the reservoir of acquired and congenital essence. It also has specific responsibilities for human growth and development, and the capacity for reproduction, all closely related to kidney essence.

Essence is what is essential for life. The kidney stores the "earlier heaven," or congenital essence, the genetic endowment of the parents nurtured by the nutritional events of gestation. This "earlier heaven" provides the support for healthy development, particularly of bones, teeth, marrow, nervous tissue, the brain, and hair, and of the organs and body in general. Growth is driven by the impetus of the congenital essence, puberty arrives under its in-

fluence, and conception relies on it (see quote on p.83). The congenital essence may be supplemented but not replenished throughout life. Carefully husbanded congenital essence, a balanced lifestyle, and diet engendering acquired essence *qi*, allows the kidney to store and distribute the essence in a balanced way throughout life. Together, congenital and acquired essence or "essence *qi*" (or "essential *qi*") constitute the basis for both kidney *yin* and kidney *yang*.

"The kidney governs *qi* absorption," refers to the fundamental role of the kidney in supporting the respiratory functions of the lung; insufficiency of kidney essential *qi* can lead to respiratory problems such as shortness of breath or panting on exertion.

"The kidney governs water," reflects the role of the kidney in water metabolism. As fluids are diffused and downborne by the lung and separated from the digestate by the stomach, small and large intestines, the kidney manages their elimination by the urinary bladder, its *yang* partner.

Clinically the kidney manifests insufficiency in areas of reproductive function, chronic fatigue, enuresis, hair loss, hearing disorders, dental problems, low back pain, knee pain, osteoporosis, spinal stenosis, and chronic respiratory tract conditions such as asthma. Presentations such as dizziness, mental dullness, poor memory, and slow healing of fractures, can all be related to insufficiency of the kidney's essential *qi*.

| *Yin* viscus: | kidney |
| *Yang* bowel: | urinary bladder |

Water Phase Correspondences	
Season	Winter
Climate	Cold
Direction	North
Development	Dormancy
Color	Black
Taste	Salty
Viscus	Kidney
Bowel	Urinary bladder
Sense organ	Ears
Tissue	Bones
Mind	Fear
Odor	Putrid
Vocalization	Sighing
Body fluid	Urine
Manifestation area	Head hair

Critical Principles

"The kidney stores essential *qi* and is responsible for growth development and reproduction."

"The kidney governs water."

"The kidney opens into the ears and the two *yin* and its bloom is in the hair of the head."

"Kidney governs earlier heaven."

"Kidney governs reproduction."

"Kidney governs *qi* absorbtion."

"Kidney governs bones and engenders marrow."

"Teeth are the surplus of the bones."

"The brain is the sea of marrow."

"Kidney *yin* and kidney *yang* are the root of the *yin* and *yang* of all the organs."

"The two kidneys are not both kidneys."
"The concept of the life gate first appears in the Nan Jing: The thirty-sixth difficult issue: each of the depots is a single [entity], except for the kidneys which represent a twin entity. Why is that so?
It is like this. The two kidneys are not both kidneys. The one on the left is the kidney; the one on the right is the gate of life. The gate of life is the place where the spirit essence lodges; it is the place to which the original influences are tied. Hence, in males it stores the essence; in females it holds the womb. Hence, one knows that there is only one kidney."

(Unschuld 1986, p. 382)

A The kidney and the urinary bladder.

The Triple Burner

The triple burner (**A**) is simultaneously a bowel and an idea. As a *yang* bowel, it is paired with the *yin* viscus and the pericardium and both have their own channel pathways. We in the West react to the triple burner with incredulity since we know of no such anatomical structure. Similarly, its ontology was debated in the Chinese classic texts where it was described as an organ "with a name, but no form." The triple burner represents the structural divisions of the body and its organs, and the functional relationships between the lung, the spleen, and the kidney as they engage in the production of *qi* from grain and water, and the distribution and excretion of fluids.

Bereft of form, the triple burner has a definite shape. The upper burner is the body (including head and chest) above the diaphragm, and contains the lung and the heart. As the dwelling of the ancestral *qi*, the upper burner is known as the "sea of *qi*." The upper burner is said to be "like a mist" and is understood through the actions of the lung in diffusion and depurative downbearing of *qi* and fluids. The middle burner lies between the diaphragm and the navel; it contains the spleen and stomach, and is known as the "sea of food and grain." The middle burner is compared to a foam, conveying partially digested grain and water churned together. The lower burner lies below the navel; it contains the liver, small and large intestines, kidney, and urinary bladder. While the physical location of the liver places it in the middle burner, its functionality, its channel pathways, and its special relationship to the kidney ("the liver and kidney are of the same source") places it in the lower burner. "The lower burner is like a sluice" and acts to drain feces and urine from the body.

The term "burner" conveys the transformative activities of the organs in each of the levels as they carry out their functions of transforming and distributing grain and water, and *qi* and fluids.

The Extraordinary Organs

The seven extraordinary organs (*qi heng zhi fu*) are the brain, marrow, bones, uterus, blood vessels, and the gallbladder. They are considered a distinct class of organs separate from the viscera and bowels discussed above because they do not decompose food or carry away waste like the bowels, nor do they produce and store essence like the viscera. The gallbladder is included here because it is both involved in the digestive process (as a bowel) and produces a clear fluid, bile, as an extraordinary organ.

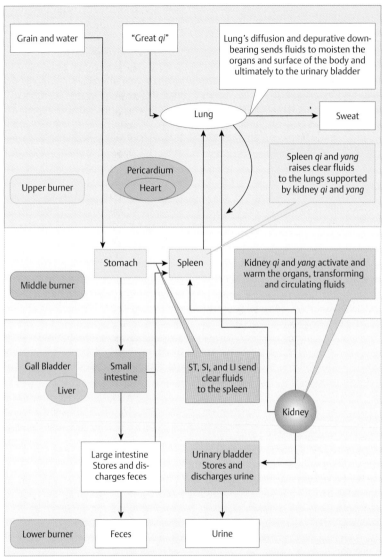

A The triple burner *(san jiao)* and the transformation, circulation and discharge of fluids. *The Yellow Emperor's Classic of Medicine* describes the *san jiao* as "the pathways for the entry and exit of grain and water."

Development, Reproduction, and Aging

The process of growth, development, maturation, reproduction, aging, and death takes place under the waxing and waning influence of the kidney *yin* and *yang* and essence. Although essence is fundamental, the body's development depends on the flourishing of *qi* and blood for its full expression. **A** and **B** summarize the insights provided by minister Qi Bo to the Yellow Emperor concerning the stages in the development and decline of men and women.

From the moment of conception as the male and female reproductive essence join, the fetus develops in dependence on the *qi* and blood of the mother. This maternal nourishment of the fetus produces congenital *qi*, the genetic and gestational endowment of the child. Assuming that this is normal and that diet, exercise, and rest are provided, the stages of development outlined by Qi Bo are typical. It should be noted that the chart in **A** reflects the importance placed on reproductive capacity in Chinese society. The cycles of seven sevens for women and eight eights for men end with the cessation of reproductive capacity, not death.

The bones and marrow form under the influence of the kidney essence, and teeth are the surplus of bone. Strong and healthy teeth and flourishing hair suggest robust kidney *qi*. Menarche occurs when two of the extraordinary vessels, the controlling and the penetrating, become filled with the surplus blood and *qi* produced by a developing body. The extraordinary vessels depend on the surplus of maturity for their full function. The spleen's role in blood production is vital to this process as is the liver's in smoothly releasing blood each month.

As the aging process advances, the first sign is the depletion of the *yang ming* channels (stomach and large intestine), which are replete with *qi* and blood through growth and maturity. As aging sets in, the *qi* and blood in these channels diminishes, leading to the loss of the surplus *qi* and blood that fills and supports the function of the controlling and penetrating vessels. When this surplus completely wanes, the vessels empty and the menses end. Some of the troubling experiences that can be associated with menopause: hot flushing, mood swings, dryness and so on, are attributed to the decline of blood, essence, and kidney *yin*, producing vacuity heat and the disruption of *qi* flow.

The development and decline of men depends on similar factors. The controlling and penetrating vessels support the abundant production of reproductive essence and as they decline so does male reproductive capacity.

In both genders the reduction of bone density, the thinning and whitening of hair, and the withering of flesh and sinew as we age are all signs of the reduction of congenital essence and the insufficiency of *qi* and blood.

Age	Men	Age	Women
8	Kidney *qi* increases, hair grows longer, teeth are renewed	7	Kidney *qi* increases, hair grows longer, teeth are renewed
16	Kidney *qi* is exuberant, reproductive function matures, essence *qi* flows, *yin* and *yang* are in harmony, and he can beget offspring	14	Fertility arrives, controlling vessel flows, penetrating vessel fills, menses flow and she can bear children
24	Kidney *qi* is even, muscles and bones are strong and firm, wisdom teeth grow vigorously	21	Kidney *qi* is even, wisdom teeth grow vigorously
32	Muscles and bones are very strong, bulk of flesh is full and firm	28	Muscles and bones are firm, hair reaches greatest length, body is powerful and strong
40	Kidney *qi* declines, hair falls, teeth dry out	35	Vessel of *yang ming* (stomach and large intestine channel) declines, face begins to wrinkle, hair begins to fall
48	*Yang qi* declines and dries up above, face becomes wrinkled, hair and sideburns whiten in places	42	Three *yang* vessels begin their decline, face wrinkles, hair begins to whiten
56	Liver *qi* declines, muscles can no longer move	49	Controlling vessel empties, penetrating vessel weakens, fertility dries up, earth passages are cut, body withers, and she can no longer have children
64	Fertility dries up, sperm becomes scarce, kidney storage declines, the body is nearing its end and teeth and hair depart		

A Kidney essence *qi* and development of men and women
(adapted from *Huang Di Nei Jing Su Wen*).

"In the *Yellow Emperor's Inner Classic Basic Questions* Chapter 1, 'The Authentic Men of High Antiquity.' The Yellow Emperor asks his minister Qi Bo about the reproductive capabilities of men and women. Qi Bo's answer delineates the waxing and waning of the kidney essence *qi*. The periods of increase and decrease are given in yang intervals for women (7 is a *yang* number) and in *yin* intervals for men (8 is a *yin* number). It is interesting to note that the shorter intervals for a woman's development accurately represent the earlier maturation of that sex."
(From Larre 1994, pp. 65–84 with some minor adaptations of the translation)

B Quote from the *Huang Di Nei Jing Su Wen*.

The Three Causes of Disease

In the 12th century Chen Yan organized disease causation into three major categories (*san yin*). These are external causes of disease, internal causes, and causes that are neither external nor internal (**A**). Fundamentally, all illnesses are due to the disruption of the smooth, harmonious, and sufficient flow of *qi* and it is important to bear this in mind as we explore ideas of etiology.

External Causes: The Six Evils

The six evils are wind, cold, heat or fire, dampness, summer heat, and dryness (**A, B**). When the body is exposed to an evil, if the defense *qi* is not sufficient, the correct *qi* is not strong, or if the evil is powerful, the evil may enter the surface of the body and, unless repelled by the correct *qi*, will progress from the surface to the interior of the body.

Each evil affects the body's *qi* in a manner similar to its environmental characteristics. Wind strikes suddenly at the upper part of the body, just as it sways tree tops. Cold slows and congeals, heat quickens and parches, damp is moist and gluey, retarding the smooth motion of *qi* and blood in the body, dryness desiccates, depriving the body of moisture. Summer heat is a seasonal event associated with conditions such as heat stroke and the prevalent infectious diseases that affect the gut in tropical climates.

Evils can combine, wind and cold can often produce the symptoms associated with the common cold: headache, aversion to cold, aching muscles and bones, fever, and a cough. Wind is expressed in the sudden onset of the symptoms and their effect on the upper part of the body, and cold is displayed in the aching muscles and bones as the free movement of *qi* is impeded by cold, causing pain. Whether the patient had a specific encounter with a cold wind shortly before the onset of the symptoms is not necessarily relevant. It is the patient's presentation that determines the nature of the evil. A patient may mention being outside on a chilly and windy day before the onset of a cold, but such exposure could be followed by signs of "wind–heat" with a sore throat, a dry mouth, and a rapid pulse.

The six evils are not detected in a lab, but are known through distinctive signs. These ideas developed in a culture where there was no thought of a bacterial or viral cause of disease. The process of careful observation of the body's response to disease provides the information necessary for treatment.

The six evils can also be produced by disruption of the internal environment and manifest in the internal landscape without a direct external cause (see also p. 240). In the 16th century Wu You Ke posited the concept of pestilential *qi* which suggested that certain diseases, those that we now know to be caused by viri and bacteria, are caused by specific, "pestilential" *qi* that produced the same effects in different individuals. He expressed this idea as one disease, one *qi* (Wiseman 1995: 78).

Neither internal nor external	Internal	External: six evils
Dietary irregularities	Affect (damage)	Wind
Sexual intemperance	Joy	Cold
Taxation fatigue	Anger	Heat/fire
External injury	Anxiety	Dampness
Parasites	Thought	Dryness
Phlegm	Sorrow	Summer heat
Static blood	Fear	
	Fright	

A Causes of disease and the six evils.

	General characteristics	External invasion	Internal development
Wind	Mobile, rapid, quick changes in symptoms. Typically seen in conjunction with heat or cold	Facial paralysis, dizziness, tremor, itching, pain that moves	Associated with disturbances of the liver *qi* producing internal wind, can present with tremor, dizziness, convulsion.
	Wind-cold	Fear of cold, headache, muscle aches, absence of sweating, no thirst	n/a
	Wind-heat	Mild aversion to wind and cold, sore throat, dry mouth, red tongue	n/a
Cold	Chills, slowed or stagnant movement of *qi*.	Aversion to cold, desire for warmth, thin clear excreta and secretions	Associated with insufficiency of the kidney *yang*, cold pain in abdomen, cold extermities.
Heat	Hot, redness, reckless movement, drying of fluids	Fever, vexation, delerium, vomiting or coughing of blood, rapid pulse, red tongue with yellow fur	Damage to or insufficiency of *yin* can produce signs of heat or fire
Dampness	Viscous, moist, and persistent	Damp, cold and wind can enter the channels causing obstruction leading to joint pain, damp heat can attack the liver or enter the intestines.	The consumption of excessive cold, greasy foods can overburden the spleen and cause the production of dampness and phlegm
Dryness	Absence of moisture causing damage to the body	Dry cough, dry nostrils, tendency to nose bleeds, little or bloody expectorate	Damage to liquid or damage to *yin*, can produce dryness.
Summer heat	Seasonally occurring disease with signs of heat or heat and dampness	Heat stroke, and sudden onset of fever, thirst, absence of sweating, agitation	n/a

B Key signs and concepts.

Internal Causes: The Seven Affects

Internal damage by the seven affects (**A**) conveys an inseparable linkage of mind and body. The seven affects expand the idea of the five minds (**B**), which are associated with the phases and organs (see also **C**). As brief exposure to wind and cold cannot damage the movement of *qi* in the body, so moments of anger, joy, and fright are not inherently damaging, but rather stimulate the *qi* and the organs. Prolonged or severe engagement with the affect can damage *qi* in the channels and organs. As exposure to wind and cold can congest the *qi* in the channels on the surface of the body, so too can giving way to violent temper disrupt the smooth flow of liver *qi*, forcing it to move upwards erratically, producing headaches.

The Embodied Mind in Chinese Medicine

"Mind" in the sense of aspects of consciousness, does not live apart from the body. The notion of a unitary Christian soul apart from the flesh that, as it merged with the legacy of Cartesian thought, gave the West its cultural predilection to separate mind and body, does not exist in Chinese medicine. Even the souls of the ancient Chinese are multifarious and lodged prosaically in the liver and lung.

Consciousness (spirit) is traditionally ascribed to the heart. However, what we would characterize as aspects of the mind and localized to the brain are distributed to and regulated by the viscera. Each organ can influence and be influenced by the psychic processes that they are linked to. Specific organs support decision (gallbladder), reflective thought (spleen), and intention (kidney). Planning, many functions of the nervous system, and the capacity for anger are all linked to the liver. The brain is not neglected; it is the "sea of marrow" supported by the kidney. Physicians in 16th-century China knew it as the "seat of original spirit" and understood that it was closely related to movement and physical function.

Chinese physicians of TCM sometimes display a disconcerting lack of interest in contemporary psychotherapy or the concerns of their patients. However, they are quick to link mental activities and emotional states to physiological process, in a manner that might intrigue a psychobiologist. Psyche and soma are inextricably linked, with "physical" processes affecting "mental" states and vice versa. This can be challenging for the Western student who, conditioned by the intellectual and cultural legacy of Western thought, seeks an explicit psychology and finds only a physiology of the psyche or an embodied mind.

The healthy and balanced function of each of the viscera plays a critical role in normal mental function and maintaining emotional balance. The practices of *qi gong* and health preservation encourage the development of mental tranquility and flexibility.

Affect	Critical Principle	Discussion
Anger	Anger causes the *qi* to rise	Excessive anger and other strong emotions can overstimulate the upbearing and effusing movement of liver *qi*, causing headache, dizziness, and pain in the liver channel
Joy	Joy causes the *qi* to slacken	Excessive joy can produce damage to the essence-spirit and can weaken the heart *qi* with palpitations, sleeplessness, and mental illness
Anxiety	Anxiety damages the lung and spleen	Anxiety can disturb the *qi* dynamic of the lung and spleen, producing depressed affect, cough, reduced appetite, lack of strength
Thought	Thought causes *qi* to bind	Preoccupation and obsessive thought can damage heart and spleen, with reduced appetite, palpitations, insomnia, and forgetfulness
Sorrow	Sorrow causes *qi* to disperse	Sorrow can produce crying, agitation, pale complexion, lack of energy. Sorrow can cause depression of lung *qi*, producing lung heat that can damage the kidney, causing incontinence, diarrhea
Fear	Fear causes *qi* to precipitate	Fear directly impacts the kidney leading to damage to kidney *yin* and *yang*
Fright	Fright causes derangement of *qi*	Fright disturbs the *qi* dynamic, disturbs movement of *qi* and blood, can disturb the heart spirit, liver, and the kidney

A The seven affects.

Five Minds		Associated Organ
△	Anger	Liver
▽	Joy	Heart
◇	Thought	Spleen
□	Sorrow	Lung
○	Fear	Kidney

B Five-phase relationships. Traditionally five-phase relationships link a specific organ and a specific mental activity. Each of the organs is linked to one of the five minds, which express essential mental processes and emotional states. Excess on any of the five minds can cause heat due to qi disturbance and damage to yin, producing a range of clinical signs including irritability, insomnia, and dizziness.

"The liver stores the ethereal soul"	If the liver blood is insufficient or disturbed the liver's ability to store the animal soul can be disturbed
	Excessive dreaming, disquieted spirit, sleep walking, and talking in the sleep can occur
"The heart stores the spirit"	The heart's blood and qi support the heart's ability to store the spirit, and permit a clear and engaged response to the environment
"The spleen stores reflection"	The ability to think depends on the spleen and excessive or obsessive thought can produce spleen damage
"The lung stores the corporeal soul"	The corporeal soul exists in the body from birth and dies at death
	It is closely related to essence and supports movement and the sensation of pain and itching
"The kidney stores the will"	The kidney is associated with willpower and memory of purpose

C The critical principles—the embodied mind.

Neither Internal Nor External Causes

These disease causes do not result directly from environmental influences or mental states. All have the effect of depleting *qi*, or obstructing its movement. "Dietary irregularities" refers to malnourishment, or diets containing excesses of food that imbalance the internal landscape. Spicy foods, shellfish, and alcohol can lead to the congestion of heat internally. In food stagnation, gastrointestinal tract obstruction from eating too much or poorly prepared or spoiled food, the food acts as a physical obstruction to the normal flow of *qi* (see chapter 7).

"Excessive sexual activity" is the overuse of reproductive capacity, resulting in damage to essence. Frequent emission of semen can deplete kidney essence, which is vital to the body's function. Women can damage the essence through bearing children too frequently, or when too young or too old.

"Taxation fatigue" (see **A** for the five taxations) expresses the dangers of engaging in repetitive or demanding activities for prolonged periods. Both overexertion and inactivity as possible causes of disease are captured here. Taxation fatigue reflects the essential thought that moderation is the key to health. Lying down for prolonged periods damages the *qi*, and prolonged standing damages the bones. Both the couch potato and the marathon runner, although their activities are very different, are subject to taxation fatigue (see p. 250).

Trauma directly impacts the movement of *qi* and blood from a simple blow or fall causing a bruise (static blood) to sprains, broken bones, and lacerations. In all cases, the healing process is carefully managed to avoid long-term obstructions to the movement of *qi* and blood from occurring (see p. 248).

The accumulation of worms in the gut can act on the body in several ways. The first is that the worms compete for nutrition with the host, diminishing the production of *qi* and leading to malnutrition. The second is that the worms themselves can form an obstructive mass blocking and interfering with the *qi* flow in the digestive tract (see p. 258).

When the organs are not functioning properly, the body may form pathological products: phlegm-rheum (**B**) and static blood (**C**, see also pp. 246 and 248). Like food stagnation or worms, phlegm and static blood produce a direct obstruction to the movement of *qi* and blood in the body. Depending on their location these products can disrupt organ function. Both can be caused by the six evils and any condition producing *qi* stagnation can cause these products to occur as well. Phlegm is often seen as wind–cold entering the lung, but it can be produced when an overburdened spleen fails to transform fluids, leading to dampness and then to phlegm formation. Blood stasis is produced by trauma. It is often seen in gynecological conditions where liver *qi* constraint, blood vacuity, or cold has caused blood to fail to flow smoothly.

- Prolonged vision damages the blood.
- Prolonged lying damages the *qi*.
- Prolonged sitting damages the flesh.

- Prolonged standing damages the bones.
- Prolonged walking damages the sinews.

A Damage by the five taxations.

Pattern	Symptoms
Phlegm congesting in the lung	Coughing up large amounts of phlegm
Phlegm lodging in the stomach	Nausea and vomiting
Phlegm confounding the orifices of the heart	Delirium, disturbance of spirit-mind, unconsciousness
Phlegm lodging in the channels	Phlegm nodules (lipoma)

B Presentations involving phlegm. Phlegm is the viscous mucus produced by the respiratory tract and a pathologic product that can occur throughout the body. When the movement and transformation of fluids by the lung, spleen, or kidneys is impaired or when interior heat evil cook fluids, phlegm will occur.

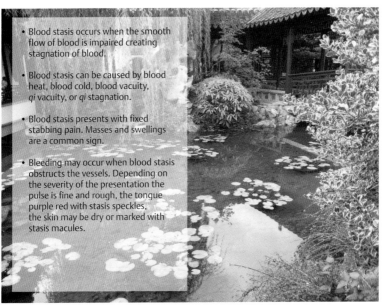

- Blood stasis occurs when the smooth flow of blood is impaired creating stagnation of blood.

- Blood stasis can be caused by blood heat, blood cold, blood vacuity, *qi* vacuity, or *qi* stagnation.

- Blood stasis presents with fixed stabbing pain. Masses and swellings are a common sign.

- Bleeding may occur when blood stasis obstructs the vessels. Depending on the severity of the presentation the pulse is fine and rough, the tongue purple red with stasis speckles, the skin may be dry or marked with stasis macules.

C Blood stasis.

The Healthy Body as an Orderly Landscape

In Chinese medicine the healthy body is an orderly landscape, a terrain harmoniously adapting to sleeping and waking, eating and drinking, the rhythms and influences of the seasons, and the development and decline of the human organism. As we have seen, the social metaphors available to the ancient Chinese from an agrarian economy, and a society organized around an emperor, informed the body of Chinese medicine.

The body in Chinese medicine is an economy of substances transacted between organs. *Qi*, the vital substance that pervades the body and is created from the transformation of grain and water, is almost inseparable from blood. Together they flow through the channels nourishing the organs and supporting all bodily functions. Each of the organs have specific functions in Chinese medicine and these functions express a fundamental physiology that is, in many respects, distinctive to Chinese medicine.

While the ancient scholars of China investigated human anatomy, they never did so with the systematic energy of the Renaissance and the Enlightenment. Instead, anatomical structures were understood in general terms, but close observation was made of living systems and attributions of physiological function were made to anatomical structures. For this reason the spleen is a fundamental organ of digestion with functions that relate to a wide variety of anatomical structures, including the pancreas. The heart is clearly implicated in circulation, but also serves as an organ of consciousness. The kidneys are associated with the production of urine, but also with a range of endocrine functions. It is important to understand that the physiology of Chinese medicine is neither metaphysics, nor error. It is a collection of observations concerning anatomy organized in a fashion that exhibits a genius for generalizing about complex systems using a carefully structured language.

There is no boundary between psyche and soma in Chinese medicine. Classical Chinese concepts concerning mind are exceptionally sophisticated (from a psychobiological perspective) in that there is no Cartesian error, no "ghost in the machine." Psyche is embodied and reflects physiological processes.

The body of Chinese medicine is both a microcosm in its own right and a responsive inhabitant of its own environment. The body can fall sick due to the influences of various types of evil *qi*, which attack and penetrate its defenses. Or, fatigue, stagnation of vital substances, or lack of proper nourishment can cause disruptions of the inner landscape and produce illness. Ultimately, therapy in Chinese medicine is the restoration of internal and external balance achieved through dispelling pathological substances (evils) and restoring the normal functions of the channels and organs.

Health and longevity are found in a lifestyle that is moderate and obedient to the laws of *yin* and *yang*. Qi Bo explains this in **A**.

"In ancient times people patterned themselves upon *yin* and *yang*: The Yellow Emperor asks Qi Bo to explain the relationship between the observation of the laws of nature and declining life spans. He observes,

'I have heard that in ancient times the people lived to be over a hundred years, and yet they remained active and did not become decrepit in their activities.' Qi Bo explains, 'In ancient times those people who understood Dao patterned themselves upon *yin* and *yang* and lived in harmony with the arts of divination. They were temperate in eating and drinking. Their hours of rising and retiring were regular and not disorderly and wild. By these means the ancient kept their bodies united with their souls, so as to fulfill their allotted span completely, measuring unto a hundred years before they passed away.

'Nowadays people are not like this; they use wine as a beverage and they adopt recklessness as usual behavior. They enter the bedchamber in an intoxicated condition, their passions exhaust their *qi*; their cravings dissipate their essence; they do not know how to find contentment within themselves; they are not skilled in the control of their spirits. They devote all their attention to the amusement of their minds, thus cutting themselves off from the joys of long life.'"

(Adapted from Veith 1972, p. 98)

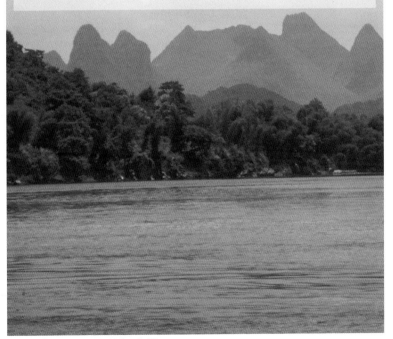

A Quote from *Huang Di Nei Jing Su Wen*.

3

Diagnosis in Chinese Medicine

Kevin V. Ergil

Signs of a Disrupted Landscape

If the healthy body is a harmonious landscape, then the body in disease is a disrupted landscape. The aim of the clinician is to understand the nature of the disruption and conceive of a plan for restoring harmony. The steps in this process are the examination of the patient, the organization of the information collected in the course of the examination into a meaningful context for the patient's complaint(s), and the development of a general plan for treatment based on established principles. In one sense, the practice of Chinese medicine is like the practice of any clinical medicine; signs and symptoms are evaluated so that the clinician can understand the nature of the patient's problem and then attempt to correct it. However, the practice of Chinese medicine depends on both the recognition of disease and the identification of the pattern of signs and symptoms that convey the way in which the bodily landscape of substances and organs has been disrupted. This pattern of signs is known as a disease pattern (*bing zheng* 病症) or pattern (*zheng* 证 or *zheng hou* 证候). The organization of these signs is the process of pattern identification or disease evil pattern identification.

It is this process that gives Chinese medicine its unique character. The premise of this approach is that bodies respond to the disease process differently and that as the illness progresses, the strength of the correct *qi*, the exu-

berance of the evil, and other factors, such as the patient's constitution or pre-existing disease processes, will cause different bodies to respond differently. Thus, a patient whose difficulty in sleeping is produced by an insufficiency of heart blood, would present different signs and receive different treatment than one whose insomnia stems from effulgent *yin* fire. In both cases, the disease "insomnia" is the same, but the pattern diagnosis and treatment is different. This situation gives rise to the famous saying "one disease many treatments, many diseases one treatment." This is the case because effulgent *yin* fire (a condition in which heat rises, particularly at night due to a vacuity of kidney *yin*) can also produce hearing problems, night sweats, menopausal symptoms, and so on, which will all be treated in a similar fashion due to the underlying similarity of the disease pattern. A patient with heart blood vacuity insomnia might present with pallor, palpitations, blurred vision, and so on, all stemming from the insufficiency of blood.

This chapter provides a systematic overview of the fundamental elements of the diagnostic process: the four examinations and disease patterns, and through the use of case studies provides examples of the way in which a clinician reasons from fundamental theory in examining signs, perceiving a pattern, and identifying a treatment method (**A**).

Diagnosis Outline	Topics discussed
The four examinations	Inspection – Body and color – Tongue Listening and smelling Inquiry Palpation – Pulse – Body areas
Pattern diagnosis	Eight principles Six excesses Six-channels and four-aspects patterns – Cold damage – Warm disease *Qi*, blood, and body fluids Organ patterns – Heart and pericardium – Lung – Spleen, stomach, and intestines – Liver and gallbladder – Kidney and bladder
Patterns and diseases	
Principles and treatment methods	
Analysis of case studies	Kidney *yang* vacuity *Qi* and blood stasis in liver and gallbladder Wind–cold

A Diagnosis outline: topics discussed in this chapter.

Collecting and Organizing Information

Forming a diagnosis and treatment plan relies on collecting and organizing information. Depending on the experience of the practitioner and the situation of the patient the process is comparatively systematic. However, it is also driven by the patient's presentation, his or her chief complaint, and the information provided by the patient. While certain aspects of the diagnostic process are common to all patient encounters, not all aspects of all examinations are used with every patient. The ability to select and use appropriate aspects of the examination process is a product of clinical experience.

One of the key differences between the orderly and linear presentation of diagnostic principles presented in this and other texts is that the forest of information obscures the trees of individual patient encounters. In order to illustrate this aspect of the diagnostic process, we have used composite examples of three patients from clinical practice who will help illustrate aspects of the diagnostic process. They will make appearances where their signs and symptoms can help elucidate the diagnostic process. At the end of the chapter, we will look at them in detail and examine how their presentations guide us to a pattern diagnosis. As you read the coming chapters on Acupuncture and Traditional Chinese Pharmacotherapy you will again encounter *John*, *Alice*, and *Jeremy* as examples of how treatment emerges from a diagnosis (**A**).

The Four Examinations

The four examinations: inspection, listening and smelling, inquiry, and palpation, are the tools used to collect information. These are traditionally organized according to the progressive intimacy of the encounter with the patient: one first sees the patient, listens to the sound of their voice, asks them questions, and finally touches their body. The actual clinical encounter may deviate from this rubric depending on circumstance.

Inspection (*wang* 望) refers to the visual assessment of the patient, including the spirit, form and bearing, and the tongue. The second aspect of diagnosis, **listening and smelling** (*wen* 闻), refers to listening to the quality of speech, breath, and other sounds, as well as being aware of the odors of breath and body. The third aspect of diagnosis, **inquiry** (*wen* 问), is the process of taking a comprehensive medical history. **Palpation** (*qie* 切) includes palpation of channels, points, areas of the body and the pulse.

All four of these diagnostic methods must be used in order to come to a complete and correct diagnosis. While sometimes pulse or tongue appear to be given greater importance, their usefulness is only in the context of the other methods. No one diagnostic method is sufficient for reaching a diagnosis.

→ **Case Study**

John

John is a 69-year-old Caucasian man who stands 5´8˝ (176 cm) and weighs about 250 lb (113.4 kg). He has experienced chronic low back and knee pain for 12 years. His face is pale and he has large, puffy, white and slightly edematous bags under his eyes. The low back and knee pain developed gradually with no initial injury. The pain is a constant, low-level, fixed aching that is worse with exertion and fatigue and better with warmth and rest. It begins at the level of the second lumbar vertebra and spreads over the left side of the back. *John* is overweight and has been diagnosed with diabetes, for which he takes insulin. He has difficulty controlling his glucose levels, and due to the diabetes, there is numbness in the toes and he gets toe blisters that take months to heal; recently an unhealed cut on his right foot required amputation of the toe.

Alice

Alice is 23-year-old Caucasian female who has had dysmenorrhea for 8 years. She is 5´5˝ (167 cm) tall and weighs 125 lb (56.7 kg). Her body is compact and wiry. Her overall complexion is slightly dark. She began menstruating at age 13 and her cycle is very consistent. Her menses arrive every 29 days and last for 5 days. The blood is dark red with large purple-red clots. Bleeding is heavy for the first 3 days. Every month, on day 27, she gets a very bad headache, located in her temples, that lasts for 4 days. The first 2 days of menstruation are extremely painful. She takes painkillers but still experiences pain. About 1 week prior to menstruation, she experiences breast tenderness, a feeling of tightness in her chest, and extremely labile emotions.

Jeremy

Jeremy is 45 years old and a thin 5´10˝ (178 cm). He weights 140 lb (63.6 kg). He has been receiving acupuncture for treatment of fatigue due to overwork. On this visit he arrived with an acute cold. His symptoms included a sore throat, a sensation of heat that easily transformed into cold after sweating. His nose was stuffy, but it was difficult to expel any phlegm. When there was visible phlegm, it was slightly yellow. His body was sore, his eyes red, and he was fatigued.

A Three patients from clinical practice.

Inspection (*Wang Zhen* 望诊)

The first of the four diagnostic methods, inspection, refers to the visual assessment of the patient, particularly the spirit, form, and bearing, the head and face, and substances excreted by the body. The color, shape, markings, and coating of the tongue are inspected. Inspection uses an established body of empirically derived information and theoretical perspectives.

Observing Spirit

The observation of the spirit, considered very important in assessing the patient's prognosis, relies on assessing the overall appearance of the patient, especially the eyes, the complexion, affect, and the quality of the patient's voice. Good spirit, even in the presence of serious illness, indicates a good prognosis.

Form and Bearing

The inspection of form is the examination of the *yin*, or substantive aspects of the body, where the size and shape of the body are examined. Emaciation suggests *yin* vacuity. Corpulence suggests overeating and the breakdown of the spleen's ability to transport and transform. Bearing refers to the *yang* aspect of bodily movement. Tremor and quivering suggests wind. Somnolence and a curled up posture suggest *yang* vacuity cold.

Inspecting the Color of the Face and Body

While the examination of the color of the body (**A**) is primarily applied to the face, the principles can be used in the inspection of any area. The inspection of color is not a matter of evaluating skin pigmentation. Instead, the clinician is looking at the hue and sheen of the skin produced by circulation of blood and the relative moisture and health of the skin and underlying tissue. The physician considers the color from the perspective of what is normal for the patient. A healthy color is appropriate for the patient's background and is said to have a healthy sheen, which refers to the skin being appropriately moist and lustrous.

Colors inspected are produced by both subtle and dramatic shifts in circulation and moisture. Colors such as black and blue-green reflect the changes in circulation produced by blood stasis. Red is produced by increased blood circulated to the surface of the body and is often a sign of increased body temperature.

Color and sheen of the face are the outward manifestation of the *qi* and blood of the viscera and bowels. Observing the color and sheen of the face reveals the health of the *qi* and blood and whether the disease progression is changing in a positive or negative way.

Color has prognostic value. If the color and sheen remain bright and moist and color changes associated with disease are not substantial, the disease is considered lighter and the prognosis is good. If the color and sheen is darkened and withered and the normal color of the patient is hard to see, the disease is considered serious and the prognosis is poor.

- Blue-green governs cold, blood stasis, or pain:

  - Pale blue-green = cold

  - Dark dusky blue = *yang qi* vacuity

  - Green-blue or purple lips, grayish green-blue complexion = heart blood stasis

- Red governs heat:

  - The entire face is red = repletion heat

  - Deep red cheeks with a pale complexion or tidal reddening of the cheeks = vacuity heat

- White governs vacuity or cold:

  - Pale white, lusterless white, or light, white color = *qi* and blood not flourishing

  - Desertion of *qi* and blood

  - Bright white with edema = *yang* vacuity cold

  - Sudden loss of large amounts of blood and *qi* with cold limbs, cold sweat, faint pulse = *yang qi* desertion

- Yellow governs spleen and stomach, or damp:

  - Desiccated yellow = debilitated stomach *qi*

  - No yellow color on the face = absence of stomach *qi*. Likely means death.

  - Yellow body, yellow face, yellow eyes = dampness

  - In an overweight patient = phlegm damp in the spleen/stomach

  - In a withered, desiccated body = stomach fire with heat damaging the fluids

  - Bright yellow like an orange = *yang* jaundice

  - Dark and dusky yellow, smoky yellow = *yin* jaundice

- Black governs the kidney, pain, or water rheum:

  - Dark, dusky black complexion, swelling, and distention of the skin and muscles, possible dark purple lips = kidney *yang* vacuity cold

  - Dark black, dusky purple lips, dry skin = blood stasis

  - Tip of the nose is black, complexion is black and below the eyelid is slightly swollen = water rheum

A Inspection of color.

Inspecting the Tongue

The tongue is a rich source of information concerning the *qi* and blood of the organs, the extent of heat and cold in the body, the progress of disease, and how deeply disease has penetrated. The tongue is the sprout of the heart and the external sign of the spleen. Many channels traverse the tongue. The stomach is considered to manifest its activity through the quality and color of the tongue fur.

Tongue examination is a routine part of assessing a patient. Care needs to be taken with regard to the quality of light during this examination since variations in the color of ambient light can cause errors in evaluating tongue color (**A**). It is also important to be aware of the patient's diet and hygiene habits since dark coffee, carrots, colored candy, or the routine scraping or brushing of the tongue can change the color or quality of tongue fur (**B**).

Findings from the tongue are always considered in relation to all the information gleaned from examining the patient. This is especially important because in some cases the findings from tongue examination may not accurately reflect the condition of the patient.

The tongue's form is evaluated in terms of size and other specific changes in its appearance (**C**). An enlarged tongue with impressions of the teeth on its margins can be a sign of *qi* vacuity or the accumulation of dampness in the body. A tongue that is thin or shrunken can indicate damage to the body's *yin*. Fissuring of the tongue can be considered as signs of damage to *yin* fluids or as a sign of heat in the body.

The examination of the bearing of the tongue involves looking for signs of abnormal movement: stiffness, limpness, tremor, deviation, contraction, and repetitive worrying movement. These abnormal movements are often signs of serious disease and may indicate wind, phlegm obstruction, and damage by heat. Wind evil, because of its sudden effects, is often implicated in tremor and seizure disorders, where the tongue becomes stiff or deviated.

The normal color of the tongue is pale red and describes a normal balanced hue. Changes in normal tongue color can be evenly distributed throughout the tongue body, but are often localized, which can add to their diagnostic significance. Shifts toward a paler color suggest insufficiency of blood and *qi*. A pale tongue can also be a sign of cold. A red tongue suggests heat and can be seen in patterns of both vacuity and repletion heat. When the red color is deep this is called a crimson tongue and suggests either extreme heat or heat at deeper levels in the body.

Normal tongue	A normal tongue is described as pale red
Pale tongue	Paler than a normal pale red Indicates a vacuity of *qi* or blood Pale and enlarged accompanied by cold signs indicates a *yang* vacuity
Red tongue	Deeper red than a normal tongue Red indicates heat. Seen in vacuity heat and replete heat conditions
Crimson tongue	A crimson tongue is even deeper in color than a red tongue Indicates heat in the construction or blood aspect of the four aspects
Purple tongue	A purple tongue or a tongue with purple macules indicates blood stasis. Macules indicate a less severe condition. Generalized purple is severe blood stasis

A Tongue colors.

Normal fur	Normal tongue fur is thin and white, and appropriately moist
White fur	Glossy or excessively moist, white tongue indicates cold Dry, white tongue fur indicates cold transforming into heat or insufficiency of fluids Thick, slimy, white fur indicates phlegm damp
Yellow fur	Yellow fur indicates heat Thin, dry, yellow fur indicates damage to the fluids by heat Slimy, yellow fur indicates damp–heat Mixed white and yellow fur indicates a cold evil transforming into heat Thick, yellow fur indicates repletion heat
Thin fur	Indicates a weak evil. If a thick fur thins, the condition is improving
Thick fur	Indicates a strong evil. If a thin fur thickens, the evil is advancing
Peeled fur	Indicates an insufficiency of *yin* and stomach *qi* If the entire tongue is peeled, *yin* vacuity is severe; described as "mirror-like"
Moist fur	Indicates damp phlegm or cold–damp
Dry fur	Indicates heat or damage to fluids, or poor circulation of fluids

B Tongue fur.

Enlarged	Indicates *qi* vacuity or water damp
Shrunken	Indicates insufficiency of fluids, *yin*, or blood
Fissured	Indicates fluid vacuity
Scalloped	Dental impression on the tongue indicate *qi* vacuity
Red speckles	On the tip or margins indicate replete heat

C Tongue form.

Purple hues suggest blood stasis, impaired flow of *qi* and blood. Purple shading to red-purple suggests stasis and heat. Blue-purple suggests blood stasis cold resulting from the failure of *yang qi* to move the blood.

Tongue fur is also closely observed. A normal fur is thin, slightly moist, and white. It is produced by the upward steaming of stomach *qi* and is a manifestation of the healthy function of the stomach. Thickening of the tongue fur suggests an evil penetrating into the body. Scant or absent fur may suggest damage to the *yin* fluids leaving insufficient moisture for the stomach *qi* to steam upwards. Yellow fur indicates heat; greasy, slimy fur can suggest phlegm damp; film of fluid covering the entire tongue suggests damp, or cold–damp.

Changes in the color of the tongue as well as certain abnormalities in its form such as fissuring, stasis macules, or heat speckles are interpreted based on their location using a general model of the tongue surface in relation to the organs (**A**). The model uses the three-burner organization of the body in the tongue: the tip and upper third represent the upper burner, heart and lungs; the center, the middle burner and spleen and stomach; and the back the lower burner, kidney and urinary bladder. The liver and gallbladder are observed along the sides of the tongue, which is consistent with their channel and burner distribution. This model is considered heuristic and is not applied in a rigid fashion (**B**).

John, our 69-year-old low back pain patient, presents with a swollen and pale tongue with toothmarks and thick white fur. Pallor here is a sign of cold. The enlarged tongue with toothmarks shows failure of fluids to be transformed and is usually directly attributed to the spleen. In this case it is a sign of damp, as is the thick, white fur, suggesting dampness accumulating internally.

Alice, our 23-year-old dysmenorrhea patient, presents with a slightly purple tongue with stasis macules on the sides and normal thin, white fur. Here the slightly purple tongue color suggests blood stasis and the localization of the stasis macules in the region of the liver and gallbladder is consistent with blood stasis in the liver and gallbladder (organs and channels), producing menstrual irregularity and emotional distress. The normal tongue fur suggests that no evil has penetrated or developed interiorly.

Jeremy, our 45-year-old with an acute cold, presents with a pale, swollen, and toothmarked tongue. This tongue is consistent with his original diagnosis of fatigue due to spleen *qi* vacuity. At the present stage of the disease progression of his acute cold his tongue would not be expected to show significant changes since the evil has not interiorized.

A Correlation between the tongue, the three burners, and the organs.

Kidney, urinary bladder, intestines
Lower burner

Liver, gallbladder
Middle burner
Spleen, stomach

Lung
Upper burner
Heart, pericardium

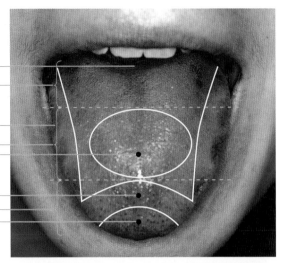

B Inspection of the tongue is frequently used in Chinese medicine to evaluate the condition of the patient's *qi*, blood, and fluids, the status of the organs, and the progression and severity of disease (© Marnae Ergil).

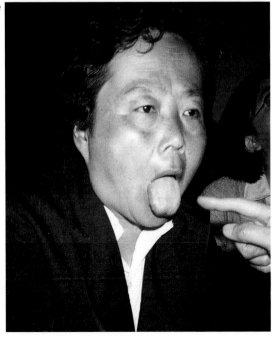

Listening and Smelling
(*Wen Zhen* 闻诊)

The second examination, listening and smelling, refers to listening to the qualities and sounds of the patient's speech, breath, and other noises that they might make, and smelling the odors of breath, body, and excreta. The classical saying "The sage is one who knows by listening and smelling" (Deng 1999, p.62) points out the potential value of these examinations. This examination can be quite important depending on the clinical circumstances and the criteria applied for examination. Traditionally, the strength of sounds and odors are used as a general rubric for *yin* and *yang* classification. Five-phase theory can also be incorporated into this assessment of the patient's condition (**A**, **B**, **C**). As was discussed in the preceding chapter and as seen to the right, each phase and its viscus have a corresponding vocalization and smell.

The assessment of sounds and smells is by no means limited to a narrow set of criteria. Instead, clinical experience fills the void of static theory and associates specific sounds and smells with specific clinical issues. Simply listening to the sound of the patient's voice gives the clinician insight into the quality of the patient's lung *qi* and by extension, the overall situation of the original *qi*. If the voice is soft and hard to hear, the

qi may be insufficient. The "shouting" sound of a patient whose liver *qi* is ascendant is a clinical commonplace, as is the incessant conversation of the patient who manifests with signs of heart fire. Liver *qi* constraint is traditionally understood to manifest with long or short sighs and is frequently associated with presentations of emotional depression.

The place of smelling in diagnosis is determined in part by the patient's presentation as well as by the goals of the practitioner. Contemporary bathing practices and the widespread use of deodorants has reduced the characteristic smells produced by the bacteria that live on the human skin. However, the odors that surround a patient in the hospital or a sick room, distinctive individual odors, and the odors of the severely ill support this diagnostic process. In an outpatient setting, patients report on the smells of their excreta where this is relevant.

The smell of ammonia on the patient's breath reflects the metabolic changes associated with the final stages of chronic renal failure. In Chinese medicine this is characterized as the vanquishing and debilitation of the viscera and bowels. Ketosis, the acetone sweet scent presented by the uncontrolled diabetic patient, is described as the smell of rotten fruit and associated with patterns of wasting and thirsting in Chinese medicine.

Sounds	
Types of sounds: crying, groaning, speech, breathing, panting, wheezing, shortness of breath, coughing, vomiting, hiccough, belching, and sneezing	
Yin	Weak, low sounds expressed without force are signs of insufficient correct *qi*
Yang	Rough, forceful, full or loud sounds suggest an exuberant evil

A Sounds in *yin* and *yang* perspective.

Smells	
Types of odors: breath, sweat, expectorated phlegm, nasal secretions, urine, feces, menstruum, and vaginal discharge	
Yin	Fishy smells suggest cold and insufficiency of correct *qi*
Yang	Foul, rotten, strong smells suggest and exuberant heat evil

B Smells in *yin* and *yang* perspective.

Category	Wood ▽	Fire △	Earth ☐	Metal ◇	Water ○
Viscus	Liver	Heart	Spleen	Lungs	Kidney
Odor	Goatish	Scorched	Fragrant	Raw fish	Putrid
Vocalization	Shouting	Laughing	Singing	Weeping	Sighing

C Sounds and smells in five-phase perspective.

Inquiry (*Wen Zhen* 问诊)

The third diagnostic examination, inquiry, is the process of taking a comprehensive medical history (**A**). This process is often referred to as "the 10 questions" based on a rubric of 10 areas for clinical inquiry presented by Zhang Jie Bin in the Ming dynasty and his assertion that that the medical history was the most critical aspect of clinical practice (Wiseman and Ellis 1996, p. 104). Based on Zhang's model, the classical areas of inquiry are: 1) cold and heat, 2) sweating, 3) head and body, 4) stool and urine, 5) food and drink, 6) chest, 7) deafness, 8) thirst, 9) old illness, and 10) the causes of present illness (**B**). Over the years, many minor variations of the "10 questions" have been described.

The use of the expression "10 questions" has sometimes led to a misconception that only 10 questions are asked in Chinese medical diagnostics, or that the "10 questions" represents the limit of inquiry diagnosis. Neither idea is true. In fact, areas specified in the "10 questions" are designed to form a comprehensive mnemonic of areas of bodily function that can be affected by the six evils, the seven affects, and by pathological processes affecting the viscera and bowels. The outline presented to the right from the work of the highly regarded contemporary diagnostician, Tie Tao Deng, illustrates the breadth of inquiry in diagnosis (**C**).

Inquiry is considered critical to creating a complete and accurate diagnosis. The findings of inspection, listening and smelling, and palpation fall into place according to the results of clinical inquiry. Questioning begins with eliciting the nature of the presenting complaint, its history, and cause. Then specific questions concerning bodily processes and regions are asked to determine the nature and characteristics of the disease process.

Cold and Heat

The patient's experience of cold and heat are critical to understanding the progression of disease and the nature of the disease process in terms of *yin* and *yang*. An evil invading the body's surface may produce sensations of fever and chills; often the patient will be averse to drafts and cold. All of these signs indicate an engagement of the evil with the correct *qi* on the surface of the body.

Yang vacuity can produce a sense of cold on the part of the patient and a desire for warm clothing. An interior cold evil presents with similar signs. Heat evils can produce the subjective sensation of warmth or actual fever. A replete heat presents with high fever, no fear of cold, sweating, and thirst. Where the heat is produced by vacuity of *yin* and is the manifestation of the body's unbalanced *yang* (its own natural heat) there is only a low-grade fever or what is termed "tidal fever," which is a fever that arrives in the late afternoon.

"If, in conducting the examination, the practitioner neither inquires as to how and when the condition arose, nor asks about the nature of the patient's complaint, about dietary irregularities, excesses of sleeping and waking, and poisoning, but instead proceeds immediately to take the pulse, he will not succeed in identifying the disease."

(From the *Huang Di Nei Jing Su Wen*, in Wiseman 1995, p. 107)

A Quote from *Huang Di Nei Jing Su Wen*.

"First ask hot and cold, second ask sweat, third ask head and body, fourth ask stools and urine, fifth ask food and drink, sixth ask chest, seventh ask hearing, eighth ask thirst, ninth ask old disease, tenth ask cause."

(*Zhang Jing Yue* in Deng, p. 64)

B "Ten Questions Song" ("*Shi Wen Pian*" 十问篇).

- Collecting information with regard to patient's age, gender, relationship status, ethnicity, profession, place of birth, and residence

- Taking the history of the present disease and asking about causes of the complaint as well as any previous treatment and changes produced by it

- Inquiring into specific areas:
  - Cold and heat
  - Sweat
  - Head and body
  - Stools and urine
  - Drink, food, and taste
  - Chest, rib-side, stomach duct, and abdomen
  - Ears and eyes
  - Thirst and intake of beverages
  - Sleep
  - Inquiry pertinent to women or children

- Previous medical history

- Life circumstances

- Family medical history

C Contemporary organization of Chinese medical history.

Sweat

Sweat is a direct manifestation of the body's *yang qi* diffusing fluids to the surface. The defense and healthy moistening of the body's surface depends on a well-regulated relationship between the construction (*ying qi*) and the defense (*wei qi*). All abnormalities of sweating reflect a disruption of this relationship. External cold evils often manifest with lack of sweating, reflecting an obstruction of the defense or by sweating without any relief of symptoms, indicating that the defense *qi* is vacuous. External heat evils present with sweating, which temporarily relieves symptoms.

Head and Body

This broad inquiry elicits specific findings related to dizziness, headaches, and the nature and location of pain or numbness (**A**, **B**). These can be very helpful in understanding the nature of the disease as well as the channels that are affected.

Drink, Food, and Taste

The dietary habits, preferences, and experiences of the patient give a clear sense of the disposition of the spleen and stomach, *yin* or *yang* characteristics of the disease, and, through five-phase associations, the disposition of individual organs. In many instances, treatment begins with modification to the diet.

Chest, Rib-side, Stomach Duct, and Abdomen

This broad area of inquiry is designed to elicit information about sensations of oppression or pain in the chest, feelings of distension or fullness in the epigastrium, pain in the rib-side or flanks (along the course of the gallbladder channel), and the presence or absence of abdominal masses. By carefully asking about the presence of these types of symptoms and their presentation, a wide range of clinical patterns can be assessed.

Ears and Eyes

The ears are the sprout of the kidney and hearing impairment is frequently associated with the insufficiency of kidney *yin* or *yang*. Replete conditions such as liver gallbladder damp–heat can also, because of the tendency of fire to rise up and the pathway of the gallbladder channel around the ears, cause disturbances of the hearing. The eyes are the sprout of the liver, and so liver blood, as well as blood in general, is critical to the nourishment and healthy function of the eyes. Loss of visual acuity or dryness of the eyes is often attributed to liver blood vacuity. Redness of the eyes may indicate heat in the liver.

Channel	Headache pain
Grater *Yang* Headache Urinary Bladder/Small Intestine	Pain radiates to the neck and back
Yang Brightness Headache Stomach/Large Intestine	Pain in the forehead, eyebrows, sub maxillary sinuses
Lesser *Yang* Headache Gallbladder/Triple Burner	Pain in the temples and sides of head
Greater *Yin* Headache Spleen/Lung	Pain and heaviness of the head with abdominal fullness
Lesser *Yin* Headache Kidney/Heart	Pain radiates into the brain and teeth
Reverting *Yin* Headache Liver/Pericardium	Pain is felt at the vertex of the head and may move to the temples, nausea may be present

A Headache pain, sinus pain, and other pain presentations on the head and neck are considered in relation to the distribution of the channel pathway. This information is useful in diagnosis and in planning acupuncture treatment.

Head or body pain presentaion	Diagnostic implication
Headache and body pain without fixed location, or pain radiating to the neck and back, accompanied by fever and chills, aversion to cold, and a scratchy throat	External evil
Heaviness and numbness of the low back and limbs	Dampness evil
Piercing pain with a fixed location that is swollen and resists pressure	Blood stasis
Impediment patterns on *bi* involve pain throughout the body particularly in the joints and low back. Traditionally this presentation is referred to generically as wind damp cold impediment, but is often differentiated with more precision:	
Pain moves from place to place and different joints hurt at different times	Moving impediment with wind being the primary evil
Pain is fixed in location, the body feels heavy and the patient fatigued	Fixed impediment with dampness being the primary evil
Sharp and persistent pain that is slightly diminished by warmth	Painful impediment with cold being the primary evil
Joint pain with fever, redness of the affected area, pain that is slightly diminished by cold	Heat impediment

B Head and body pains are categorized according to their distinctive manifestations.

Stools and Urine

Because the activities of the spleen, stomach, intestines, kidney, bladder, and liver all pertain to the orderly process of digestion and excretion, information about the appearance and frequency of the patient's feces and urine is considered fundamental to any interview (**A**).

Thirst and Intake of Beverages

Questions concerning thirst and the desire for liquids can indicate a great deal about the status of the body's fluids as well as the nature of the disease process. Hot conditions produce a desire for cold beverages, cold diminishes thirst, and if thirst is present there is a desire for warm beverages. Dampness, because it is associated with the failure of fluid transformation and the accumulation of fluids, is characterized by thirst due to the failure of fluids to perfuse the body, and yet no wish to drink, because fluids are congested.

Sleep

Normal sleep cycles are produced by a healthy balance between the *yin* and *yang* elements of the body, particularly the *yin* blood and the original *qi*. Where the body's *yin* or blood is insufficient, the *yang qi* cannot enter the *yin* to rest and so sleeplessness occurs. Sorrow and anxiety can damage the heart blood and the spleen *qi*'s ability to produce blood, resulting in insomnia and vivid dreaming. *Qi* vacuity can produce difficulty in falling asleep or early rising. Both replete and vacuity heat can rise in the body and harass the heart, disturbing the spirit and causing restlessness at night.

Women and Children

Inquiry must take into account the special situations of female patients, children, as well as the elderly and other special populations. Women are always asked about their age at menarche, the nature of their menstrual cycle, reproductive history, menopause and so on, because these processes indicate a great deal about the movement of *qi* and blood and the status of the liver and kidney. As the developmental process discussed in the preceding chapter shows, the waxing and waning of the menses is closely linked to other bodily processes and so is critical for understanding a female patient's constitution.

For children, questions pertaining to their gestation, development, childhood illnesses, vaccinations, and dietary habits over time are asked, in addition to those discussed above. A child's constitution and development reflects the condition of the congenital essence and the health of the mother during gestation. During the early years, development is rapid and dynamic. Bodily changes in response to disease and therapy often occur quickly and easily.

Summing Up

While there is no fixed rule about the order of the four examinations, it is generally understood that inquiry precedes palpation, since the information provided by inquiry helps the practitioner focus their tactile attention on certain areas, understand what must be ruled out, and helps to form the basic idea of the diagnosis. Subsequent to, or during palpation further questions may be asked to help clarify matters for the practitioner.

Presentation	Pattern association
Constipation	
Constipation with abdominal fullness that is exacerbated by pressure, fever, thirst; tongue fur is yellow	Repletion heat where an exuberant heat evil is present and the bowel *qi* is obstructed
Constipation with abdominal fullness that is exacerbated by pressure, aversion to cold, cold limbs, and other cold signs	Repletion cold where a cold evil ostructs the *yang qi* and the bowel *qi* is stagnant
Constipation where the stool is dry and pellet like and defecation is difficult	Vacuity of blood and fluids, and *qi* and *yin* where moisture and *qi* is insufficient and free movement of *qi* not permitted
Diarrhea	
Diarrhea that starts quickly, of great volume, foul smelling, and presents with abdominal pain, intestinal gurgling, and burning of the anus	Damp–heat
Watery diarrhea with only a little fecal matter that is pale yellow and foul smelling; the tongue body is pale	Cold–damp
Diarrhea presents with vomiting. The diarrhea and vomit are foul smelling. Fever and abdominal pain are present	Food stagnation casued by overeating, dietary irregularity, inappropriate, or unclean food
Diarrhea with thin and sloppy stools or with undigested food visible in the stool. The diarrhea persists over several days	Spleen *yang* vacuity
Diarrhea occurs at dawn each day	Kidney *yang* vacuity

A Pattern association for abnormal bowel movements.

Palpation Examination (*Qie Zhen* 切诊)

While pulse diagnosis comes to mind immediately as the most well-known aspect of palpation, all areas of the body may be palpated to assist the practitioner in achieving a diagnosis and planning a treatment. The channels and collaterals, and specific points are pressed diagnostically and any region may be pressed to assess whether it is hot or cold, dry or moist, hard or soft, or whether or not lumps or pain are present. Certain regions are particularly important in palpation: the forearms, the abdomen, the hands and feet, the transport points, and the reflex regions of the ear.

Pulse Examination

The examination of the pulse has a long history and approaches to pulse palpation have varied. The body affords a number of locations where an arterial pulsation can be detected and easily palpated. *The Yellow Emperor's Classic of Medicine (Huang Di Nei Jing)* described nine specific pulse points on the body that might be palpated to assess the progress of disease and the health of the patient.

Today, while the palpation of regional pulses is still used in some instances, the most common method of pulse diagnosis is palpation of the radial artery at both wrists. The patient may be seated or lying down and should be calm and relaxed. The practitioner should also be relaxed and mentally focused. The amount of information gathered by this diagnostic method is dependent on the sophistication of the diagnostic model used by the practitioner, their experience, and the time spent in directly palpating the patient's pulse.

The simplest method is to conduct a general assessment of the rate and overall quality of the pulsations. The table to the right shows 13 of the 28 standard pulse terms that describe typical pathological variations in the level, rate, force, rhythm, and form of the pulse (**A**). These qualities help the practitioner to organize the sensations felt under their fingers and so characterize the condition of *qi* and blood in the body.

A normal pulse is said to have spirit, stomach *qi*, and root. This means that it has a smooth flow and a regular rhythm, and a rate that, for an adult, ranges from 60 to 80 beats per minute. Stomach *qi* refers to a healthy fullness of the vessels and should be detectable as a slightly slippery quality in the pulse. Root refers to the pulse having force and resilience under the fingers. The 28 pulses reflect the impact of the disease process on the normal pulse.

Although the pulse qualities define pathology, some may be present in health. The slow pulse of a trained athlete, or the slippery pulse when produced by exuberant *qi* and blood may both signify vigorous good health.

Name	Pulse Image	Clinical Implications
Level: superficial		
Floating	Clearly felt with light pressure, weaker with pressure	Exterior evil
Level: deep		
Deep	Not clearly felt with light pressure, clear when pressed deeply	Interior evil, *qi* depression, water swelling
Rate: slow		
Slow	Less than 60 beats per minute	Cold
Rough	Arrives roughly, slowly, and hesitantly, like a knife scraping bamboo	Essence damage, blood depletion, *qi* stagnation, blood stasis
Rate: fast		
Rapid	More than 80 beats per minute	Heat pattern (racing pulse governs extreme heat, yin exhaustion, floating *yang*)
Slippery	Arrives smoothly, the fingers feel roundness and slipperiness	Phlegm, food accumulation, repletion heat
Force: forceless		
Vacuous	Lacks force and does not push back when pressed	Dual vacuity of *qi* and blood
Weak	Deep, fine, without force	Insufficient *qi* and blood
Force: forceful		
Replete	Forceful when pressed	Repletion pattern, heat pattern
Tight	Feels tight and forceful under the fingers, like a twisted rope	Cold, pain, food storage
Abnormal rhythm		
Skipping	Rapid with irregularly skipped beats	Flourishing *yang* repletion heat, phlegm flourishing, food stagnation
Abnormal form		
Fine	Narrow in diameter like a thread and clearly felt	Vacuity taxation detriment with *yin* vacuity as primary, governs damp
String-like	Straight and long, sensation of pressing on the string of an instrument	Liver gallbladder disease, pain pattern, phlegm rheum

A Pulse qualities. 13 of the 28 abnormal pulse qualities divided according to level, rate, force, rhythm, and form. These five divisions characterize major differences in the tactile quality of the pulses.

The **level** at which the pulse is felt conveys the degree to which the movement of *qi* and blood is engaged at the interior or the exterior of the body. A superficial pulse is readily felt at the surface of the skin and may be a sign of an invading external evil. A pulse that is felt only at a deep level with finger pressure can be a sign of an interiorized evil.

The **rate** of a normal pulse is considered to be 60 to 80 beats per minute. A pulse rate at the lower end of this range may indicate cold or insufficiency of *qi*. A rate of 80 beats or more is often indicative of heat.

The **arrival force** of the pulse indicates the strength of the patient's *qi* or the exuberance of the evil. Forceful or replete pulses are seen in conditions where the evil is strong; forceless, or vacuous pulses where the correct *qi* is insufficient.

The **rhythm**, when disturbed, can reveal abnormalities in the function of the heart and emotional disturbance.

The **form** of the pulse speaks to the overall condition of *qi* and its response to the disease process. A large pulse feels big and broad under the fingers; it can be a sign of healthy *qi* and blood. In illness, if forceful, it is associated with entry of disease into the interior. If forceless, it signifies damage to *yin* and blood. A "small" or fine pulse suggests insufficiency of *qi* and blood or dampness preventing the *qi* and blood from getting to the extremities.

Precise assessment of the status of *qi* and blood in specific regions of the body can be made by palpating areas of the radial artery that are associated with specific organs or body regions. The artery is divided into three regions. The middle, adjacent to the styloid process of the radius is the "bar" position; the "inch" is distal to it, and the "cubit" is proximal. Each position is felt by one finger of the practitioner's hand (**A**). The inch, bar, and cubit positions indicate the upper, middle, and lower burners respectively and are associated with specific organs. **B** shows the relationships typically used in China today.

C describes the pulse assignments made by the *Nan Jing (The Classic of Difficulties)*, the first text to describe the division of the radial artery into three areas (see p. 30). This schema is still used in some clinical contexts particularly outside China. This pattern of pulse associations is particularly useful in relation to five-phase models of diagnosis and treatment.

A Palpating areas of the radial artery.

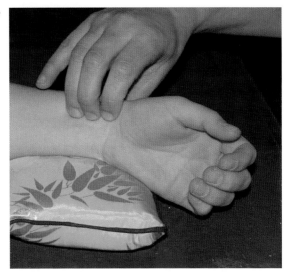

	Left		Right	
Cun/inch	Heart		Lung	
Guan/bar	Liver	Gallbladder	Spleen	Stomach
Chi/cubit	Kidney (yin)	Bladder, intestines (reproductive organs)	Kidney (yang)	Bladder, intestines (reproductive organs)

B Association of organs and positions on the radial artery according to classical and contemporary pulse diagnosis.

	Left		Right	
Position	Deep	Superficial	Deep	Superficial
Cun/inch	Heart	Small intestine	Lung	Large intestine
Guan/bar	Liver	Gallbladder	Spleen	Stomach
Chi/cubit	Kidney	Bladder	Pericardium	Triple burner

C *Nan Jing* pulse.

Channels, Abdomen, and Other Regions

The channels and networks and specific points are pressed diagnostically and any region may be pressed to assess whether it is hot or cold, dry or moist, hard or soft, or whether or not lumps or pain are present. Certain regions are particularly important in palpation: the forearms, the abdomen, the hands and feet, the transport points, and the reflex regions of the ear.

As an example, the alarm (*mu*) points are a group of points, one associated with each of the viscera and bowels, that are all located on the ventral aspect of the trunk (**A**, see also p. 188f). When palpated, these points are used diagnostically to help to determine the location of disease. They are also used to make up one of several diagnostic maps of the abdomen. In some traditions outside of China, abdominal diagnosis has developed to a much greater degree.

Palpation and observation of channels is also very important. Vacuity and repletion of channels can be assessed through palpation, as can the channel location of pain. Palpation of a patient requires that the practitioner be attuned to the patient's response. Small responses that the patient does not actually verbalize may be seen in the face. Additionally, the practitioner's hands must be able to perceive differences in texture, tension, and temperature.

Palpation Examination in Clinical Cases

John who came to us with chronic back and knee pain displays several critical findings on palpation. His knees are cold to the touch suggesting cold or *yang* vacuity. The tender regions on his back suggest obstructed movement of *qi* in the urinary bladder channel pathway. His pulse rate (62 bpm) is suggestive of cold, it is deep, indicating an interiorized evil, and the slippery quality, in this case, suggests dampness.

Alice who presented with severe dysmenorrhea has a pulse rate well within the normal range. Its string-like quality suggests pain and *qi* stagnation, the rough quality is strongly suggestive of blood stasis, and the force felt on palpation suggests that *qi* and blood are significantly obstructed. For *Alice*, one could also palpate the abdomen for areas of tenderness and the possibility of fibroid masses.

Jeremy's pulse is slightly rapid, suggesting that heat is part of his clinical picture, the floating quality is typically a sign of the entry of an external evil, and a floating pulse at the lung position, especially in the presence of signs of a slight respiratory tract infection and a slightly rapid pulse rate suggest wind–heat.

In all three cases, palpation would be important in planning and confirming the selection of specific acupuncture points prior to treatment.

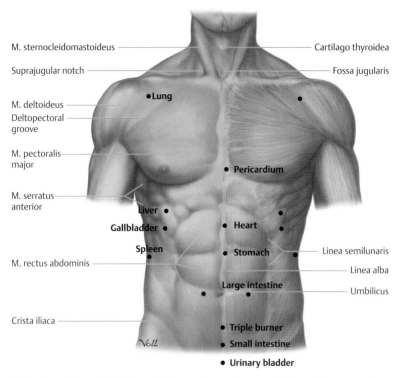

A Front *mu* points on the chest and abdomen. Shown above are all but one of the acupuncture points that function as alarm points. These points are all located on the chest and abdomen, in proximity to the organ with which they are associated, though not necessarily on the channel associated with that organ. The points may be palpated to assess the condition of *qi* and blood in their associated organs and/or needled to treat the associated organ. The points and their associations are: lung / LU-1; large intestine / ST-25; stomach / CV-12; spleen / LR-13; heart / CV-14; small intestine / CV-4; urinary bladder / CV-3, kidney (not shown because it is located further posterior than is visible in this image) / GB-25; pericardium / CV-17; triple burner / CV-5; gallbladder / GB-24; liver / LR-14. (From Atlas of Anatomy, (c) Thieme 2008, Illustration by Marcus Voll.)

Pattern Diagnosis

In the formal presentation of the diagnostic process, patterns (*zheng* 证 or *zheng hou* 证侯) are explored after the four examinations, since the process of the four examinations produces the information, signs, and symptoms* (*zheng* 症 or *zheng zhuang* 症状), required by the clinician to form a diagnosis of a specific pattern. In a clinical setting this process of the four examinations and pattern identification is inextricably linked and is continuous from the moment the physician encounters the patient. Lines of inquiry and examination are pursued and discarded as the clinical encounter reveals more information about the patient and their condition. The goal of the clinician is to establish a complete view of the patient's situation by staying focused on collecting relevant information while being sure that no critical information is overlooked. This is a complex skill and one that is developed in the course of clinical training and practice.

The concept of pattern identification is a distinctive aspect of Chinese medicine diagnosis since it structures the presentation of pathological processes into an integrated understanding of the patient's constitution and can result in highly individualized diagnoses. A diagnostic pattern manifests the nature of a disease. It conveys its nature, location, and cause (Huang 1987). The pattern is constituted out of a meaningful constellation of signs and symptoms that portray the disease process and suggest a method of treatment (**A**).

It is sometimes said that Chinese medicine does not diagnose a disease, but rather a "pattern of disharmony." In actuality, the concept of disharmony (*bu he* 不和) in Chinese medicine refers to the functional disturbance of any bowel, viscus, or vital substance. In fact, Chinese medicine makes extensive use of the concept of disease (*bing* 病) as a collection of specific types of afflictions characterized by typical signs and symptoms. Common cold, painful menstruation, wasting and thirsting disease, smallpox, goiter and so on, would all be examples of disease names. This topic is discussed in greater detail at the conclusion of this chapter.

For this reason pattern identification is typically concerned with determining the disease pattern (*bing zheng* 病证), which describes the distinct process by which the disease is manifesting. As discussed at the beginning of the chapter a specific disease such as insomnia or painful menstruation can arise from many patterns and so one disease could elicit many different treatment methods depending on the presenting pattern.

---

* The matter of symptom (subjective) versus sign (objective) is a comparatively recent distinction in the West and does not formally obtain in TCM where both subjective and objective findings are highly valued.

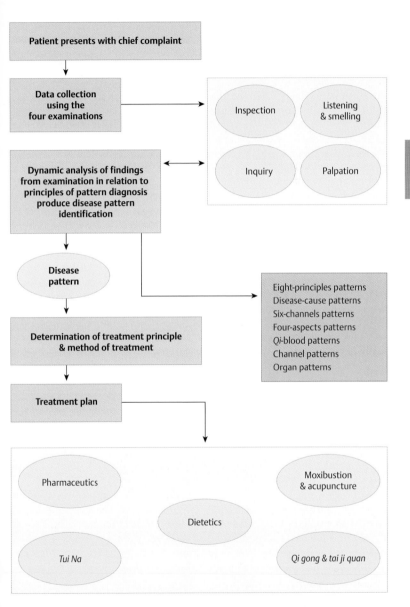

A Steps in pattern diagnosis.

Eight-principles Pattern Diagnoses

The first step of pattern identification is the evaluation of the disease process in *yin* and *yang* terms, using the eight principles or "*ba gang*"(八纲). The basis for this approach to organizing a diagnosis is found in the earliest texts such as *Shang Han Lun (On Cold Damage)*. The idea was continuously developed but was explicitly stated in the Ming dynasty by Wang Zhi Zhong who wrote, "In the treatment of disease, there are eight words, vacuity, repletion, *yin*, *yang*, exterior, interior, cold, hot. If [the physician] does not vary from these eight words, then people will not be killed" (Deng 1999, p.165). Wang's statement expresses the fundamental importance of understanding and applying eight principle diagnosis in order to avoid serious mistakes.

The eight principles rarely provide a final diagnosis. They are the gateway to a more detailed diagnosis using other patterns such as six-evils or organ pattern identification. The eight principles do not organize information with enough specificity to fully guide a treatment. Instead, the eight principles prevent clinical error, establish the nature and location of the disease, and characterize the relative strength of both the evil and the correct *qi*.

Jeremy, who has recently come down with a cold, manifests a combined clinical pattern. His cold is an exterior, hot, replete, and *yang* condition. It is an exterior condition because there are only signs of surface involvement, particularly fever, the floating pulse, and body aches. The condition shows heat signs such as a sore throat, red eyes, rapid pulse, and yellow phlegm. With respect to vacuity and repletion, *Jeremy*'s cold is a repletion condition since there are signs of exuberant heat and his bodily response, sweating, is strong enough to diminish the sensations of heat, and the evil itself is exuberant. However, *Jeremy*'s clinical presentation is complex because his fatigue from overwork (previously diagnosed as spleen *qi* vacuity) suggests an underlying pattern of interior vacuity.

John, with chronic low back and knee pain as well as diabetes is also a complex case, although straightforward in terms of eight-principles analysis. His presentation is one of interior, cold, vacuity, and so is a *yin* pattern. *John* has no signs of exterior involvement. All of his clinical manifestations speak to internal disease processes. His body shows signs of cold and his pain is relieved by warmth. Finally, the chronic nature of the condition, the fatigue, and the slowness of wounds to heal all suggest that the correct *qi* is vacuous.

Depending on the presentation of the patient and the progression of the disease the use of eight-principles terms can be complex, allowing for mixed patterns and the simultaneous presence of hot and cold or vacuity and repletion. The tables to the right illustrate basic applications of eight-principles ideas (**A, B**).

Principle	Fundamental Characteristics
Hot	Signs of heat, red tongue, rapid pulse
Cold	Signs of cold, pale tongue, clear copious secretions, slow pulse
Exterior	Signs of surface involvement, indicating a contest between the defense *qi* and the evil; changes in sweating may be seen, floating pulse
Interior	Signs that the evil has become interiorized, tongue fur becomes thickened or damaged, deep pulse
Repletion	Signs that the evil is exuberant and/or that the correct *qi* is strong enough to forcefully engage it, forceful, replete pulse
Vacuity	Signs that the correct *qi* is insufficient and cannot successfully engage the evil, forceless, vacuous pulse
Yang	The terms *yin* and *yang* are seen as generally imprecise unless the *yin* factors of cold and vacuity, or the *yang* factors of heat and repletion are both present. A *yang* vacuity pattern, where the body's *yang* warmth is insufficient is both cold and vacuous, while a pattern where an exuberant heat evil has invaded and is strongly contested by the correct *qi* is both hot and replete and so is a *yang* pattern
Yin	

A Fundamental eight-principles clinical signs.

Examples of the Eight Principles in Combination	
Exterior repletion cold	Exuberant cold evil contesting the correct *qi* on the surface of the body: aversion to cold, fever chills, glossy, white tongue fur, floating, tight pulse, no sweating
Exterior vacuity cold	Vacuous correct *qi* unable to resolve a cold evil on the surface of the body: aversion to cold, floating, moderate pulse, sweating without relief of symptoms
Exterior repletion heat	Exuberant heat evil contesting the correct *qi* on the surface of the body: aversion to cold, fever and chills, sweating with subsequent coolness, sore throat, red tongue body, floating rapid pulse
Exterior vacuity heat	Vacuous correct *qi* unable to resolve a heat evil on the surface of the body: aversion to cold, fever, and chills
Interior repletion cold	Interiorized exuberant cold evil: aversion to cold, cold limbs, abdominal pain, slimy, white tongue fur, deep, tight, pulse
Interior vacuity cold	Insufficient *yang qi* to warm the interior: aversion to cold, cold limbs, with pale complexion, fatigue, clear copious urine, watery diarrhea, forceless, slow, fine pulse
Interior repletion heat	Interiorized exuberant heat evil: fever, vexation thirst, abdominal fullness, red tongue with yellow fur, rapid, slippery, replete pulse
Interior vacuity heat	Insufficient *yin* to restrain the yang: tidal fever, night sweating, red tongue with little fur, rapid and fine pulse

B The eight principles in combination.

Disease-cause Pattern Identification—Six Excesses

Disease-cause pattern identification uses patterns associated with the external, internal, and neither internal nor external causes of disease to form a diagnosis. Six-excesses pattern identification is the most commonly used. It organizes signs and symptoms into patterns based on manifestations of the influence of a particular evil or combination of evils. The excesses are external in origin and progressively enter the body, moving from surface to interior depending on the ability of the correct *qi* to repel them. As they move from exterior to interior eight-principles analysis governs the observation of signs that indicate whether an evil remains on the surface or has interiorized. Once in the interior, evils can transform. For example, wind–cold moving into the body can transform into heat. Or a dampness evil can become bound and depressed and produce heat.

While this method of pattern diagnosis focuses on diseases of external origin, it should be remembered that, with the exception of summer heat, all of the evils can be produced internally due to imbalances of the internal landscape produced by disease processes and so this method can be applied to a range of internal diseases as well.

The six evils can appear singly and in combination (**A**) and reflect the influences of the season and the prevailing climate. Their precise manifestation depends on whether they rest on the exterior or move inward, and on the state of the patient's correct *qi*.

Wind is said to be the lord of the 100 diseases because it strikes suddenly and can carry and drive other evils such as heat, cold, damp, and dryness into the body. Thus, wind is a fundamental factor in understanding external disease.

Jeremy, who presented with an acute cold, has many of the clinical signs of wind–heat. His acute presentation suggests an evil that arrived suddenly with wind, as does the discomfort of his throat. The body aches suggest wind evil attacking the surface and congesting the channels. His sore throat, red eyes, and the production of scant, but yellow mucus all suggest heat. The disease pattern diagnosis would be one of exterior wind and heat.

In contrast, a wind–cold patient would present with aversion to exposure to cold, headache, body aches, absence of thirst, a moist tongue with a thin white coating, and a floating and tight pulse. Wind–cold–damp impediment involves the simultaneous entry of these evils into the channels, from where they move into the limbs and joints, producing the aches, pains, and degenerative changes that we associate with osteoarthritis. Depending on which of the three evils predominate clinical signs will vary slightly (see also pp. 240 and 268).

Evil or Combination of Evils	Signs and Symptoms
Wind	– Fever – Aversion to cold – Sweating – Dizziness – Headache – Nasal congestion – Itching throat – Cough – Floating pulse
Wind–cold	– Marked aversion to cold – Headache – Aching bones – No thirst – Moist – White tongue fur
Wind–heat	– Slight aversion to cold – Sore throat – Dry mouth – Red tongue
Wind–cold–damp impediment	Joint or muscle pain that may be fixed, sharp, or mobile, and is relieved by warmth
Damp–heat	– Fever, pain, and distension in the chest and rib-side – Abdominal fullness – Nausea and vomiting – Anorexia – Thirst without great desire to drink – Constipation or diarrhea – Rapid and slippery pulse – Tongue fur that is thick, yellow, and slimy
Dryness	– Aversion to cold – Fever – No sweating – Headache – Dry mouth, throat, lips, and nose – Dry cough – Sticky phlegm – Nosebleed – Dry skin – Dry hard stools
Fire–heat	– High fever – Aversion to heat – Irritation – Concentrated reddish urine – Red face – Red eyes – Red tongue – Yellow tongue fur – Rapid pulse

A Common disease patterns of the six evils.

Six-channels and Four-aspects Disease Patterns

Cold Damage

The work of Zhang Ji (Zhang Zhong Jing) in 220 CE produced an important text, *Shang Han Lun (On Cold Damage)*, which described the way in which cold evil entered the body, moving from the exterior to the interior and from bowels to viscera, producing different clinical signs as it penetrated the body (see also pp. 30 and 226).

The six channels refer to the *yin/yang* nomenclature applied to the channels in *The Yellow Emperor's Classic of Medicine (Huang Di Nei Jing)*. Each term is used for the combination of one of the six channels that travel along the arms and hands, and one of the six that travel along the legs and feet. Thus, the stomach channel and the large intestine channel are both *yang* brightness channels of the foot and hand respectively. These terms were used by Zhang Ji to describe stages of disease progression, not as a discussion of channel theory.

The clinical observations and strategies developed by Zhang Ji inform many contemporary systems of pattern diagnosis, particularly six-excesses pattern identification and organ pattern identification. The model of the six channels also stands as a system of pattern identification in its own right (**A**). It is considered particularly important in managing infectious disease, and as a resource for clinically challenging presentations. The close linkage between the therapeutic strategies developed by Zhang Ji and his diagnostic insights make this system quite important, particularly in herbal medicine.

Since wind and cold attack the exterior of the body and strike the greater *yang* (*tai yang*) channel at the neck where it is exposed; the first stage of the entry of a cold evil is the greater *yang*. The clinical signs of the greater *yang* stage are exactly those of external wind–cold discussed above. If the cold evil is not resolved at the greater *yang* stage then it may move to another channel, such as the lesser *yang* (*shao yang*). The lesser *yang* is considered to be neither exterior nor interior and so the clinical signs manifest with alternating fever and chills, fullness and congestion along the lesser *yang* channel pathways, a bitter taste in the mouth, nausea, and vomiting. Clinically, conditions such as malaria or later stages of a cold may manifest with this pattern.

While Zhang Ji's model implied progression from the exterior to deeper *yin* organs, it did not mandate it, so the diagnostic pattern of each "channel" in the disease process can be considered in its own right. Evil in the greater *yang* may also progress to the *yang* brightness (*yang ming*) instead of the lesser *yang*. Yang brightness patterns are characterized by the transformation of the cold evil into heat as it penetrates and interacts with the copious *qi* and blood of the *yang* brightness channel.

Channel	Disease process	Signs and symptoms
Greater *yang* *Tai yang*	Cold evil enters the exterior obstructing the greater yang channel. The evil congests the channels and is battled by the correct *qi*.	Fever, mild aversion to wind or to cold, head ache, dry mouth, scratchy throat, cough, red tongue, rapid and floating pulse
Lesser *yang* *Shao yang*	The evil enters the gallbladder and triple burner interfering with the free movement of *qi* in these channels. Characterized as „mid-stage" the evil is trapped between the interior and the exterior of the body.	Alternating fever and chills, bitter taste in the mouth, painful distension of the chest and rib-side, irritation, vomiting, and a string-like pulse
Yang brightness *Yang ming*	The evil enters the stomach and large intestine channels which are replete with *qi* and blood. Here the evil transforms into dryness and heat, which scorches the interior producing a range of heat signs.	Fever, aversion to heat, thirst, bitter taste in the mouth, concentrated possibly reddish urine, rapid pulse, thick yellow or white tongue fur. Where the evil enters the channel there can be the clinical sign of the „four greats": great fever, great thirst, great sweating, and a large pulse
Greater yin *Tai yin*	Either cold damage progresses and *yang* transforms into *yin* as the evil damages the correct *qi*, or cold directly attacks the spleen damaging the *yang qi* of the spleen and producing interior cold and damp	Abdominal fullness, vomiting, inability to swallow food, diarrhea, abdominal pain, white tongue fur, and a slow weak pulse
Lesser *yin* *Shao yin*	Where a cold evil progresses to or directly enters lesser *yin* and damages the heart or kidney causing differing clinical signs depending on preexisting conditions. Cold patterns due to damage of heart and kidney *yang* are typical, but heat patterns can occur as well	Aversion to cold, cold limbs, clear diarrhea, a desire for warm liquids, a pale tongue with white glossy fur, and a deep and slow pulse
Reversal *yin* *Jue yin*	Disease enters the liver causing disturbance to the *yang* (ministerial fire) of that organ and producing signs of both heat and cold in alternation as the evil and the correct *qi* struggle with each other	Heat in the upper burner, cold in the lower burner manifest primarily with sensations of either cold traveling up the limbs (reversal cold) or heat. The severity and prognosis of the disease is determined by the degree of heat or cold

A Six-channels—stages and symptoms (based on *Shang Han Lun*).

A *yang* brightness pattern can vary in its presentation depending on whether the evil remains lodged in the *yang* brightness channel where the heat manifests as a pattern of interior repletion, heat with the "four greats": great fever, great sweating, great thirst, and a large pulse. If the evil progresses into the *yang* brightness bowel (stomach and large intestine) there are signs of repletion dryness with abdominal fullness, pain, and constipation in addition to other signs of heat.

The next three channels of six-channels theory involve the later stages of disease where the unchecked or unsuccessfully treated evil has begun to damage the correct *qi*. At this point, the disease progresses into the *yin* organs where the impact of the evil manifests primarily with signs of vacuity and cold or mixed hot and cold presentations as the cold evil and the body's *yang qi* struggle.

Warm Disease

Warm disease theorists offered a model of disease progression, diagnosis, and therapeutics that emerged from the 11th to the 16th century as a response to the model expressed by six-channels theory (see also pp. 42, 226, and 270). This model considered the progression of a warm or heat evil into the body and described four stages or "aspects" of its progression. These fours aspects used the concepts of defense *qi*, *qi* construction, *ying qi*, and blood to describe a process of penetration and pathology

in which heat moves from the most external and *yang* aspect of the body (the defense) to the most internal and *yin* (the blood) (**A**). Clinically, warm disease theory has been very important in the management of epidemic infectious disease and as a resource for developing clinical approaches to newly encountered disease processes. Warm disease theory played an important part in creating treatment models in the United States and on the continent of Africa when Traditional Chinese Medicine practitioners encountered and treated large numbers of patients with HIV and AIDS during the 1980s and 1990s.

The defense aspect presents as an external wind–heat pattern. *Jeremy* would be described as having a defense aspect presentation, in which the defense is actively engaging the evil on the surface of the body. A *qi* aspect pattern is closely comparable to the *yang* brightness channel pattern of six-channels theory and manifests with exuberant heat and the four greats. However, warm disease theory elaborates several patterns at this stage of disease progression. The next two aspects portray the penetration of the heat evil deep into the body. As heat progresses into the construction there are cardinal signs of a crimson tongue, disturbances of the spirit, and skin conditions. Finally, heat enters the blood, with signs of damage to blood, *yin*, and body fluids, and possibly bleeding.

Aspect	Disease process	Signs and syptoms
Defense *wei fen* 卫分	Warm evil enters the exterior or the defense aspect. The evil congests the channels and is battled by the correct *qi*	Fever, mild aversion to wind or to cold, head ache, dry mouth, sore throat, cough, red tongue, rapid and floating pulse
Qi *qi fen* 气分	Exuberant heat evil in the *qi* aspect. The warm evil has penetrated interiorly and will manifest in different ways depending on the organs affected. Exuberant heat of the lung and stomach, great *qi* aspect heat, and great binding of the stomach and intestines are among the patterns that can occur	High fever, profuse sweating, thirst, red face, irritation, a red tongue with yellow fur and a large and rapid pulse. Great *qi* aspect heat, similar to the *yang* brightness channel pattern, produces the sign of the "four greats": great fever, great thirst, great sweating, and a large pulse
Construction *ying fen* 营分	A warm evil has penetrated to the construction and begins to damage the yin aspects of the body. In severe cases heat can enter the pericardium and cause spirit clouding and delirium	High fever at night, vexation of the heart, sleeplessness, delirium, lack of thirst (due to steaming of the *yin*), a crimson tongue, and a fine and rapid pulse
Blood *xue fen* 血分	When heat penetrates from the construction or emerges directly in the blood aspect the heart and liver are affected. This is a serious disease presentation and signs can vary depending on the degree of vacuity or repletion present	Repletion patterns present with fever, agitation, spirit clouding and delerium. Vacuity patterns present with dry mouth, dry crimson tongue, hot palms of hands and soles of feet

A Four-aspect symptoms.

Patterns of Qi, Blood, and Body Fluids

Diagnostic patterns of *qi*, blood, and body fluids overlap substantially with other models of pattern diagnosis. Just as the eight-principles patterns describe fundamental aspects of the disease process, so these patterns describe the damage and disrupted movement of the body's vital substances. The consequences of vacuity of *qi*, blood, or body fluids can be well understood in a general way (see pp. 68–69 in Chapter 2) and will be examined further in this chapter where they impact the function of an associated organ (see p. 134).

Qi stagnation is a very important idea as the blockage or impeded flow of *qi* is fundamental to every disease process (see also p. 248). It is said that where *qi* flows smoothly there is no pain and when it is obstructed there is pain. An effect, for example, of an external evil is to obstruct the flow of *qi* within the channels on the surface of the body, causing body aches. All pain and dysfunction associated with disease processes are ultimately the result of the obstructed movement of *qi*. While fundamental, this idea is so general that it offers little diagnostic power.

However, there are two very important ideas that emerge out of both disease causation pattern diagnosis, and *qi*, blood, and body fluid pattern diagnosis: the idea of static blood and phlegm as pathological products (**A**, **B**). Both blood and fluids are vital parts of the internal economy of the organs and the triple burner. However, when obstructed, or congealed by evils or by vacuity, they can form barriers to the movement of *qi* and blood and to the normal functioning of the organ, creating disease in their own right.

Static blood is produced in many ways. Trauma, with its attendant bruising, is the most obvious and visible example of blood stasis; however, any process that impedes the free flow of *qi* and blood, such as cold that congeals, heat that cooks, *qi* stagnation that impedes, can produce static blood. Blood stasis produces sharp stabbing pain, such as that seen in *Alice's* case of dysmenorrhea. Blood stasis interrupts the free flow of *qi* and blood and impedes the nourishment of tissue. A wide range of conditions associated with aging, including premature senescence, are attributed to blood stasis (see also p. 248).

Congested fluids arise when the transformative function of the *qi* is diminished. This can occur due to vacuity or because the organs are encumbered by cold or dampness evil. The progressing congestion of fluids and the accumulation of damp eventually produce phlegm, which has many manifestations. Phlegm is clearly seen as the visible expectorate associated with the lungs. Phlegm is also seen in intractable disease, and its presence is inferred in disease processes where obstruction of organs and openings occurs (see also p. 246).

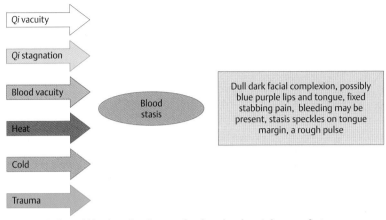

A Non-pathological blood can be obstructed and rendered static by many factors.

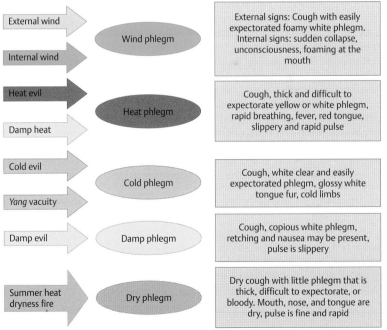

B Non-pathological fluids can be congested and congealed by many factors producing the "five phlegms."

Organ Patterns

Disease Patterns of the Heart and Pericardium

The heart has the office of the sovereign. It governs blood and vessels and stores the spirit. The heart manifests in the face and tongue. While the heart controls the vital functions of the body and stores the most critical aspect of consciousness, it is dependent on all of the organs, particularly the spleen and kidney for the vital substances that sustain its functions: *qi*, *yang*, *yin*, and blood. When pathology affects the heart, or disturbs the organs on which it relies, the functions of the heart are disrupted, producing signs such as irregular heartbeat, chest pain, disturbance of the spirit, and alterations of consciousness.

The heart is susceptible to affect damage either through direct damage to its *yin* and blood, or when emotions disturb the free coursing of the liver, producing heat that disturbs the spirit. The heart's function is often disturbed through patterns of insufficiency, but heat produced either by febrile disease, replete heat patterns of other organs, and vacuity heat conditions can rise and disturb the heart and the spirit that it stores (**A**).

The heart has a close relationship to the pericardium (literally heart wrapper), which is considered to act as the protector of the heart and as its intermediary or envoy. Also important to understanding pathology of the heart is the concept of orifices. In this context, the orifices refer to the portals through which the spirit stored in the heart engages the world. The concept of orifice, pericardium, and heart are all closely linked in the mediation of the conscious experience of the world. When heat rises and disturbs the spirit, producing irritability, vexation, or, in extreme cases, mania, this is heat harassing the heart or heat entering the pericardium. When phlegm is driven upwards by wind or fire and blocks the orifices, producing alterations of consciousness (delirium, coma) this is phlegm confounding the orifices of the heart, phlegm turbidity clouding the pericardium, or phlegm misting the orifices. These expressions show the synonymous character of the heart and pericardium in the role of mediating consciousness.

Although the digestive functions of the small intestine are traditionally subsumed under the role of the spleen and stomach, as the heart's *yang* bowel the small intestine has a special role in relation to the heart. Because of their shared phase and channel relationships, heart heat can easily shift to the small intestine, disrupting its ability to separate the clear and the turbid and producing distinctive patterns of reddish painful urination (urinary tract infections) accompanied by signs of heart fire.

Pattern	Etiology	Clinical Signs May Include
Heart *qi* vacuity	Chronic disease, insufficiency of spleen or kidney, loss of fluids and blood with concurrent loss of *qi*, affect damage due to emotional distress	Palpitations, difficulty in falling asleep, forgetfulness, easily frightened, spontaneous sweating, fatigue, pale, white complexion, pale, white tongue, a forceless pulse
Heart *yang* vacuity	*Yang* vacuity of heart and kidney, often subsequent to heart *qi* vacuity, can be produced by shock, severe fluid loss, or blood loss leading to *yang* desertion	Palpitations, difficulty in falling asleep, forgetfulness, easily frightened, spontaneous sweating, fatigue, fear of cold, cold limbs, pale, white complexion, pale and moist tongue, copious sweating and cold limbs may also be present, a weak and slow pulse
Heart *yin* vacuity	Emotional distress, thought, and anxiety and heat and dryness patterns, *yin* vacuity of any associated organ	Palpitations, irritation, insomnia, low-grade fever, heat of the five centers, night sweats, dry lips, dry throat, red tongue, fine and rapid pulse
Heart blood vacuity	Loss of blood, damage to blood from external evils or from internal heat, emotional distress, liver failing to store blood, or spleen failing to manage blood	Palpitations, irritation, insomnia, vivid dreaming, forgetfulness, dizziness, lusterless white face, pale lips, pale nails, pale, white tongue, a fine pulse
Heart fire flaming upward	Sequela of warm disease, eating hot and spicy food, alcohol, transformation of seven affects into fire	Irritation, red face, red lips, thirst, eroded and painful tongue tip, red tongue, with yellow fur, rapid pulse
Heart impediment	Damage to *qi*, cold or other causes produce blood stasis, phlegm produced by poor diet or *qi* depression	Dull, dark, or cyanotic complexion, palpitations, shortness of breath, stifling sensation and oppression in the chest, pain in the chest center and shoulder, sweating, dull, red tongue, fine, rough, or irregular pulse
Phlegm confounding the heart orifices (phlegm turbidity clouding the pericardium)	*Qi* stagnation produced by affect damage or damage to fluids by heat engendering phlegm, anger transforming into fire	Coma, delirium, thick, slimy tongue fur, vomiting of phlegm drool, gurgling of phlegm in the throat, slippery or string-like pulse

A Heart disease patterns.

Disease Patterns of the Lung

The lung dwells in the sea of *qi*, the chest. It governs *qi*, and the depurative downbearing and diffusion of *qi* and fluids. It manifests in the skin and body hair. The lung's function is vital to the production of *qi*, the protection of the body, and the orderly distribution of fluids. The lung depends on the spleen *qi* and the *yin* and *qi* of the kidney to support its functions.

The lung is a tender organ with great susceptibility to damage by external invasion, especially heat, cold, and dryness. These evils can depress the lung *qi* and interfere with downbearing and diffusion. Wind–heat travels directly to the lung and can scorch the lung *yin*. Wind–cold can enter the lungs and inhibit diffusion or transform into heat, doing further damage.

The lung stores phlegm. If lung diffusion and downbearing is inhibited by heat or cold, fluids can congest and create phlegm, producing patterns of hot or cold phlegm.

Dryness and heat can damage lung *yin*. In febrile disease, the replete heat of a *yang* brightness or *qi* aspect pattern can scorch the *yin* and leave the *qi* debilitated, producing patterns of lung *qi* and *yin* vacuity. All of these assaults can inhibit diffusion, producing cough. From a biomedical perspective the lung suffers under the impact of conditions such as bronchitis, pneumonia, and tuberculosis, all of which can do lasting damage to the *qi* and *yin* of the lung.

Lung *qi* and lung *yin* vacuity can have the same cause, either physical weakness or frequent damage to lung *qi* diffusion and depuration. Because the lung likes moisture and dislikes dryness and because of the criticality of lung function to the orderly movement of *qi* and fluids, damage to lung *yin* can harm the lung *qi* and vice versa. This clinical picture is known as dual vacuity of *qi* and *yin* and presents with fatigue, cough, shortness of breath, perspiration, reddening of the cheeks, red tongue, and a forceless, rapid pulse

Lung pathology can disturb other organs. The kidney *yin* and *yang* are the root of the *yin* and *yang* of the entire body. Insufficiency of lung *yin* can tax the kidney *yin* and produce clinical signs of kidney *yin* vacuity. Chronic coughing and panting can harm the *qi* and *yin* of the entire body, damaging the kidney, spleen, liver, and heart.

Pathologies of other organs can disturb the lung. The lung is the upper receptacle of phlegm, easily bogged down in moisture when the lower source of phlegm, the spleen, fails to transform and transport fluids effectively. Damage to the *yin* or *qi* of the kidneys can cause lung dryness or panting and wheezing (**A**).

Pattern	Etiology	Clinical Signs May Include
Non-diffusion of lung *qi*	Wind–heat or wind–cold entering the lung or obstructing the exterior, heat evil obstructing the lung, and phlegm-rheum	Cough, productive cough with varying amounts of phlegm, loss of voice and scratchy throat, if associated with heat there is high fever, flaring nostrils, panting, rough breathing and sticky, yellow phlegm. If associated with cold, the phlegm is white and foamy and the tongue has glossy white fur
Impaired depurative down-bearing of lung *qi*	Heat from the transformation of external evils (dryness, heat, cold), phlegm damp	Cough, if associated with heat and damp: dry cough, dry throat, and hoarseness or loss of voice; if associated with phlegm damp: productive cough, thick, viscid phlegm, and chest oppression
Lung *qi* vacuity	Chronic cough or asthma, spleen *qi* vacuity	Shortness of breath, soft voice, fatigue, weakness, spontaneous sweating, thin, clear sputum, easily attacked by external evils, pale tongue, and a weak pulse
Lung *yin* vacuity	Warm evil damaging the lung, chronic cough damaging lung *yin* and the *yin* of other organs	Emaciation, dry cough, dry throat and mouth, low voice, rapid breathing

A Lung disease patterns.

Spleen, Stomach, and Intestine Disease Patterns

The spleen and stomach are synonymous with the middle burner. The spleen and stomach are considered the root of the acquired essence. Together with the stomach and intestines, the spleen begins the process of transforming food and drink into *qi* and blood. As the spleen conveys the clear essence of grain and water upwards, the stomach conveys turbid digestate downward, continuing a transformative process that culminates with excretion.

The spleen governs upbearing and dislikes dampness, while the stomach governs downbearing and dislikes dryness. Disease patterns of the spleen and stomach often present signs and symptoms that exhibit the disruption of these tendencies. The two organs are directly linked and function as a pair and many of their disease processes are closely connected. However, it is helpful first to consider the disease patterns that primarily affect the spleen and then those affecting mainly the stomach and intestines.

Disease Patterns
Primarily Related to the Spleen

Spleen *qi* vacuity can be caused by irregular diet, mental and emotional disturbance, especially sustained mental effort, by weakness following illness, by taxation fatigue, blood loss weakening the *qi*, injury to the spleen from nausea and vomiting, and by liver disorders. Fundamental *qi* vacuity signs are fatigue, weakness, pallor, abdominal pain, and loose stools.

Spleen *qi* vacuity patterns can manifest with signs of impairment to the upbearing of the spleen function (center *qi* fall). Failure of the spleen *qi* to support upbearing is seen in conditions where organs "fall": distended sagging of the stomach and prolapse of the kidneys, uterus, and rectum. Because the spleen manages blood and is responsible for its containment, bleeding disorders such as bloody stools or urine, purpura, and abnormal uterine bleeding can be produced by spleen *qi* vacuity.

Because the spleen is so fundamental to the production of blood and original *qi*, a spleen *qi* vacuity can directly or indirectly affect the *qi* and blood of the other organs. Lung *qi* vacuity, heart *qi* vacuity, liver blood vacuity, and heart blood vacuity are all treated with reference to supporting the functions of the spleen. Longstanding vacuity of spleen *qi* can weaken the kidneys as well since the role of the spleen is both supported by and supportive of the kidney *yang*.

Dampness signs appear when the spleen's ability to transform fluids is impaired by vacuity or by an evil. Spleen *qi* vacuity, cold–damp encumbering the spleen, and damp–heat of the spleen and stomach, show signs of abdominal discomfort and digestive disturbance due to dampness. Most spleen disease patterns involve vacuity presentations. However, some, such as cold–damp encumbering the spleen, and damp–heat of the spleen and stomach are produced by replete evils (damp, cold, and heat) (**A**).

Pattern	Etiology	Clinical Signs May Include
Spleen *qi* vacuity	Irregular diet, mental and emotional disturbance, weakness following illness, and taxation fatigue	Abdominal discomfort or pain, loose stools, diarrhea, discomfort after eating, rumbling stomach, dull or lusterless facial complexion, fatigue, weakness, pale tongue with white fur, and a forceless, soggy pulse
Spleen *yang* vacuity	Advanced spleen *qi* vacuity, underlying kidney *yang* vacuity, or eating cold and raw foods	Bright, white complexion, cold body and limbs, bland taste in the mouth, no thirst, lack of appetite, clear urine, sloppy stools, clear and thin vaginal discharge, pale tongue with white, slimy fur, and a weak and slow pulse
Center *qi* fall	Spleen *qi* vacuity from taxation fatigue, enduring disease, or other cause	Sagging distention of the stomach duct and abdomen, distension after eating, diarrhea, rectal prolapse, uterine prolapse
Spleen not controlling the blood	Spleen *qi* vacuity from taxation fatigue, enduring disease, or other cause	Blood in the stools, profuse menstrual and uterine bleeding, easy bruising, dull, white complexion, fatigue, dizziness, palpitations, pale tongue, and a fine, soggy pulse
Cold–damp encumbering the spleen	Cold and damp evils invading the interior, eating cold and raw foods, or internal damp overcoming spleen *yang*	Heavy head, bland, slimy taste in the mouth, epigastric oppression, abdominal distension, desire for warmth, heavy limbs and body, loose stools, slimy, white tongue fur, and a slow, moderate, or soggy pulse
Damp–heat of the spleen and stomach	External damp–heat, or internal damp–heat produced by greasy food or alcohol, or damp turbidity produced by failure of splenic transformation	Bright yellow body and eyes, bitter taste in the mouth, rib-side pain, abdominal fullness, nausea and vomiting, diarrhea, lack of appetite, yellow, slimy tongue fur and a rapid pulse

A　Spleen disease patterns.

Disease Patterns
of the Stomach and Intestines

The stomach and intestines are bowels and as such are said to discharge, but not to store. Their nature is to be filled, but not to be full. Typically, the stomach and intestines function well when they are not burdened with excessive amounts of food and drink and when cold, raw, spicy, and hot foods are not consumed in immoderate amounts. Spoiled food is also injurious. Conditions such as food stagnation arise from challenging the digestive tract with inappropriate types or amounts of food. Cold, sweet, or fatty foods can cause stomach cold. Hot, spicy foods or alcohol consumed to excess can engender heat in the stomach, drying it and causing disease. The aftermath of a heat evil entering the body and causing febrile disease can leave the stomach *yin* (its natural moistness) impaired and the stomach dry. All of these process can act on the stomach and interfere with the normal downward movement of its *qi*.

Hiccough, belching, nausea, and vomiting are all movements of *qi* that are against or "counter" to the normal movement of stomach *qi*, thus they are part of a pattern that is commonly seen in many stomach conditions, "counterflow ascent of stomach *qi*." This can occur when an evil such as heat or cold, or the consumption of inappropriate types or amounts of food have damaged the *qi* dynamic of the stomach, causing the *qi* to move counterflow.

Just as patterns of the spleen present with signs of dampness and impaired upbearing, produced by the effects of *qi* vacuity or a replete evil impairing the natural tendencies of the spleen, so stomach patterns can easily present with conditions that counter its role in downbearing and its dislike of dryness.

The large intestine is adversely impacted by heat and improper diet. Intestinal humor depletion occurs after febrile disease or in the aged when lack of moisture due to insufficient blood and fluids leads to hard dry stools. Intestinal vacuity efflux desertion is longstanding diarrhea that saps the spleen *qi*, interfering with its ability to upbear. Intestinal welling abscess, understood biomedically as appendicitis, is said to result from damp–heat produced by stagnating food.

Large intestine cold–damp and large intestine damp–heat may both be caused by the ingestion of unclean foods, causing acute diarrhea. Large intestine cold–damp may also be a consequence of internal cold due to spleen or kidney *yang* vacuity. Large intestine damp–heat may also occur as a result of summer heat damp (**A**).

Pattern	Etiology	Clinical Signs May Include
Food stagnating in the stomach duct	Eating unclean food or excessive consumption of cold, sweet, or fatty food	Aversion to food, sour vomiting, belching, abdominal pain and distension, diarrhea containing food, yellow or white, slimy tongue fur and a slippery pulse
Stomach *qi* vacuity cold	Excessive consumption of cold, sweet, or fatty food or emotional disturbance leading to liver overwhelming the spleen	Stomach duct pain relieved by eating or warmth, lusterless facial complexion, aversion to cold, cold extremities, pale and large tongue, soggy pulse
Stomach heat	Exterior heat evil, eating excessive amounts of rich or hot and spicy foods, or liver fire invading the stomach	Quick digestion, constant hunger, stomach pain, vomiting, hard stools, gum disease, bad breath, red tongue with dry, yellow fur and a slippery pulse
Stomach *yin* vacuity	Warm heat scorching *yin* fluids or yin vacuity from other causes	Dry mouth and tongue, thirst, either no or voracious appetite, abdominal pain, dry retching, mirror tongue, a fine and rapid pulse
Counterflow stomach *qi*	Cold, heat, phlegm, foul turbidity, food stagnation, *qi* stagnation	Nausea, vomiting, belching, hiccough, with signs indicating cold, heat, phlegm, or food or *qi* stagnation
Intestinal humor depletion	Insufficient fluids and blood, due to postpartum blood vacuity, aging, taxation, or damage to fluids by disease	Hard, dry stools, difficult defecation, fatigue, and a weak pulse
Intestinal vacuity efflux desertion	Longstanding diarrhea reduces ability of the spleen's *yang qi* to uplift	Chronic diarrhea with either incontinence or rectal prolapse during defecation, and abdominal pain, fatigue, debility, aversion to cold, desire for warmth, and forceless and slow pulse
Large intestine cold–damp	Cold evil, cold or unclean foods, spleen or kidney *yang* vacuity	Intestinal rumbling, abdominal pain, clear and thin diarrhea, white, glossy tongue fur, and moderate pulse
Large intestine damp–heat	Summer heat damp, unclean food, or fatty, sweet, cold, raw foods	Abdominal pain, diarrhea with pus and blood, urgency to defecate, burning anus, foul stools, red tongue, slippery and rapid pulse

A Disease patterns of the stomach and intestines.

Disease Patterns
of the Liver and Gallbladder

Disease patterns associated with the liver and gallbladder emerge when the liver blood or *yin* becomes insufficient, or when the free flow of liver *qi* is impaired.

Vacuity of liver blood can arise due to chronic bleeding problems or from diseases that damage the ability of the spleen and lung to produce blood. Lack of liver blood affects the eyes, the sinews, and the reproductive system, leaving them unnourished and disturbing their function.

These patterns exemplify *yin* and *yang* relationships in a very distinct way. The liver's *qi* flows smoothly when it is unobstructed and when the liver's *yin* blood is sufficient to balance the *yang qi*. Since the liver is the only viscera that produces surplus *qi* (which is stored in the gallbladder as bile), its pathologies often involve disturbances of its *yang qi*, which lead it to move erratically. This can occur when the *yin* blood fails to balance the liver *yang qi*, or when the *qi* becomes depressed (trapped and obstructed) or stagnant. These disturbances can result in the erratic, often upwards movement of liver *qi*.

Binding depression of liver *qi* results when the smooth flow of liver *qi* is disturbed by strong emotions, a lack of the *yin* blood needed to allow it to flow smoothly, or by an evil such as damp–heat. Binding depression of liver *qi* is commonly encountered in clinical situations and can give rise to a wide variety of symptoms. Left uncorrected, binding depression of liver *qi* can give rise to upflaring of liver fire, which can be thought of as the smoldering heat of depressed liver *qi* bursting into flame and rising to disturb the upper part of the body.

The liver channel runs to the top of the head and connects to the eyes, and the gallbladder channel runs along the flanks and through the eyes and ear. When the *yang qi* of the liver is disturbed it typically ascends, causing headache, visual disturbance, dizziness, ringing in the ears, and other upper body symptoms. In severe cases, the disturbed liver *yang* can produce "internal wind," which produces tremor, alterations in consciousness, convulsions, and other wind-like symptoms. Stagnant or depressed liver *qi* moves "cross-counterflow" to disturb the spleen, causing diarrhea and other digestive disturbances associated with patterns such as liver overwhelming the spleen. Because of the close relationship of the liver blood and the liver channel to the genitals and reproductive system both insufficiency of liver blood and depressed liver *qi* can produce disturbances of the menstrual cycle and other aspects of reproductive function. In relation to biomedical disease, liver patterns are often present in depressive disorder, hypertension, epilepsy, irritable bowel syndrome, cerebral vascular accident, amenorrhea, dysmennorrhea, and tinnitus (**A**).

Pattern	Etiology	Clinical Signs May Include
Liver blood vacuity	Long-term illness, chronic bleeding disorders, including profuse menstruation	Dizziness, insomnia, blurred vision, frequent dreaming, muscle weakness, scant menses, irregular menses, pale tongue, and fine and forceless pulse
Binding depression of liver *qi*	Mental or emotional disturbance, *yin* blood insufficiency, or damp–heat	Depression, emotional lability, impatience, flank and rib-side pain, chest oppression, and string-like pulse
Liver gallbladder damp–heat	External damp–heat, or internal damp–heat produced by greasy food or alcohol	Jaundice, rib-side pain, abdominal fullness, nausea and vomiting, constipation or diarrhea, lack of appetite, yellow, slimy tongue fur and a rapid pulse
Upflaming of liver fire	Depressed liver *qi* transforming into fire, severe emotional disturbance, or damp–heat evil	Irritation, impatience, severe headache, red face, red eyes, sudden hearing problems, nosebleed, heavy menstrual flow, vomiting, dry stools, red tongue with yellow fur, and a rapid, forceful, string-like or slippery pulse
Ascendant hyperactivity of liver *yang*	Liver *yin* and liver *yang* imbalance produces upward movement of liver *yang*	Excitation, irritability, dizziness, headache, blurred vision, red eyes, tinnitus, insomnia, red tongue, and a fine string-like pulse
Liver wind stirring internally	Liver and kidney *yin* insufficient to balance liver *yang qi*, producing internal wind	Severe dizziness and headache, neck rigidity, numbness of limbs, tremor and spasm, aphasia, convulsion, red tongue with dry fur, and a fine string-like pulse

A Liver and gallbladder disease patterns.

**Disease Patterns
of the Kidney and Bladder**

The kidney has its home in the lower back and is the primary organ of the lower burner. The kidney supports all reproductive function. It is fundamental to the growth and development of the body and to the functioning of the viscera and bowels. The kidney stores essence, governs bone, engenders marrow, governs water, and absorbs *qi*. The kidney is connected to the brain, manifests in the hair, and opens at the ear.

The body relies on the kidney to directly support the production of *qi* and to indirectly support the function of all the organs and so the kidney is constantly taxed. Patterns of the kidney involve vacuity of *qi*, *yin*, *yang*, or essence. Diseases associated with the kidney involve insufficiency of the essence-marrow, deficient reproductive functions, and disorders of fluid metabolism. Because the other organs depend on the kidney *yin* and *yang* to support their functions, dual patterns involving both the kidney and the supported organ are common. Spleen and kidney *yang* vacuity, non-interaction of the heart and kidney, lung and kidney *yin* vacuity, and liver and kidney *yin* vacuity all describe patterns where kidney vacuity simultaneously affects a dependent organ or where that organ has overused the resources of the kidney.

Kidney *yin* has a critical role in counterbalancing the kidney *yang*. The kidney *yin* may become insufficient due to chronic illness damaging fluids, or damage to *yin* and fluids from aging,

emotional distress, or immoderate lifestyle. When this occurs, the kidney *yang* (life gate fire) has no substance to anchor it and its heat rises. The rising *yang* heat may produce low-grade fever, ringing in the ears, night sweating, and other signs of *yin* vacuity heat.

Kidney *yang* vacuity patterns can result from longstanding retention of water–damp causing *yang* damage, chronic illness, excessive sexual activity, constitutional weakness, and so on. The pattern manifests with lumbar soreness and weakness of the knees, the areas of the body specifically associated with the kidneys, and the pathway of the associated urinary bladder channel. Ringing in the ears, dizziness, and a bright, white facial color are all signs of the absence of sufficient *yang* to nourish and support the upper areas of the body. Other signs result from the absence of warming *yang* and include coldness of the body and limbs and disturbance of the kidney *yang*'s restraint of stools and urine.

Kidney *yang* is critical to the function of the spleen in transforming and transporting grain and water. Diarrhea with undigested food is a cardinal sign of combined insufficiency of spleen and kidney *yang*.

While the kidney is not typically associated with repletion patterns, its associated organ is the urinary bladder. The urinary bladder is often subject to repletion patterns involving damp–heat or damp turbidity, including strangury patterns. Strangury may present in many different ways, but painful urination is always the primary sign (**A**).

Pattern	Etiology	Clinical Signs May Include
Kidney *yin* vacuity	Chronic illness damaging fluids, aging, damage to fluids by febrile disease, affect damage, immoderate sexual activity	Sore and weak lower back and knees, dizziness, tinnitus, emaciated body, seminal emission, five-center heat, low-grade fever, night sweats, malar flush, dry mouth, dry throat, red tongue with scant fur, fine and rapid pulse
Lung and kidney *yin* vacuity	Chronic illness damaging fluids, damage to lung and fluids by febrile disease, affect damage, immoderate sexual activity	Kidney *yin* vacuity signs as seen above with a hoarse voice, and a dry cough with no, little or blood-streaked phlegm
Kidney *yang* vacuity	Chronic illness, constitutional weakness, immoderate sexual activity, retained water–damp damaging *yang*, consumption of raw and cold foods	Sore and weak lower back and knees, dizziness, tinnitus, bright, white face color, fatigue and weakness, drowsiness, cold body and limbs, impotence, clear urine and watery stools, pale, enlarged tongue, moist, white tongue fur, a slow and weak pulse
Insufficiency of kidney essence	Seen in children or adults where congenital essence is insufficient, or where chronic illness has damaged essence	In children: delayed development, diminished intelligence, weakness, or impaired development of bones; in adults: premature senescence, white hair or hair loss, sore and weak lower back and knees, dizziness and tinnitus
Insecurity of kidney *qi*	Insufficient kidney *qi* due to constitutional insufficiency, debilitation by aging, poor nutrition, chronic illness, or immoderate sexual activity	Sore and weak lower back and knees, dizziness, tinnitus, seminal emission, premature ejaculation, frequent, clear copious urination with dribbling, pale tongue, white tongue fur with a deep and fine pulse, spotting and threatened miscarriage during pregnancy
Non-interaction of the heart and kidney	Kidney *yin* vacuity leading to insufficient heart *yin* and hyperactivity of heart fire	Sore and weak lower back and knees, dizziness, tinnitus, seminal emission, emaciation, five-center heat, palpitations, insomnia, low fever, night sweats, irritation, malar flush, red tongue, yellow tongue fur, a fine and rapid pulse

A Kidney and bladder disease patterns.

Patterns and Diseases: Understanding and Integrating TCM Pattern Diagnosis

As discussed earlier, the idea of "disease" is important in Chinese medicine (**A**). Traditionally identified diseases in Chinese medicine include a wide range of entities. There are the biomedically identified disease entities such as the common cold, diphtheria, mumps, malaria, measles, eczema, and asthma that are clearly recognizable between medical traditions. Parasitic infestations such as pinworm, tapeworm, and roundworm are also mutually recognizable. Then there are distinctive Chinese medicine disease concepts such as strangury, chest impediment, suspended rheum, lung taxation, goose palm wind. Many of these capture biomedical disease entities or processes or intersect with them. "Sudden turmoil" can refer specifically to cholera. "Leg *qi*" can express the idea of beriberi, vitamin B12 deficiency. Finally, there are the diseases that, from a biomedical point of view, would be considered technically as symptoms, such as cough, headache, low back pain, menstrual pain, constipation, and diarrhea. In fact, a standard list of Chinese disease conditions would seem, at least in part, like a list of presenting complaints or symptoms.

That all of these diseases (*bing* 病) can be evaluated and managed through the lens of a "disease pattern" (*bing zheng* 病证) is, as discussed earlier, a distinctive feature of Chinese medicine (**B**). Intriguingly it is this aspect of Chinese medicine that allows it to be a good fit in settings where clinical co-management or integrative medicine is a goal. Just as the traditionally identified disease entities of Chinese medicine are evaluated and managed through the lens of pattern identification, so too are biomedically defined diseases (**C**).

Since the 1950s, TCM has been functioning in China as a parallel medical model, accepted, funded, and supported in its research, clinical, and educational endeavors by the state. Part of this support included initiatives such as the Integration of Chinese and Western Medicine (*Zhong Xi Yi Jie He*), a research initiative to develop approaches to integrating Chinese and Western medicine. In addition, TCM physicians were treating patients with clearly identified biomedical diseases and finding that the application of pattern identification using the lens of TCM was entirely appropriate to the management of these conditions. Over the years, their work has generated a substantial literature on pattern identification in relation to biomedical disease entities.

From this perspective, pattern diagnosis is critical in the successful integration of Chinese medicine into biomedical environments, since the pattern identification paradigm evaluates pathophysiology in individualized ways regardless of the disease name applied. The challenge is addressing the comparatively reductionist model of the biomedical approach to disease, which typically posits one model of etiology, as it confronts the notion born of pattern diagnosis that one disease has many treatments and one treatment has many diseases.

A Selected TCM disease terms.

Abdominal pain	Impediment
Amenorrhea	Impotence
Asthma	Insomnia
Common cold	Jaundice
Constipation	Lateral costal pain
Cough	Lower back pain
Diarrhea	Painful menses
Dizziness and vertigo	Palpitations
Dribbling urinary block	Scrofula
Drum distension	Sprain
Dysentery	Stomach pain
Eczema	Strangury
Edema	Uterine bleeding
Epilepsy	Vomiting
Goitre	Wasting and thirsting
Headache	Whooping cough
Hiccough	Windstroke

Painful menses
Cold damp coagulation
Liver *qi* stagnation
Descent of damp–heat
Yang vacuity internal cold
Liver kidney vacuity
Qi and blood vacuity

Strangury
Stone strangury
Qi strangury
Blood strangury
Unctuous strangury
Taxation strangury

B Examples of TCM diseases and associated patterns.

Aplastic anemia
Qi and blood vacuity
Spleen and kidney insufficiency
Liver and heart blood vacuity

Coronary heart disease
Qi stagnation and blood stasis of the heart
Qi and *yin* vacuity
Yang qi vacuity
Yang qi collapse
Chest impediment

Influenza
Wind–cold
Wind–heat
Summer heat damp
Replete lung heat
Damp–heat obstructing the middle *jiao*

C Examples of biomedical diseases and associated patterns.

Principles and Methods of Treatment

While later chapters will discuss different techniques of treatment in detail, the linkage between diagnosis and approaches to treatment rests on the concepts of treatment principles and methods. The process of diagnosis leads to the determination of the disease pattern, which is the basis for identifying the correct principle and method of treatment. A treatment principle expresses the broad therapeutic context for the treatment, a philosophy of treatment designed to address the needs of the specific patient. Should we address fundamental problems with the patient's constitution that are causing the disease pattern to occur? If we do, this is to treat the "root" of the disease. However, not all patients like their suffering to remain unaddressed while we correct the root. Perhaps we should then treat the presenting symptoms, the "tip," and reduce the patient's discomfort.

Is it best to expel evils quickly or should the patient's correct *qi* be strengthened first? Should this be done simultaneously according to the principle of "dispelling evil and supporting right?" While beyond the scope of this text these considerations revolve around the state of the correct *qi* versus the evil. After all, if the patient has dampness in the spleen and lower burner it would be good to disperse dampness, but the failure of fluid metabolism that has produced dampness accumulation has resulted in some *yin* damage in various organs.

Treatment methods refers to a collection of methods used to treat the disease pattern such as dispelling evils: clearing heat or moistening dryness; dispersing accumulations of pathologic products: transforming phlegm or quickening blood to dispel stasis; supplementing vacuity: supplement *qi*, nourish *yin* (**A**, **B**). At its heart, Chinese medicine is an allopathic system of medicine in that it uses treatment methods that oppose and counter the pathology. Heat is cleared with cold agents, vacuity is supplemented, that which has accumulated is dispersed, and so on.

The determination of the treatment method is fundamental to creating a treatment plan. All diagnoses propose a pathological process to be corrected by a treatment method. The concept of a method of treatment is applied to all modalities. In the chapters on Acupuncture and Traditional Chinese Pharmacotherapy we shall see how this applies to the treatment of *John*, *Alice*, and *Jeremy*. The formal progression from diagnosis, to disease pattern, to treatment principle, to method of treatment is often implicit in the therapeutic choices made by the clinician. "Distinguishing patterns of disharmony [disease pattern] takes the physician just so close to a particular disharmony; the attempt is completed in treatment—in particular combinations of herbs and/or acupuncture points. In fact, it could be said that any pattern of disharmony [disease pattern] is actually defined by the treatment prescribed for its rebalancing" (Kaptchuk 2000, p. 253).

A Eight methods of treatment. The eight methods of treatment originally proposed by *Cheng Zhong Ling* was very concise.

| Sweating |
| Clearing |
| Ejection |
| Precipitation |
| Harmonization |
| Warming |
| Supplementation |
| Dispersion |

Method	Purpose
Resolving the exterior	Eliminating an evil from the surface of the body
Clearing	Clearing heat
Ejection	Inducing vomiting to eliminate congested food or phlegm
Precipitation	Freeing the stool
Harmonization	Restoring balance between organs, substances, and areas of the body
Warming	Treating cold with warmth
Supplementation	Nourishing and invigorating the *qi*, blood, *yin*, and *yang*
Abductive dispersion and transforming accumulation	Gradually removing accumulations of pathological substances
Expelling worms	Killing and eliminating worms
Dispelling dampness	Removing dampness evil from the body
Moistening dryness	Restoring healthy moisture
Rectifying *qi*	Correcting abnormal movement of *qi* (stagnation and counterflow)
Rectifying blood	Correcting abnormal movement of blood (stasis and bleeding)
Dispelling phlegm	Removing phlegm
Quieting spirit	Calming the mind
Dispelling wind	Eliminating both internal and external wind
Orifice opening	Restoring normal consciousness
Securing astriction	Preventing leakage of vital substances

B Contemporary methods of treatment. The outline of methods of treatment shown here is not exhaustive and does not include specific subcategories.

→ *Case Study John:*
   69-year-old Male with
   Chronic Low Back and
   Knee Pain for 12 Years

John presents with chronic low back and knee pain that developed gradually with no initial injury. The pain is a constant, low-level, fixed ache that is worse with exertion and fatigue and better with warmth and rest. It begins at the level of the second lumbar vertebrae and spreads over the left side of the back. There is one spot about 4 in (10 cm) lateral to the spine, at the level of L4 that is particularly tender to palpation. The knee pain is in the anterior medial aspect of both knees. The knees are cold to the touch. *John* is overweight and has been diagnosed with diabetes, for which he takes insulin. He has difficulty controlling his glucose levels, and due to the diabetes, there is numbness in the toes and he gets toe blisters that take months to heal. *John*'s face is pale and he has large, puffy, white bags under his eyes. His pulse is 62 bpm, deep and slippery. The tongue is swollen and pale with toothmarks and a thick, white fur.

John has been diagnosed with kidney *yang* vacuity and dampness, causing low back and knee pain. The kidneys are the root of *yin* and *yang* in the body. The home of the kidneys is the lower back, therefore, disharmony of the kidneys often manifests as low back pain. The fact that there is no history of trauma or any direct cause of the back pain helps us to understand this pain as being a result of the normal waning of the kidneys that occurs as we age. We know that this is a *yang* vacuity because of the cold signs, signs of a relative *yin* repletion. These signs include the pain improving with warmth and that the knees are cold to the touch. The puffy bags under the eyes, pale face, and puffy tongue with thick, white fur also point to the kidney, to cold, and to damp. Because the *yang* is depleted, the kidney and spleen are unable to warm the fluids and separate the clear from the turbid, thus damp accumulates and causes *John* to be overweight, which exacerbates his back pain. Scallops on the tongue always refer to spleen *qi* or *yang* vacuity. The deep pulse is indicative of a deeper internal condition and the slippery quality of the pulse is indicative of damp.

Based on the diagnosis (**A**), our treatment method is to warm and invigorate kidney *yang*, transform damp and stop pain. We will see the application of these treatment methods when we look at this case again in the Acupuncture and Traditional Chinese Pharmacotherapy chapters.

➡ **Case Study**

Eight-principles Diagnosis: Internal, Cold, Mixed Vacuity, and Repletion		
Internal/External	Hot/Cold	Vacuity/Repletion
Internal	Cold	Mixed/primarily vacuity
Chronic condition (12 years)	Pain is better with warmth	Vacuity:
No history of trauma or external invasion	Knees are cold to the touch	Pain worse with exertion and fatigue, better with rest
Back and knees home of the kidney	Pale face	Pain is an ache, not acute
Large, puffy, white bags under the eyes	Large, puffy, white bags under the eyes	Chronic, non-healing sores
Deep pulse	Pale tongue	Pale face
		Deep pulse
		Pale tongue with toothmarks
		Repletion = presence of damp
		Overweight
		Numbness of toes
		Large, puffy, white bags under the eyes
		Slippery pulse
		Thick, white tongue fur

Qi, Blood and Body Fluids Diagnosis: *Qi* Stagnation, Blood Stasis and Damp
Although not included as a part of *John's* initial diagnosis, the presence of pain indicates that the flow of *qi* and/or blood is disturbed, resulting in stagnation

Qi stagnation:	Constant, low-level achy pain
Blood stasis: blood stasis is in part as a result of the cold	Fixed location, specific pinpoint spot lateral to the spine
Disruption of body fluids/damp:	Overweight, numbness of toes, large, puffy, white bags under the eyes, slippery pulse, thick, white tongue fur
Qi vacuity:	Pain worse with exertion and fatigue, better with rest, pale face, pale tongue

Viscera and Bowel (*Zang Fu*) Diagnosis: Spleen and Kidney *Yang* Vacuity

Kidney: back and knee pain with no history of trauma; insidious onset, large, puffy, white bags under the eyes, deep pulse

Spleen: scalloped tongue, pale face/tongue, puffy tongue, presence of damp is associated with a spleen *qi* vacuity

A Analysis of signs and symptoms for Case Study *John*.

→ *Case Study Alice:*
23-year-old Female with Severe
Dysmenorrhea for Eight Years

Alice began menstruating at age 13 and her cycle is very consistent. Her menses arrive every 29 days and last for 5 days. The blood is dark red with large purple-red clots. Bleeding is heavy for the first 3 days. Every month, on day 27, she gets a very bad headache, located on her temples, that lasts for 4 days. The first 2 days of menstruation are extremely painful. She takes painkillers but still experiences pain. About 1 week prior to menstruation, she experiences breast tenderness, a feeling of tightness in her chest, and extremely labile emotions. Her bowels and urine are normal and she denies any other complaints. The tongue is slightly purple and has stasis macules on the sides with a normal, thin, white fur. The pulse is 72 bpm, string-like, rough, and forceful.

Based on her presentation, *Alice* is diagnosed with *qi* and blood stagnation in the liver and gallbladder channels causing menstrual pain (**A**). The free flow of *qi* and blood is dependent upon smooth coursing of the liver. As a woman goes through her monthly cycle, there are two occasions when the *qi* is most likely to stagnate, at ovulation and prior to or during menstrua-

tion. *Qi* stagnation at ovulation may present with lower abdominal pain and irritability. *Qi* stagnation prior to menstruation will present as breast tenderness, tightness in the chest and emotionality, typical pre-menstrual signs. If only the *qi* is depressed, then the period will arrive and although there may be slight cramping, in general the woman will feel better. If the blood is also stagnant, then there will be severe cramping, clotted, dark menstrual blood, and often headaches. Because of the location of *Alice*'s headaches, on the sides of the head, we know that the gallbladder channel is also involved in her presentation.

This is a very common diagnosis for women suffering from menstrual pain. One of the things that must be considered in treating a patient like *Alice* is that treatment will change depending upon where she is in her menstrual cycle. The focus remains on moving the *qi* and blood to stop pain, but this is mediated by whether she is about to begin menstruating or has just completed menstruating. After menstruation the treatment principle is on building blood while gently moving *qi*. After ovulation, but prior to the beginning of symptoms, treatment will focus more on moving *qi* and blood. Just prior to menstruation, the primary focus is on moving blood.

→ Case Study

Eight-principles Diagnosis: Internal, Neither Hot nor Cold, Replete		
Internal/External	Hot/Cold	Vacuity/Repletion
Internal	Neither	Repletion
Chronic condition (8 years' duration) No exterior signs	*Alice* does not present with any clear heat or cold signs; with her diagnosis, there is probably more of a tendency to heat	Acute pain Purple tongue with stasis macules Normal bowels and urine Rough, string-like, and forceful pulse Absence of vacuity signs

Qi, Blood and Body Fluids Diagnosis: *Qi* Stagnation and Blood Stasis	
Qi stagnation:	Breast tenderness, tightness in the chest, labile emotions, string-like pulse
Blood stasis:	Severe pain, dark, red blood with large clots, heavy bleeding, rough pulse, slightly purple tongue with stasis macules

Viscera and Bowel (*Zang Fu*) Diagnosis: Liver *Qi* Stagnation and Blood Stasis	
Liver:	Pain associated with menstruation (the liver is responsible for the free flow of the menses), breast tenderness, tightness in the chest, labile emotions, normal bowels and urine, normal tongue fur, string-like pulse
Gallbladder:	Internally/externally paired organ with the liver; headache on the sides of the head/temples

A Analysis of signs and symptoms for Case Study *Alice*.

→ *Case Study Jeremy:*
45-year-old Male
with an Acute Cold

Jeremy had been receiving acupuncture for treatment of fatigue due to overwork. On this visit he arrived with an acute cold. His symptoms included a sore throat, a sensation of heat that easily transformed into cold after sweating. His nose was stuffy, but it was difficult to expel any phlegm. When there was visible phlegm, it was slightly yellow. His body was sore, his eyes red, and he was fatigued. His tongue had not changed from its previous presentation, which was slightly pale, swollen, and toothmarked, but his pulse was slightly rapid (82 bpm) and floating at the lung position.

Jeremy's original diagnosis was spleen *qi* vacuity causing fatigue. Individuals with *qi* vacuity are often susceptible to catching frequent colds. Unfortunately, when this occurs, the fight between the right and evil may exacerbate the pre-existing *qi* vacuity, thus it is important to give the patient prompt and correct treatment in order to expel the evil and support the right. If the evil is not expelled, the acute signs of common cold may resolve, however there may be lingering cough or the patient may get sick again shortly afterwards, indicating that the original evil has lodged in the body. Over time, the evil may cause further problems or, may eventually emerge as a much more serious condition.

When a pre-existing patient presents with an acute condition, the diagnosis may be temporarily changed to address the presenting condition. However, the initial diagnosis should not be ignored or forgotten when giving treatment as it may be affected by the new condition. In this instance, we changed our diagnosis to an external invasion of wind–heat causing common cold. We know that this is an exterior condition because of the acute nature accompanied by the floating pulse, the lack of change in the tongue image, and the sensation of heat accompanied by cold, indicating the presence of a battle between the right and evil. The differentiation of wind–heat from wind–cold is made clear by the presence of the sore throat, the red eyes, the yellow phlegm that was difficult to expel, and the rapid pulse. Sweat, although commonly viewed as an important sign to differentiate wind–heat from wind–cold in fact does not do so. There are times, when, in an exterior wind–cold pattern a patient may present with sweating. In *Jeremy*'s case, the other heat signs, accompanied by the sweating are sufficient to diagnose wind–heat rather than wind–cold (**A**). At this visit we must resolve the exterior by promoting sweat and expel the wind–heat from the exterior. Because our patient has a pre-existing *qi* vacuity, we will also boost the *qi* slightly to aid the right *qi* in expelling the evil.

→ **Case Study**

Eight-principles Diagnosis: External and Internal, Hot, Mixed Replete and Vacuous		
Internal/External	Hot/Cold	Vacuity/Repletion
External (with pre-existing internal condition)	Hot	Repletion (with pre-existing vacuity)
Acute onset	Sore throat	The presence of an external evil is inherently a replete condition; the evil is replete, but the body is vacuous
Sensations of heat and cold	Yellow phlegm	
No change to tongue	Red eyes	
Floating pulse	Slightly rapid pulse	

Six-excesses Diagnosis: Wind–Heat	
Wind:	Acute onset, stuffy nose, floating pulse, alternating heat and cold
Heat:	Sore throat, yellow phlegm, red eyes, rapid pulse

Four-aspects Diagnosis: Defense *(Wei)* Aspect	
In this instance, the use of four-aspects diagnosis is more appropriate than six-channels diagnosis because this is a condition where heat has invaded	
Defense aspect	Acute onset, sensations of heat and cold, floating pulse, slightly rapid pulse, sore throat, yellow phlegm, red eyes

A Analysis of signs and symptoms for Case Study *Jeremy;* in this case, analysis is only of the acute condition.

4

Acupuncture

Marnae C. Ergil

Introduction

Acupuncture and moxibustion can be used together or independent of each other. They are so closely associated that the term for this therapy is *zhen jiu* 针灸, meaning "needle moxibustion." In fact, moxibustion appears to have been the form of therapy first used on the channels to treat problems of the body. Both techniques provide stimulus to points that lie along channel pathways or other appropriate sites.

Acupuncture 针法

The therapeutic goal of acupuncture is to regulate the *qi*. *Qi* and blood flow through the body, its organs, and the channel pathways. When they flow freely, the body is healthy. When some cause, an evil, an emotion, trauma, and so on, disrupts the flow of *qi*, illness or pain can result. Acupuncture may be used to help the body to remove the evil, to direct *qi* to where it is insufficient, to move obstructions and allow *qi* to flow, or to boost the functions of organs to produce more *qi* or blood.

The *Spiritual Pivot (Ling Shu)* part of *The Yellow Emperor's Classic of Medicine (Huang Di Nei Jing)* describes nine needles for use in acupuncture (**A**). With the exception of one that appears to have had a specifically surgical application, the needles are still in use, either in original or adapted form.

Today, acupuncture is performed with a wide variety of tools and methods, but the filiform needle is the most common, and it can vary significantly in terms of structure, diameter, and length (**B**).

The average needle is 30–50 mm long and 0.20–0.30 mm in diameter, with a handle of approximately 30 mm. The distinctive part of the needle is the tip, which is round and moderately sharp, much like the tip of a pine needle. The acupuncture needle is solid and gently tapered; it does not have the open lumen or the cutting edge of the hypodermic needle. Its diameter ranges from 0.18 to 0.38 mm. The most typical is 0.25 mm.

The aim of the acupuncturist is to obtain *qi* (*de qi* 得气) at the site of insertion. The practitioner seeks either an objective or subjective indication that the *qi* has arrived. The arrival of *qi* may be experienced by the practitioner as sensations felt by the hands as the needle is manipulated or through observation of color changes or of skin appearance at the site of insertion. The sensation of the arrival of *qi* is often felt by the practitioner as a gentle grasping of the needle at the site, as if one is fishing, and one's line has suddenly been seized by the fish. The patient senses the arrival of *qi* as a sensation of itching, numbness, soreness, or a swollen feeling, or they might experience local temperature changes or an "electrical" sensation.

A The nine needles of the *Nei Jing.* *The Yellow Emperor's Classic of Medicine* described nine needles. From left to right: the arrow head, used for superficial skin puncture and blood-letting, the round and the blunt needles were used to press and stimulate channels and sinews without puncturing skin, the sharp edged needle was used to let blood and to lance boils, and the sword needle was used to open abscesses. The next four vary in thickness and length. These are the round and sharp needle, the filiform needle, the long needle, and the large needle. Longer needles are used for deeper insertion, thicker needles are used for stronger techniques or in methods where the needle is heated.

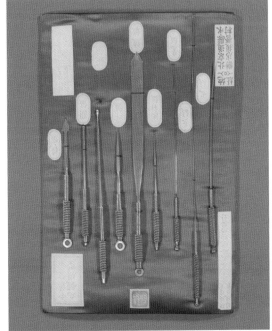

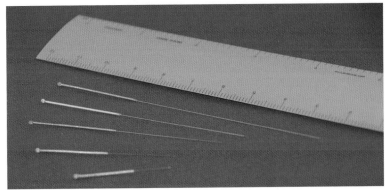

B Images of modern needles. Today, needles of various length and diameter are used. The average needle is 30–50 mm long and 0.20–0.30 mm in diameter. Longer needles are used in areas where there is more flesh (for example, the hip) or to connect two points by threading.

When a site for insertion has been determined, the needle is rapidly inserted and then adjusted to an appropriate depth. Many considerations will alter the angle and depth of insertion, methods of manipulation, and the length of retention. A 12th-century text, *Ode of the Subtleties of Flow*, states, "Insert the needle with noble speed then proceed (to the point) slowly, withdraw the needle with noble slowness as haste will cause injury" (Shanghai College of Traditional Chinese Medicine 1981).

Throughout this text, we will refer to the sites of needle insertion or stimulation as "points," however, it is important to realize that this is not, in fact, the best translation of the Chinese term. The Chinese term, *xue* 穴 is literally translated as cave or hole, thus reflecting the idea that these sites are found in depressions or holes located between bones, tendons, and so on. The concept of a hole into which the finger will naturally fall when palpating the body is not expressed by the term point, which conveys an imaginary place in space rather than a tangible location.

Once a site has been needled, and *qi* obtained, the practitioner may manipulate the needle to achieve a specific therapeutic effect. Methods of manipulation range from simply inserting the needle and leaving it, to using techniques that involve slow or rapid insertion, to deeper or shallower insertions. The needle may be withdrawn immediately after *qi* arrives, may be retained for 20–30 minutes or longer, or a very short fine needle (known as an intradermal) may be retained for several days. In all cases, the goal of the clinician is to influence the flow of *qi* (**A**, **B**, **C**).

Practitioners use different methods to select acupuncture points for a particular patient or condition. Points may be chosen on the basis of the trajectory of the channel on which they lie, on the basis of membership in a particular traditional point category, or through an empirical understanding of what points work best for a given condition, based on the experience of generations of practitioners. Points may also be selected based on the patient's sensitivity to palpation (pain, tenderness, comfort) or changes in texture that are perceived by the practitioner. Each of these methods gives the practitioner information about a particular point and should be considered when creating a treatment plan.

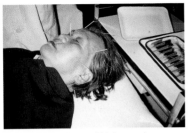

A Acupuncture in use. This image shows acupuncture being practiced in a large hospital in China. The patient is being treated for facial pain (© Marnae Ergil).

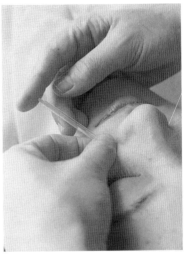

B Although not typically used in China the guide tube was developed in Japan and has become popular in the West.

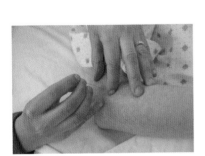

C An example of free hand needling that is typical of Chinese needle insertion methods.

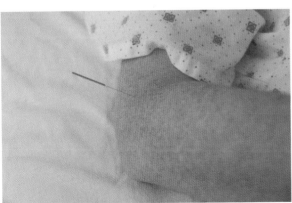

D An acupuncture needle inserted at the point LI-11, *qu chi*, Pool at the Bend.

Moxibustion (*Jiu Fa* 灸法)

Moxibustion (*jiu fa* 灸法) (**A**) refers to the burning of dried, powdered leaves of *ai ye* (Artemesia vulgaris/mugwort), either on or close to the skin, to affect the flow of *qi* in the channel. Artemesia is acrid and bitter and it warms and enters the channels. References to moxa appear in very early materials, including the Ma Wang tomb texts (Unschuld 1985).

Moxibustion can be applied to the body in many ways. Direct moxa, for example, involves burning a small amount of moxa (the size of a grain of rice), directly on the skin. The moxa can be allowed to burn directly to the skin, causing a blister or a scar, or it can be removed before it has burnt down to the skin. Indirect moxibustion involves putting a substance between the moxa and the patient's skin (**A**). This gives the practitioner greater control over the amount of heat, and helps to protect the patient from burns. Popular substances include ginger slices, garlic slices, and salt.

During pole moxa (**A** inset), a cigar-shaped roll of moxa wrapped in paper is used to gently warm an area without touching the skin. This is a very safe method of moxibustion that can be taught to patients for self-application. The warm needle method is accomplished by inserting an acupuncture needle and then placing moxa on its handle. After the moxa is ignited, it burns slowly, giving a gentle sensation of warmth to the acupuncture point and to the channel.

Any of these techniques might be used to stimulate acupuncture points, especially when warming is appropriate. For example, if a patient is suffering pain in the joints that is worse in cold, damp weather, applying moxa either directly or indirectly to the affected areas will help to relieve the pain by warming the area and thus allowing the *qi* to flow smoothly.

Cupping and Bleeding

Two additional methods that are very important to the practice of Chinese medicine, and used by most acupuncturists, are cupping and bleeding.

Cupping (**B**) involves inducing a vacuum in a small glass or bamboo cup and applying it to the skin. Cupping is often used to drain or remove cold and damp evils from the body or to assist blood circulation. For example, if a patient arrives with a common cold accompanied by cough and sore muscles of the upper back, cupping might be applied to the upper back to move the *qi* and dispel the evil.

Bleeding is done to drain a channel or to remove heat from the body. This method expresses small amounts of blood, from a drop to a few centiliters. Bleeding is commonly used on points that are located on the tips of the fingers or toes. In the example above, if the cold was accompanied by a severe sore throat, then a point located on the thumb and associated with the lung might be bled to remove heat from the lung and benefit the throat.

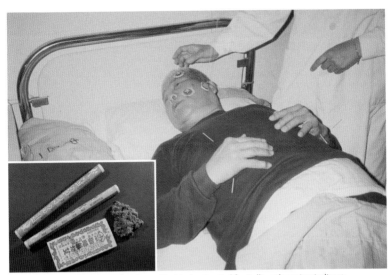

A Moxibustion. This image shows a patient being treated for Bell's palsy using indirect moxibustion and needles. The inset shows different forms of moxa (© Marnae Ergil).

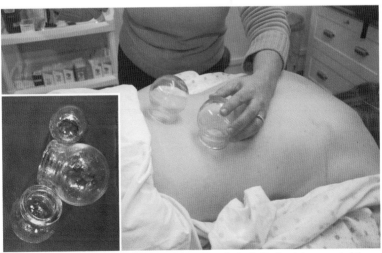

B Cupping. This image shows a patient being cupped on the back. The inset shows a set of three differently sized glass cups.

Channel and Network Theory
(Jing Luo Xue 经络学)

Although in the modern practice of acupuncture, much emphasis is placed on the acupuncture points and point functions, historically the channels and the use of channels for therapeutic purposes preceded the development of specific sites on the channels. While *The Yellow Emperor's Classic of Medicine* and the *Classic of Difficulties* are quite specific about points, their locations and even some of the point categories, early texts, in particular the texts removed from the Ma Wang tombs, discuss only the channels and the use of moxa or heated stones on the channels with no reference to points.

It is only by having a thorough understanding of all of the various types of channels, their functions and their interconnections, that an acupuncturist can understand how to select the correct points for treatment. Many of the actions of individual points are determined by the intricate connections made by the channels and their pathways. If these connections are not understood, then the actions of the points become statements that are no longer connected to their theoretical basis but must simply be accepted. Understanding the channels, their functions, and their pathways allows the practitioner to understand point selection and treatment strategies.

The theory of the channels and networks is the guiding principle of acupuncture practice. The five major functions of the channel system are transportation, regulation, protection and diagnosis, therapeutic and integration (**A**). The channels and networks (*jing luo* 经络) are the pathways that carry *qi* (气), blood (*xue* 血), and body fluids (*jin ye* 津液) throughout the body. They are the paths of communication between all parts of the body. When *qi* and blood flow through the channels smoothly, the body is properly nourished and healthy. The organs (*zang fu* 脏腑), the skin and body hair (*pi mao* 皮毛), the sinews (*jin* 筋) and flesh (*rou* 肉), the bones (*gu* 骨), and all other tissues rely on the free flow of *qi* and blood through the channels. Ultimately, it is the channels and networks that create a unified body where all parts are interacting and interdependent.

There are two types of major pathways in the body. These are the channels (*jing* 经) and the networks (*luo* 络). The channels are, for the most part, bilateral and symmetrical. They travel vertically through the body and are relatively deep within the body. The networks connect interiorly/exteriorly related organs and they connect channels. They are also bilateral and symmetrical, but they travel in all directions and are relatively superficial. A more detailed discussion of each of these pathways is found later in the chapter, beginning with the various types of channel pathways and then moving to the network pathways.

Functions	Clinical Actions
Transportation	Provides pathways for the circulation of *qi* and blood
	Carries *qi* and blood throughout the body
	Provides *qi* and blood to the organs and tissues for nourishment and moistening
Regulation	Maintains the flow of *qi* and blood through the pathways
	Maintains the balance of *yin* and *yang* to regulate the functions of the organs
Protection and diagnosis	Protects against the invasion of evils into the body
	Reflects signs and symptoms of disease:
	– observable: color change, rashes and so on
	– palpable: changes in resistance, bumps, lumps etc.
	– subjective: pain, numbness etc., along a pathway
Therapeutic	Acupuncture and Chinese herbal medicine both use the channel and network system therapeutically:
	– Acupuncture: examines the signs and symptoms of disease reflected in the channel
	– Acupuncture: treatment is based on the selection of points along the channels that have a direct impact on the affected organ systems
	– Herbal therapeutics: every medicinal substance enters one or more of the channels, and so might be selected for use to treat the organ system(s) associated with these channels
Integration	Connects the viscera and bowels with each other and with the limbs and body surface
	Connects the internal and external parts of the body, including the five sense organs, tissues, bone, sinew, muscle, and orifices into a unified organism that is viewed and treated as a whole body surface

A Five major functions of the channel and network system. These functions inform clinical practice. For example, when an evil invades the exterior of the body, it first enters the skin and body hair. If not dispelled, it may enter the channels or the network vessels, eventually even reaching the internal organs. Understanding the path that an evil may take, helps the clinician to assess where the evil is and how to treat it. The channels also may reflect signs and symptoms of internal conditions, manifesting signs such as pain, numbness, rashes, and so on. By observing these changes, their nature and location, and by palpating the channels, the clinician can choose appropriate points to treat the condition.

The Channels

There are generally considered to be two major groups of channels. The first are the 12 regular channels (*shi er jing luo* 十二经络). These all have acupuncture points through which the *qi* of the body can be accessed. The 12 regular channels have several associated channels. These are the 12 sinew channels, 12 cutaneous regions, and 12 divergent channels. Each of these channel groups will be discussed below (also see p. 185 for an overview of the channel and network system).

The second group of channels is the eight extraordinary vessels (*qi heng ba mai* 奇横八脉). Two of the eight extraordinary vessels, the controlling vessel (*ren mai* 任脉) and the governing vessel (*du mai* 督脉), have points through which the *qi* of the body can be accessed. Because there are no directly related organs for these two channels, the points on them have an effect on the area of the body or on specific organs within the area of the body covered by the channel pathway. The other six extraordinary vessels, as well as the controlling and governing vessels, all share points located on the 12 regular channels.

The 12 Regular Channels

Distribution and Nomenclature
There are six *yang* and six *yin* channels, which are distributed bilaterally on the body. The *yin* channels run along the inner surface of the limbs (three on the arms and three on the legs) and across the chest and abdomen. Each *yin* channel is associated with a viscera. The *yang* channels run along the outer surfaces of the limbs (three on the arms and three on the legs) and along the buttocks and back (with the exception of the stomach channel). Each *yang* channel is associated with a bowel.

The channels are further divided based on their relative location on the anterior, midline, or posterior aspect of the limbs. The *yin* channels include the greater *yin* (*tai yin*) (lung and spleen), located on the anterior, medial aspect of the limbs, the lesser *yin* (*shao yin*) (heart and kidney), located on the posterior, medial aspect of the limbs and the reverting *yin* (*jue yin*) (pericardium and liver), located on the midline of the medial aspect of the limbs. The *yang* channels include the *yang* brightness (*yang ming*) (stomach and large intestine), located on the anterior lateral aspect of the limbs, the greater *yang* (*tai yang*) (urinary bladder and small intestine), located on the posterior lateral aspect of the limbs, and the lesser *yang* (*shao yang*) (gallbladder and triple burner), located on the midline of the lateral aspect of the limbs (**A**).

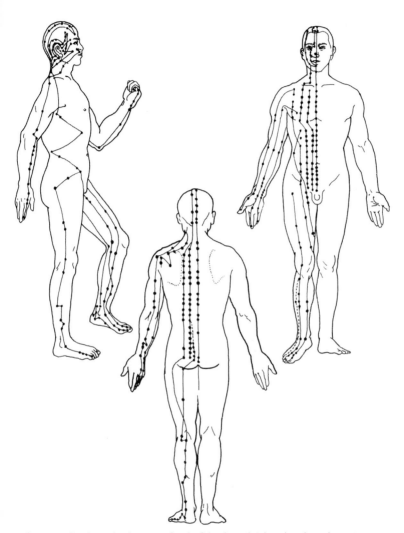

A The 12 regular channels. The name of each of the channels is based on three elements: whether the channel is distributed along the upper limbs (the hand channels) or the lower limbs (the foot channels), the *yin/yang* classification of the channel, and the organ with which the channel is associated. Thus, the channel associated with the lung is the hand greater *yin* lung channel *(shou tai yin fei jing)*.

Twelve Major Channel Relationships

Each of the six *yin* channels is paired with its interiorly/exteriorly related *yang* channel. This pairing expresses an important physiological connection between the associated viscera and bowel and an anatomical relationship between the channels. In addition, each hand channel is associated with a foot channel based on its *yin/yang* classification and location.

These two ways of pairing the channels are expressed in three circuits of the flow of *qi* through the 12 primary channels. The flow of *qi* in each circuit begins in a *yin* channel on the chest and passes to the interiorly/exteriorly related *yang* channel at the hand. It then ascends along the *yang* channel to the face where it passes into the hand *yang* channels' paired foot *yang* channel. It then descends to the foot where it passes to the interiorly/exteriorly related *yin* channel and ascends back to the chest to begin a new circuit. So, the *qi* passes from the chest to the hand, to the face, to the foot and back to the chest three times before it completes its circuit of the 12 channels (**A**).

Circulation of Qi and Blood through the Channels

As we can also see from **A**, the circulation of *qi* and blood through the body is an endless process, from one channel to the next. Before returning to the beginning of the circuit, the *qi* and blood pass through the body in three loops. Over the course of one 24-hour period, the *qi* and blood in the channels pass through the entire body in the following sequence:

LU → LI → ST → SP → HT → SI → BL → KI → PC → TB → GB → LR.

Each set of four channels creates one loop that passes from the abdomen to the hand, from the hand to the head, from the head to the foot, and then from the foot back to the abdomen, thus traversing a complete circuit through the body, covering both the *yin* (anterior) and *yang* (posterior) aspects of the body.

Diurnal Flow of Qi Through the Channels

The flow of *qi* is cyclic. Using ancient Chinese time measuring methods of 2-hour increments, at any given time of day, the flow of *qi* will be strongest in one specific organ. In the course of a day, the strength of *qi* will pass once through each of the 12 channels. When the *qi* is passing through a given channel, the organ associated with that channel is considered to be at its strongest. The *qi* of the organ associated with the channel on the opposite side of the diurnal flow is considered to be at its weakest. Thus, from 3:00 a.m. to 5:00 a.m., the *qi* of the lung is at its strongest and the *qi* of the urinary bladder is at its weakest (see p. 303).

Clinically, this information might be applied in several ways. For example, if an asthmatic patient consistently wakes between 3:00 a.m. and 5:00 a.m. in the morning with an asthmatic attack, we might think that the *qi* of the lung, which should be especially strong at this time, is, instead, exceptionally weak, creating a circumstance where the patient cannot breathe easily, and other organs, the liver in particular, take advantage of this weakness and overwhelm the lung, causing an asthmatic attack.

Viscera	Bowels
Hand greater *yin* lung channel ←→	Hand *yang* brightness large intestine channel
手太阴肺经 *shou tai yin fei jing*	手阳明大肠经 *shou yang ming da chang jing*
Chest, abdomen, anterior medial aspect of the arm →	Anterior, lateral aspect of the arm; front of the face, forehead and trunk
3:00 a.m.–5:00 a.m.	5:00 a.m.–7:00 a.m.
Foot greater *yin* spleen channel ←→	Foot *yang* brightness stomach channel
足太阴脾经 *zu tai yin pi jing*	足阳明胃经 *zu yang ming wei jing*
Anterior medial aspect of the leg; abdomen, chest ←	Front of face, trunk, anterior lateral aspect of the leg
9:00 a.m.–11:00 a.m.	7:00 a.m.–9:00 a.m.
Hand lesser *yin* heart channel ←→	Hand greater *yang* small intestine channel
手少阴心旌 *shou tai yin xin jing*	手太阳小肠经 *shou tai yang xiao chang jing*
Chest/abdomen, posterior medial aspect of the arm →	Posterior, lateral aspect of the arm, posterior aspect of the trunk and head
11:00 a.m.–1:00 p.m.	1:00 p.m.–3:00 p.m.
Foot lesser *yin* kidney channel ←→	Foot greater *yang* urinary bladder channel
足少阴肾经 *zu shao yin shen jing*	足太阳膀胱经 *zu tai yang pang guang jing*
Posterior medial aspect of the leg; abdomen, chest ←	Face, posterior aspect of the head and trunk, posterior lateral aspect of the leg
5:00 p.m.–7:00 p.m.	3:00 p.m.–5:00 p.m.
Hand reverting *yin* pericardium channel ←→	Hand lesser *yang* triple burner channel
手厥阴心包经 *shou jue yin xin bao jing*	手少阳三焦经 *shou shao yang san jiao jing*
Chest/abdomen, midline of the medial aspect of the arm →	Midline of lateral aspect of the arm, lateral aspect of the trunk and head
7:00 p.m.–9:00 p.m.	9:00 p.m.–11:00 p.m.
Foot reverting *yin* liver channel ←→	Foot lesser *yang* gallbladder channel
足厥阴肝经 *zu jue yin gan jing*	足少阳胆经 *zu shao yang dan jing*
Midline of the medial aspect of the leg, abdomen of chest ←	Lateral aspect of the head and trunk, midline lateral aspect of the leg
1:00 a.m.–3:00 a.m.	11:00 p.m.–1:00 a.m.

A The circulation of *qi* (© Marnae und Kevin Ergil). This chart depicts: ←→
1. The interior/exterior (viscera/bowel) relationships between channels. ←→
2. The hand/foot relationship between channels.
3. The flow of *qi* from one channel to the next.
4. The three loops of the body (chest–hand–face–abdomen) that the *qi* completes in one day (light, medium, dark gray).
5. The relative location of each channel on the limbs of the body.
6. The time of day during which the *qi* is said to pass through each channel (the diurnal flow).

Signs of Channel Pathology

Each of the channels has distinctive signs of pathology that are associated with either the external pathway of the channel or with its internal pathway and by extension with the associated organ. These signs guide the practitioner in determining a diagnosis and in choosing points for treatment.

External channel symptoms manifest primarily in relation to the external trajectory of the channel and are produced by congestion and obstruction along the channel, either as the result of an external invasion or due to internal factors affecting the movement of *qi* and blood in the external channel pathway. While channel patterns can be differentiated in some detail according to the presence of heat, cold, vacuity, and repletion, the basic relationships between channel and symptom are simple to characterize (**A**).

For example, many of the signs of pathology in the external pathway of the urinary bladder channel are commonly seen in the invasion of external wind cold when a replete cold evil enters the external channel and blocks the smooth movement of *qi* along its course. The symptoms of eye pain and tearing reflect the relationship of the external channel pathway to the eye. Traditionally, in certain conditions where the eye is inflamed and painful the path of the urinary bladder channel on the back might be carefully examined and channel points are treated to relieve the condition.

Pathology that is specific to the channel may present as pain, tension, rashes, and so on, that manifest along a specific channel pathway. For example, a patient presenting with pain that covers the posterior portion of the shoulder, crosses the scapula, and goes down the posterior aspect of the arm, might be diagnosed with stagnation of *qi* and blood in the small intestine channel.

Because of the internal pathways of the channels that connect directly to the associated organs, channel pathology may be a reflection of organ pathology. For example, a patient who presents with a complaint of shoulder pain along the path of the large intestine channel might also experience constipation. Through inquiry, the good diagnostician might learn that when the bowels move, the pain diminishes and both the pain and the constipation improve when there is less stress. Thus, when discussing channel pathology we refer not only to what is visible or what is manifesting along the exterior portion of the pathway, but also to the internal pathway and its organ connections.

All of the 12 regular channels have several internal pathways, along which there are no specific points that can be accessed but which must be considered in relation to diagnosis and treatment.

Channel		Major Representative Signs
Lung	External	Heat effusion and aversion to cold, nasal congestion, headache, pain along the channel
	Internal	Cough, panting, wheezing, fullness and oppression in the chest, expectoration of phlegm-drool
Large Intestine	External	Heat effusion, parched mouth, sore throat, nosebleed, toothache, redness and swelling along the channel
	Internal	Lower abdominal pain, wandering abdominal pain, rumbling intestines, sloppy stool
Stomach	External	High fever, red face, sweating, manic agitation, aversion to cold, pain in the eyes, dry nose, nosebleed, lip and mouth sores
	Internal	Severe abdominal distention and fullness, vexation and discomfort, mania and withdrawal, swift digestion, and rapid hungering
Spleen	External	Heaviness in the head or body, weak, wilting limbs, generalized heat effusion, cold along the inside of the thigh and knee, swelling of the legs and feet
	Internal	Pain in the stomach duct and sloppy diarrhea or stool containing untransformed food, rumbling intestines, retching and nausea, reduced food intake
Heart	External	Generalized heat effusion, headache, eye pain, pain in the chest and back, dry throat, thirst with the urge to drink, hot or painful palms, pain along the channel
	Internal	Heart pain, fullness and pain in the chest, rib-side, and hypochondriac region, heart vexation
Small Intestine	External	Mouth and tongue ulcers, pain in the cheeks, pain and stiffness along the channel
	Internal	Lower abdominal pain and distention with the pain stretching to the lumbus and/or testicles
Urinary bladder	External	Heat effusion and aversion to cold, headache, stiff neck, pain in the lumbar spine, nasal congestion, eye pain and tearing, pain along the channel
	Internal	Lower abdominal pain and distention, inhibited urination, urinary block and enuresis
Kidney	External	Lumbar pain, counterflow cold of the legs, weak, wilting legs, dry mouth and throat, pain along the channel
	Internal	Dizziness, facial swelling, blurred vision, gray complexion, shortness of breath, enduring diarrhea, sloppy stool, or dry stool evacuated with difficulty, impotence
Pericardium	External	Stiffness, pain, or swelling along the channel, red facial complexion, pain in the eyes
	Internal	Delirious speech, clouding reversal, heat vexation, heart palpitations, heart pain, constant laughing
Triple burner	External	Sore throat, pain in the cheeks, red eyes, deafness, pain along the channel
	Internal	Abdominal distention and fullness, urinary frequency or enuresis, vacuity edema
Gall-bladder	External	Alternating heat effusion and aversion to cold, headache, eye pain, pain under the chin, sub-axillary swelling, pain along the channel
	Internal	Rib-side pain, vomiting, bitter taste in the mouth, chest pain
Liver	External	Headache, dizziness, blurred vision, tinnitus, heat effusion
	Internal	Fullness, distention, and pain in the rib-side, chest and abdomen, vomiting, jaundice, mounting *qi*

A Signs of Channel Pathology.

The 12 Sinew Channels
(*Shi Er Jing Jin* 十二经筋)

Pathways

The sinew channels are superficial channels that follow approximately the same pathway as the external regular channel with which they share a name. They are called sinew channels because they travel across the sinews (muscles, tendons, and ligaments). The sinew channels all branch off from the regular channels at the tips of the fingers or toes, then travel up and across the body (**A**).

Functions

As surface channels, the sinew channels contain only defense *qi* and function as the body's first defense against the invasion of evils. If the defense *qi* in the sinew channels is overcome by an exterior evil, the evil may travel down the sinew channel to the tips of the fingers, and from there, enter the regular channels and travel internally. Thus, one function of the sinew channels is to defend the body against invasion.

The sinew channels also supplement transportation of the regular channels by emphasizing the circulation of *qi* and blood to the muscles, tissues, joints, and body surface. They connect the muscles, tendons, and ligaments to the joints, link the structures of the body, and facilitate articulation and normal movement and also protect the bones.

Flow of Qi

The flow of *qi* of the sinew channels differs from the flow of *qi* in the 12 regular channels. In all the sinew channels, the *qi* travels from the fingers or toes upward along the channel pathway. Also, the circuit of *qi* does not follow the same pathway as the 12 regular channels. In the sinew channels, during the day *qi* flows through the *yang* channels, and at night it flows through the *yin* channels. Our bodies are therefore more vulnerable to the invasion of an evil at night, when the *yang* sinew channels are not filled.

The pathway of the flow of *qi* through the sinew channels is as follows:

LB → ST → SI → TB → LI → SP → LU → LR → PC → KI → HT.

Pathology of the 12 Sinew Channels

The 12 sinew channels may reflect symptomatology of their associated organ, but in general, pathology of these channels manifests as impediment patterns, trauma, and muscle strain or tension that may be due to long-standing emotional or physical stressors. The primary symptom of the sinew channels is pain.

Treatment of the 12 Sinew Channels

Because the 12 sinew channels do not have their own points, points on the associated regular channel are used. Typically, points are selected on the basis of the presence of pain on palpation. Non-channel points that are painful on palpation, called *a shi* ("That's It!") points are frequently needled to release the stagnation of *qi* and blood in the sinew channels.

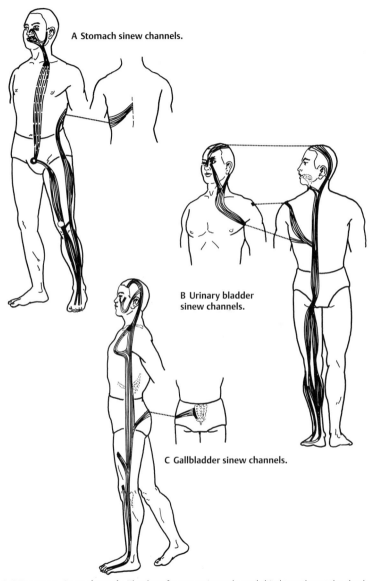

A Stomach sinew channels.

B Urinary bladder sinew channels.

C Gallbladder sinew channels.

A-C Foot *yang* sinew channels. The three foot *yang* sinew channels bind together at the cheek.

12 Cutaneous Regions
(*Shi Er Pi Bu* 十二皮部)

Even more superficial than the 12 sinew channels are the divisions created by the 12 cutaneous regions (**A**). Like the sinew channels, their distribution follows the course of the regular channels and their pathway is over the body surface. Although they do not distribute interiorly, they do communicate closely with the regular and sinew channels via the grandchild network vessels and can be used therapeutically to treat the internal organs. The cutaneous regions have no starting or terminating points, and no directional flow.

The 12 cutaneous regions circulate defense *qi* and blood to the body surface, regulate the function of the skin and interstices (pores), and strengthen the body's immunity. All of these functions are related to the functions of the lung system. Therefore, if the lung system is functioning well, then the cutaneous regions are well nourished, and there is sufficient defense *qi* on the surface of the body to keep the pores regulated, to prevent the invasion of an evil into the body or the loss of *qi* through sweat.

Clinical Application
of the 12 Cutaneous Regions
(Shi Er Pi Bu 十二皮部)

Although descriptions of the pathology of the 12 cutaneous regions do not exist, clinically, skin disorders may indicate a disorder of the related regular channel or organ. Additionally, someone who is susceptible to colds or who feels easily chilled on the exterior of the body might be showing signs of an insufficiency of defense *qi* circulating in the cutaneous regions.

Treatment via the cutaneous regions is usually accomplished with techniques such as seven-star (plum blossom) needling or *gua sha* (sand scraping) (**B, C**). Seven-star or plum blossom technique entails the use of a long-handled hammer-like tool with five to seven very small needles in its head. This hammer is lightly tapped over an area until it reddens. This technique brings *qi* and blood to the surface of the body and clears the cutaneous regions so that *qi* and blood can flow smoothly. It is often used in the treatment of numbness or tingling along a pathway. *Gua sha* entails the use of a horn tool (or a ceramic spoon or other small, smooth-surfaced tool) to scrape an area of the body. The scraping is continued until the *sha* or sand reaches the surface of the body and manifests as dark, mottled spots. If the sand is not present, no matter how hard the body is scraped, it will not manifest with *sha*. *Gua sha* might be used like cupping to release an evil from the exterior, or it might be used to bring a deeper evil to the surface or simply to move *qi* and blood in an area.

A Cutaneous regions.

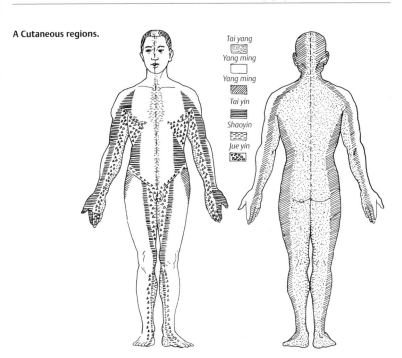

Tai yang

Yang ming

Yang ming

Tai yin

Shaoyin

Jue yin

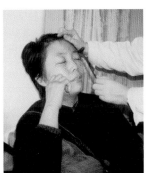

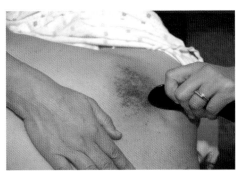

B Patient being treated with seven-star needling for facial numbness (© Marnae Ergil).

C Patient receiving *gua sha* treatment on the back.

The 12 Channel Divergences
(Shi Er Jing Bie 十二经别)

Channel divergences refer to branches of the 12 regular channels. They are distributed inside the body and have no points of their own. They are called divergences because they diverge from the regular pathway to make important internal linkages.

Distribution

The 12 channel divergences separate from the regular channel near the elbows or knees. The internally/externally related pairs merge together and enter the trunk to travel to the viscera and bowels. Together, they emerge from the body at the neck. Finally, they merge with the regular *yang* channel of the *yin yang* pair.

The point where the channel divergences separate from the regular channel and where they merge with the regular *yang* channel are important points for treatment. Called the six joinings (*liu he* 六合) (**A**), they are used to treat disorders of the paired channels. With the exception of the triple burner, which runs from the vertex of the head, down the body to the middle burner, the channel divergences run from the extremities to the trunk, face, and head.

The *qi* flow from one channel divergence to the next is as follows:
BL → KI → GB → LR → ST → SP → SI → HT → TB → PC → LI → LU.

Functions of the Channel Divergences

The channel divergences, which contain only defense *qi*, supply defense *qi* to the organs, and act as a secondary line of defense against the invasion of evil. If an evil invades the body and gets past the defense *qi* in the sinew channels, it passes to the regular channels. From here it may go directly into the organs or it may diverge and enter the channel divergences. By entering the channel divergence, it continues to battle with the defense *qi*, and thus is further weakened. From the channel divergence the evil may be pushed out of the body or it may enter the organs, but in a more weakened form.

The channel divergences strengthen the connection between *yin yang* paired organs and *yin yang* paired channels. They integrate areas of the body that are not covered by the main pathways, thus explaining the functions of certain points. For example, the urinary bladder channel divergence connects with the rectum and anus, reinforcing the BL regular channels' connection to that area (**B**).

The channel divergences share the same pathology as the regular channels. Because the channel divergences contain defense *qi* and the strength of the defense *qi* waxes and wanes, when disease enters the channel divergences, the symptoms are often intermittent or cyclic and one-sided.

Channels	Lower Joining	Upper Joining
Urinary bladder and kidney	Popliteal fossa/BL-40 area	Nape of the neck/BL-10
Gallbladder and liver	External genitalia/CV-2 area	GB-1 area/lateral aspect of eye
Stomach and spleen	ST-30 area/pubic bone	BL-1 area/medial aspect of eye
Heart and small intestine	Axilla (HT-1/SI-10 area)	Non-specific face area
Triple burner and pericardium	Non-specific middle or upper burner	Mastoid process
Lung and large intestine	Supraclavicular fossa/ST-12 area	LI-18/cheek

A The divergent channel meeting points. Lower joining: where the paired channels meet; upper joining: where the divergent channel meets the regular *yang* channel.

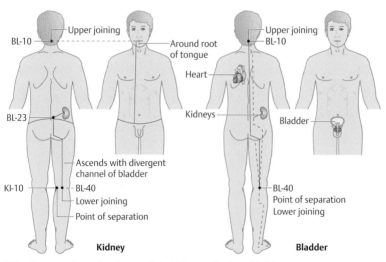

B The divergent channel pathways of the kidney and urinary bladder.

The Eight Extraordinary Vessels
(*Qi Heng Ba Mai* 奇横八脉)

Although often discussed as an entirely different category of channels, the eight extraordinary vessels are a part of the general channel system. They are extraordinary because they do not fit the pattern of the other major channels. There are two primary differences between the eight extraordinary vessels and the 12 regular channels.

First, they do not have a continuous, interlinking pattern of circulation. Although they have connections with each other and with the 12 regular channels, they do not link, one to the next, as the 12 regular channels do.

Second, they are not associated with a specific organ system. The eight extraordinary vessels are associated with specific types of disorders based upon their location and functions.

Like the regular channels, each of the eight extraordinary vessels has its own pathway. However, only two of the eight extraordinary vessels, the controlling (*ren* 任) vessel and the governing (*du* 督) vessel, have their own acupuncture points. These two channels traverse the midline of the body, and the functions of their points are often associated with the functions of the organs lying near them.

In addition to the specific points located on the controlling and governing vessels, all of the eight extraordinary vessels are associated with a specific point on one of the 12 regular channels. This point, called a confluent point, is used to access the *qi* and blood of the extraordinary vessel and make it available for use by the organ systems. Clinically, each of the eight extraordinary vessels is paired with another, making four couples. When using the confluent point for one vessel, the confluent point of its paired vessel is also used (**A**).

Functions

The eight extraordinary vessels function as reservoirs of *qi* and blood. They fill and empty as required by the changing conditions and pathologies of the regular channels or of the organ systems. All of the eight extraordinary vessels are closely related to the functions of the liver and kidney systems and also to the functioning of the uterus and the brain.

The basic functions are to provide additional interconnections among the regular channels and the organ systems and to regulate the flow of *qi* and blood in the regular channels. Surplus *qi* or blood from the regular channels may be stored in the eight extraordinary vessels and released when required (**B**).

Channel	Confluent Point	Paired Channel	Confluent Point
Governing vessel	SI-3	*Yang* springing vessel	BL-62
Controlling vessel	LU-7	*Yin* springing vessel	KI-6
Penetrating vessel	SP-4	*Yin* linking vessel	PC-6
Girdling vessel	GB-41	*Yang* linking vessel	TB-5

A The eight extraordinary vessel pairs and their confluent points.

Extraordinary Vessel	Functions	Primary Pathologies
Governing vessel *Du mai* 督脉	Sea of *yang* channels Sea of marrow Regulates *yang* channels Homes to the brain and connects to the kidney Reflects physiology and pathology of the brain and the spinal fluid	Pain and stiffness in the back, child fright reversal, heavy-headedness, hemorrhoids, infertility, malaria, mania and withdrawal, visceral agitation (mental disorders)
Controlling vessel *Ren mai* 任脉	Sea of *yin* channels Regulates the *yin* channels Regulates menstruation and nurtures the fetus	Menstrual irregularities, menstrual block, miscarriage, infertility, mounting *qi*, enuresis, abdominal masses
Penetrating vessel *Chong mai* 冲脉	Sea of the regular channels Regulates the 12 regular channels Sea of blood Regulates menstruation	Women: uterine bleeding, miscarriage, menstrual block, menstrual irregularities, scant breast milk, lower abdominal pain, blood ejection Men: seminal emission, impotence, prostatitis, urethritis, orchitis
Girdling vessel *Dai mai* 代脉	Binds all the channels running up and down the trunk Regulates the balance between upward and downward flow of *qi*	Vaginal discharge, prolapse of the uterus, abdominal distention and fullness, limp lumbus
Yang springing vessel *Yang qiao mai* 阳跷脉	Control the opening and closing of the eyes Control the ascent of fluids and the descent of *qi* Balance the *yin* and *yang qi* of the body	Eye problems, dry, itchy eyes, insomnia, poor agility, muscle spasms or tension along the lateral aspect of the lower leg combined with muscle flaccidity along the medial aspect of the lower leg
Yin springing vessel *Yin qiao mai* 阴跷脉	Control the opening and closing of the eyes Control the ascent of fluids and the descent of *qi* Balance the *yin* and *yang qi* of the body	Eye problems, heaviness of the eyes, difficulty opening the eyes somnolence, lower abdominal pain that extends into the genital area, mounting patterns, muscle spasms or tension along the medial aspect of the lower leg combined with muscle flaccidity along the lateral aspect of the lower leg
Yang linking vessel *Yang wei mai* 阳维脉	Unites all the major *yang* channels Compensates for superabundance or insufficiency in channel circulation Regulates *yang* channel activity Governs the exterior of the body	Signs of external invasion including cough, sneezing, muscle aches and heat effusion, aversion to cold, sensations of heat in the body or hyperactivity
Yin linking vessel *Yin wei mai* 阴维脉	Connects the flow of the major *yin* channels of the body Regulates *yin* channel activity Governs the interior of the body Balances the emotions	Any interior organ condition, especially those manifesting in the yin organs, or caused by emotional upset

B Functions of the eight extraordinary vessels (adapted from Ellis, Wiseman, & Boss 1991; Ni 1996).

Governing Vessel   All of the regular *yang* channels intersect with the governing vessel (**A**). It governs the *yang* channels and is called the sea of *yang*. It provides warmth to the organs and channels. It connects with the uterus, kidneys, heart, and brain. As it runs up the body, it brings *qi* and blood to the head, influencing the functioning of the brain, the head, and the sense organs. It circulates *yang qi* from the kidneys to nourish the marrow and bones, and so influences the constitution and enhances immunity. It is paired with the *yang* springing vessel and its confluent point is SI-3.

Controlling Vessel   All of the regular *yin* channels connect with the controlling vessel (**B**). It regulates the *yin* channels and is called the sea of *yin qi*. It circulates blood, essence, and body fluids to the organs and channels, and up to the face, lips, and eyes. It regulates the functions of the internal organs and of male and female reproductive function. It is paired with the *yin* springing vessel and its confluent point is LU-7.

Penetrating Vessel   This vessel (**C**) stores and regulates blood and is called the sea of blood. It regulates the circulation of *qi* and blood by regulating the 12 regular channels and is also called the sea of the 12 channels. It is paired with the *yin* linking vessel and its confluent point is SP-4.

Girdling Vessel   This is the only channel that encircles the body transversely (**D**). It controls and binds all of the longitudinal channels. It regulates the waist, lumbar spine, and lower extremities. The girdling vessel is said to regulate the gallbladder channel. It is paired with the *yang* linking vessel and its confluent point is GB-41.

Yin and Yang Linking Vessels   The *yin* linking vessel dominates the interior of the body and balances the emotions. Its paired vessel is the penetrating vessel and its confluent point is PC-6. The *yang* linking vessel dominates the exterior of the body, balances the *yang qi* and the emotions. It is paired with the girdling vessel and its confluent point is TB-5.

Yin and Yang Springing Vessels
These vessels balance the *yin* and *yang qi* of the body. In the lower body, they balance the movement of the lower extremities, allowing for an even and balanced gait. In the upper body, they regulate the opening and closing of the eyes. They regulate and balance the function of the brain, especially in relation to activity and quiescence. The *yang* linking vessel is paired with the governing vessel and its confluent point is BL-62. The *yin* springing vessel is paired with the controlling vessel and its confluent point is KI-6.

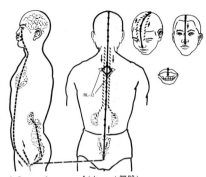

A Governing vessel (*du mai* 督脉).

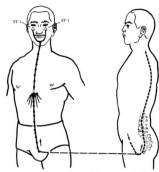

B Controlling vessel (*ren mai* 任脉).

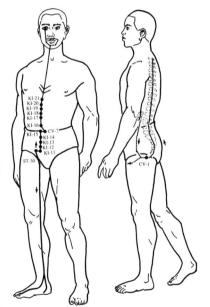

C Penetrating vessel (*chong mai* 冲脉).

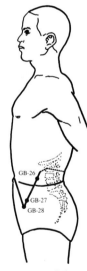

D Girdling vessel (*dai mai* 代脉).

The Network Vessels (*Luo Mai* 络脉)

As mentioned earlier, there are two types of major pathways in the body. We have just reviewed the channels. The second major group is the network vessels (**A–D**; also see p. 185 for an overview of the channel and network system). The network vessels connect interiorly/exteriorly related organs and channels. They are bilateral and symmetrical, but they travel in all directions and are relatively superficial. With the rest of the channel system, the network vessels form a network of pathways that integrate the entire body and distribute *qi* and blood, especially to the surface of the body.

There are two sub-sets of network vessels. These are the 16 network divergences (*bie luo* 别洛), and a series of very small vessels that traverse the entire body, with no particular pathways. The first set includes the transverse network vessels and the longitudinal network vessels. The second set includes the minute network vessels, the superficial network vessels (*fu luo* 浮络), and the blood network vessels (*xue luo* 血络).

Characteristics of the Network Vessels

Each of the 12 regular channels has a network vessel, which connects the regular channel to its paired channel in a direct pathway, and which has a longitudinal branch with specific pathology. Additionally, the controlling vessel has a network vessel that breaks off from CV-15 (just below the zyphoid process of the chest) and disperses over the chest and abdomen. The governing vessel has a connecting vessel that breaks off at GV-1 (the tip of the coccyx) and disperses over the back. The spleen channel has a second network vessel (the great network vessel of the spleen) that breaks off from SP-21 and disperses over the sides of the body, and the stomach channel has a second network vessel (the great network vessel of the stomach) that breaks off from ST-18 and disperses over the area of the heart.

General Clinical Applications of the Network Vessels

The 16 connecting points of the network vessels are used to treat three basic types of disorders. These are: disorders of the internally/externally related channels; whole body disorders, such as overall body pain, itching of the skin or back pain (this applies especially to the network vessels of the controlling and governing vessel and the great network vessels of the spleen and stomach); and disorders of the longitudinal network vessels.

Sixteen Network Divergences

According to *The Yellow Emperor's Classic of Medicine*, the transverse and longitudinal network vessels are one vessel with two or more different pathways. Both vessels break off from the connecting (*luo* 络) point of their associated channel; however, because their pathways are quite distinct, and the functions and symptomatologies differ, from a clinical perspective, it is useful to separate them for discussion.

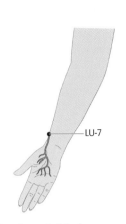

LU-7

A Network vessel of the lung.

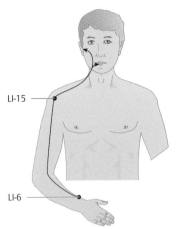

LI-15

LI-6

B Network vessel of the large intestine.

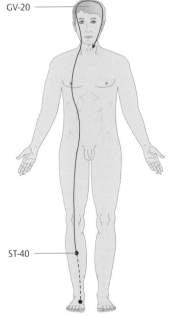

GV-20

ST-40

C Network vessel of the stomach.

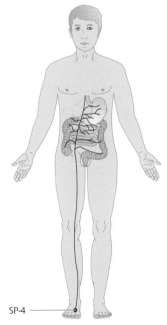

SP-4

D Network vessel of the spleen.

Transverse Network Divergences

There are 12 transverse network vessels. They are often very short pathways, running from the connecting point on each channel to its interiorly/exteriorly related channel. Clinically, through the use of the connecting and source points of the paired channels, the *qi* in a channel can be balanced or harmonized. Essentially, these rather short and specific pathways serve as a direct connection between the *yin* and *yang* channel of an internally/externally related pair, strengthening the relationship between paired channels. Through a "source-connecting point" (aka guest-host) treatment, the *qi* of the two channels can be harmonized and disease affecting both channels treated.

Longitudinal Network Divergences

As with the transverse network vessels, these vessels break off from the connecting point of their named channel. However, they have a specific pathway and specific pathology that differs from the pathology of the related regular channel. Awareness of these pathways and their associated symptoms can aid the acupuncturist in determining appropriate treatment. Like the transverse network divergences, these pathways are treated using the connecting points of the affected channel. These treatment strategies are discussed in detail later in this chapter under Point Selection Strategies (see p. 186).

Minute, Superficial, and Blood Network Vessels

The minute network vessels are very small, non-specific branches of the network divergences. They carry *qi* and blood to all of the areas of the body that are not covered by any other channel, forming a net that covers the entire body. The superficial network vessels, also called the grandchild network vessels, are the small branches of the network divergences that are sometimes visible on the surface of the skin. These are closely associated with the minute vessels, but are thought to be somewhat more superficial. The blood network vessels appear as very small blood vessels near the surface of the skin. Should the blood network vessels change in color, and become dark or stagnant, a technique called network vessel pricking is used. Here, a three-edged needle is used to prick the blood network vessels and release blood.

Having now discussed all of the various types of channels and the network vessels, we will move on to point selection strategies. Because this text is not meant to be a point location text, we will not review all of the points on the body and their individual functions but rather will present several case studies to present how an acupuncturist might think about how to select points.

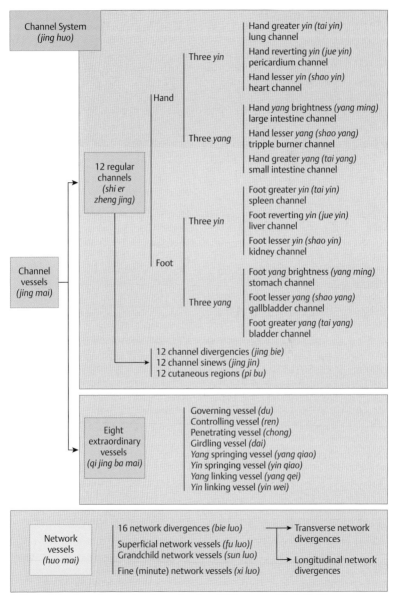

A Chart of the channel and network vessel system (© Marnae and Kevin Ergil).

Point Selection Strategies

General Principles of Creating a Point Prescription

Before determining the specific points to be used in a treatment, several things must be considered. First, a correct diagnosis must be reached. Without a correct diagnosis, points may be chosen to treat the presenting symptoms of a condition, but these points will not treat the root cause of the symptoms. For example, if a patient presents with chronic shoulder pain, there are many points that might be chosen to treat the shoulder pain without ever having come to a Chinese medicine diagnosis. While the shoulder pain may be somewhat relieved, the root of the problem has not been addressed and so the pain is likely to return.

Once a diagnosis is reached, the process of choosing a set of points to treat the condition can begin. The process begins with point matching (**A**), which requires that the practitioner be aware of all of the points that might possibly be appropriate for the given condition. The large set of points is chosen based on an understanding of channel theory and knowing the areas that different channels affect, on knowing point categories and how points in specific categories affect areas of the body, on knowledge of specific channel points and how they differ, and on knowledge about empirical points that might be appropriate for a given diagnosis or condition.

Once the large set of points has been created, two to three smaller acupuncture prescriptions may be devised. This is the process of point selection (**A**). It is important to have two to three prescriptions in mind so that the same treatment is not used all the time. Different treatments might include treatment on the front or the back of the body or treatments to be alternated each visit.

Point Selection

First, a point prescription (**A**) must address both the tip and the branch of the problem. For example, if a patient arrives with a chief complaint of headaches, the practitioner must develop a point prescription that will treat the root cause of those headaches but will also address the presenting symptoms. If the focus is entirely on the root, it may be that for several weeks there will be no improvement in the headaches, a situation that is not conducive to building a successful clinical practice.

Second, a point prescription must be balanced. Balance includes balancing points between the upper and lower portion of the body, balancing points between the left and right of the body, and balancing points on *yin* and *yang* channels (**B**). Returning to our example of headache, if points only on the upper body are chosen, this may cause the *qi* and blood to move too quickly or too forcefully to the upper body, actually causing a headache.

Point matching: choosing the set of points that might be used in treatment

1. Correct diagnosis.
2. Correct treatment principle and method.
3. Choosing a set of points to fulfill the treatment principle and method based on:

a. Channel theory
b. Channel pathways
c. Areas of effect
d. Point categories
e. Empirical points

Point selection: creating the specific point prescriptions

1. Address tip and branch.
2. Balance:
   a. *Yin* and *yang* channel points
   b. Front and back of the body
   c. Top and bottom of the body
   d. Left and right sides of the body.
3. Select local, adjacent, and distal points.
4. Understand the overall function of each point prescription.
5. Keep each point prescription to an appropriate size.
6. Determine if any adjunctive therapies are to be used:
   a. Moxibustion
   b. Cupping
   c. Seven-star needling
   d. *Gua sha*
   e. Bodywork

A Principles of point matching and point selection.

Channel	Name	Common Applications	Individual Applications
Three hand *yin* channels	Lung	Chest disorders	Lung, throat, nose, exterior patterns
	Pericardium		Mental, heart, stomach
	Heart		Mental, heart, eye
Three hand *yang* channels	Large intestine	Face, head, sense organs, febrile diseases	Front of the face and head
	Small intestine		Occipital area/nape, scapula, mental
	San jiao		Temporal region, sides of the head/face, hypochondriac region
Three foot *yin* channels	Spleen	Urogenital, abdomen and chest disorders	Spleen and stomach
	Kidney		Kidney, lung, and throat
	Liver		Liver and gallbladder
Three foot *yang* channels	Stomach	Mental disorders, febrile diseases, eye problems	Front of the face/head, digestive system
	Urinary bladder		Occipital area/nape, back and lumbus
	Gallbladder		Temporal regions, side of the head and face, hypochondriac region, hip

B The clinical applications of points on the four limbs (adapted from Ellis, Wiseman, & Boss 1991, p. 57).

Third, point selection is based on selecting local, adjacent, and distal points to treat any given condition. For headaches, one might choose a point directly at the site of the headache. Additionally, one would choose points near the site of the headache (adjacent) and finally, one would choose points on the four limbs as distal points. This process gives a balance to the prescription and the *qi* moves in such a way that it will address both the clinical problem or symptom (the tip) and its cause (the root).

Fourth, the elements of function and size of the treatment must be considered. While each individual point chosen will have its own functions and indications, the overall point prescription should also have a function. If the cause of the headaches is liver *qi* stagnation, then the points chosen should act together to move the *qi* of the liver and to treat the headache. Essentially, the function of the point prescription should match the treatment method that is determined by the diagnosis.

Finally, one must also consider the number of needles that are being inserted. Some practitioners say that no more than eight needles should be inserted. Others say that eight bilateral points (16 needles) should be used. While there is no absolute rule about the number of needles used, it is generally better to keep an acupuncture treatment small, and so choosing points that might work on several aspects of treatment is always more effective than choosing points that act only on one symptom. However, there are many exceptions to this rule, and some treatment strategies may employ far greater numbers of needles.

Issues such as the frequency of treatment to be received as well as the techniques to be used must also be addressed. In China, a typical course of treatment is considered to be 10 treatments. These treatments are generally given every day or every other day for 10–20 days. There is then a break for 10 days, and then if necessary, treatment recommences. In the West, while 10 treatments is generally considered an appropriate course of treatment, we tend to treat once a week for 10 weeks. This approach is not always useful as many conditions respond better to more frequent treatment. Techniques will also vary widely depending upon the system in which one is trained, whether it be TCM, one of the many systems coming out of Japan or Korea, or one of the systems developed outside of Asia.

One of the most important parts of the point matching/point selection process is to understand the clinical significance of point categories (**A**) (see also pp. 120–121).

Category	Description
Five transport points	Points that are located on the arms and legs, below the elbow or knee, and associated with one of the five phases. There are five on each channel (see tables on p. 191)
Source points	Points on each of the 12 regular channels where the source *qi* collects. The source *qi* is stored by the kidneys and spread throughout the body by the triple burner Used to promote the flow of source *qi* and regulate the function of the internal organs
Network points	The site where the network vessel splits from the regular channel Used to treat interiorly/exteriorly related organs and the longitudinal network vessel. Frequently, these points are combined with source points, referred to as a guest-host treatment
Alarm points	Sites on the chest and abdomen where *qi* collects. There is one alarm point for each of the 12 organs. They are palpated for tenderness, lumps, gatherings, depressions, and so on, and used to treat their associated organ
Back transport points	Points located on the urinary bladder channel, lateral to the spine. There is one back transport point for each organ and the *qi* of that organ runs through the point. Used to treat the associated organ. Back transport points are frequently combined with alarm points to treat diseases of the viscera and bowels
Eight meeting (influential) points	Points that are effective in the treatment of disorder in a specific tissue or substance. These are very general points and can treat any aspect of disharmony in their related tissue or substance. They are generally combined with other points to increase their specificity
Four command points	Points that are especially effective in treating disorders located in a particular anatomical area of the body
Eight confluent points	Each of the eight extraordinary channels has a single point on one of the 12 regular channels that is said to be confluent with the associated extraordinary channel and to open or access that channel
Cleft points	As *qi* and blood circulate through the channels they accumulate in the cleft points. These points reflect repletion or vacuity in the channel. Sharp or intense pain on pressure or redness and swelling indicates repletion, and dull or mild pain, or a depression indicates vacuity
Crossing points/intersection points	Points where two or three channels meet, they have a strong therapeutic effect on all of these channels, often eliminating the need for using multiple points
A shi points/ "That's It!" points	Points that are particularly sensitive to palpation, these are most often used to treat disorders in their immediate vicinity

A Point categories.

Transport Points (Five Phase Points)

Perhaps the most powerful, and certainly the most commonly used points on the body are the transport points. These points, located on the arms and legs, below the elbow or knee, are associated with the five phases (see also pp. 60–64). Beginning at the tip of the finger or toe, and moving up to the elbow or knee, there are five points on each channel that are associated with the five phases, for a total of 60 points. The five points are the well, spring, stream, river, and uniting (sea) points. The points that fall into this category on each channel, and their phase relationship are shown in **A**. The category name for each of these points is associated with the flow of water, which is used as a metaphor for the flow of *qi* through the body. The *qi* flows from the tip of the mountains, at the well points, located on the tips of the fingers or toes, where the *qi* is said to be "shallow and meek" through the spring, where the *qi* has a "gushing quality." From the spring, the *qi* flows to the stream points where the flow pours from shallow to deep. From the stream, flow continues to the river where the force has become more powerful. Finally, the *qi* flows into the uniting points at the knees and elbows. Here the *qi* unites with its home organ, just as a river reaches the sea. The names of

the points thus describe the nature of the *qi* at each of the points. It should be noted that this description of the nature of the *qi* is not the same as the directional flow of *qi* through the channels. There are two major ways in which these points are used clinically and that inform point selection.

First, they are employed based on the presenting condition. First discussed in the *Classic of Difficulties*, and further theoretically elaborated over the years, each of these point categories have been shown to be effective in treating certain types of conditions. Well points are especially effective in reviving a clouded spirit, and, when bled, in clearing heat. Spring points are indicated for externally contracted heat conditions. Stream points treat pain in the joints. River points treat cough and panting, and uniting points treat bowel patterns. Thus, the appropriate point on a given channel might be selected to treat any of these conditions manifesting in a particular organ (**B**).

Second, these points are selected according to their five-phase correspondences. Each of the transport points is related to a specific phase (as is the organ of the channel on which the points lie). These relationships can be utilized in theory-based treatment models of escalating complexity.

Location	Yin Channel Phase Relationship	Point Category	Yang Channel Phase Relationship	Representation of Qi
Near the end of finger or toe	Wood ▽	Well	Metal	The shallow and meek nature of *qi*
The second most distal point	Fire △	Spring	Water	*Qi* is slightly larger, like a small spring
Usually the third point on the channel, at the wrists and ankles	Earth □	Stream	Wood	*Qi* is described as like pouring down from a shallow place to a deeper one
On the forearm or calf	Metal ◇	River	Fire	*Qi* is free-flowing like the water in a river
Around the elbow or knee	Water ○	Sea	Earth	*Qi* is said to flow large and deep here as it unites with the organ of the home channel

A The natures, location and phase relationsphips of the transport points.

Point Category	Clinical Applications
Well	Revive clouded spirit Clear heat
Spring	Externally contracted heat conditions
Stream	Pain in the joints
River	Cough and panting
Sea	Bowel patterns

B The historical clinical applications of the transport points.

On a very basic level, it is understood that vacuity conditions can be treated by supplementing the mother, and repletion conditions can be addressed by draining the child of the affected organ. Thus, if there is a vacuity in the earth phase, then the mother point on the earth channel might be supplemented (the fire point on the spleen channel). Additionally, one could choose to supplement the same phase points on the mother channel (the fire point on the heart channel).

Alternatively, if there were a repletion condition in the earth phase, a condition that more commonly occurs in the stomach, then one could drain the child point on the earth channel (the metal point on the stomach channel) or the same phase point on the child channel (the metal point on the large intestine channel).

Classic Chinese compendia of point selection strategies discuss several variants of these techniques, originally suggested by the theoretical discussions in the *Classic of Difficulties*. These approaches became very popular in the 1930s and again in the 1950s as acupuncture in Japan saw periods of revived interest in the acupuncture theories from the *Classic of Difficulties*. Contemporary schools of clinical thought in Japan such as Japanese Meridian Therapy utilize transport points extensively based on a five-phase paradigm. This approach to acupuncture point selection is also practiced in Korea (notably the Korean four-point method) and elaborated in China with the six-point method (**A**). Essentially, the approach posits the notion that if a particular phase is vacuous or replete, then the relationships of the engendering and restraining cycle can be exploited to supplement or drain the affected phase as needed.

For example, where a patient presents with a stomach repletion pattern with clamorous hunger and foul breath, ST-45, the metal point (Child of Earth) on the affected channel would be drained and LI-44 the metal point of the child channel (large intestine is a metal phase channel and so again the Child of Earth) would be drained. Thus, the engendering or mother–child relationship would be used here to draw the replete *qi* from the mother by draining the child. Simultaneously the wood points (wood restrains earth) would be supplemented to increase the restraining effects of the wood phase on earth, in this case ST-43, the wood point of the affected channel, and GB-41, the wood point (the phase point) of the gallbladder (wood) channel. See the system's application to *Alice* in **B**.

These approaches to treatment have had a substantial influence on some portions of the English and US acupuncture communities through the work of J. R. Worsley, whose studies with exponents of Japanese Meridian Therapy led him to develop an approach to acupuncture diagnosis and treatment based almost exclusively on five-phase correspondences and transport points.

Vacuity Conditions	
Korean four-point	Supplement the mother point on the channel of the affected organ
	Supplement the phase point on the mother channel
	Drain the controlling phase point (the grandmother point) on the affected organ's channel
	Drain the phase point on the controlling phase (the grandmother) channel
Chinese six-point add:	Drain the phase controlled by the affected phase (the grandchild point) on the channel of the affected organ
	Drain the phase point on the channel controlled by the affected phase (the grandchild channel)
Repletion Conditions	
Korean four-point	Drain the child of the affected phase on the channel of the affected organ
	Drain the phase point on the child channel of the affected organ
	Supplement the phase point on the channel that controls the affected organ (the grandmother channel)
	Supplement the control point (the grandmother point) on the channel of the affected organ
Chinese six-point add:	Supplement the phase controlled by the affected phase (the grandchild point) on the channel of the affected organ
	Supplement the phase point on the channel controlled by the affected phase (the grandchild channel)

A Korean four-point and Chinese six-point treatment strategy rules.

→ **Case Study**

Alice, 23-year-old female with severe dysmenorrhea (see Chapter 3, pp. 152–153 and pp. 200–201 at the end of this chapter)

Diagnosis	*Qi* and blood stagnation in the liver and gallbladder channels causing menstrual pain		
Affected phase: wood	Child phase: fire	Grandmother phase: metal	Grandchild phase: earth
Drain	Fire point on wood channel		LR-2
Drain	Fire point on fire channel		HT-8
Supplement	Metal point on metal channel		LU-8
Supplement	Metal point on wood channel		LR-4
Supplement	Earth point on wood channel		LR-3
Supplement	Earth point on earth channel		SP-3

B Application of the phases to the treatment of Alice.

Acupuncture Microsystems

All of the various microsystems that are used in Chinese medicine are relatively modern developments, although some of them are based on classical theory. Essentially, maps of the body or of the organ systems are drawn on various body parts and then these body parts can be used to treat the entire system. They may be used in one of three ways: Chinese medicine theory may be applied to the choice of points (that is, for a diagnosis of spleen *qi* vacuity, the spleen and stomach points in a given system might be chosen); biomedical knowledge may be applied to the choice of points (that is, if there is a problem with the endocrine system, then the endocrine point in a given system might be chosen); or, they might be used symptomatically (that is, if there is pain in the back and knees then the back and knee points in a given system might be chosen). Many different microsystems have been developed. Below, four of the more commonly used systems are discussed.

Scalp Acupuncture

Standard acupuncture theory posits that all of the *qi* of the organs rises to the head via the various different channel pathways, thus the flourishing of *qi* and blood is reflected in the head. In the 1950s and 1960s, using knowledge gained from cerebral cortex mapping, a system of acupuncture was developed to treat central nervous system conditions. The system, shown in **A**, is one of the earliest systems to be developed. Over the past 50+ years, other systems have also developed. This system appears to be quite useful for conditions such as post-stroke paralysis, Parkinson disease, and other conditions related to balance and movement.

Hand and Foot Acupuncture

We already know that all of the hand *yin* channels run from the chest to the hand where they meet the hand *yang* channels to return to the head, and that all of the foot *yang* channels travel from the head to the feet where they meet the foot *yin* channels and return to the chest and abdomen. Thus, the hands and feet are an important gathering and meeting place for *qi* and blood. The acupuncture systems of the hands and the feet use this information and, based on empirical evidence, areas of the hands and feet have been identified as especially beneficial for the treatment of specific symptoms. For example, on the hand, there is a toothache point, a heel point, and an oral ulcer point. The hand also has organ points and condition points (common cold, cough, and so on). These points are primarily used for acute conditions, but may, in combination with standard channel points, be used for chronic conditions (**B, C**).

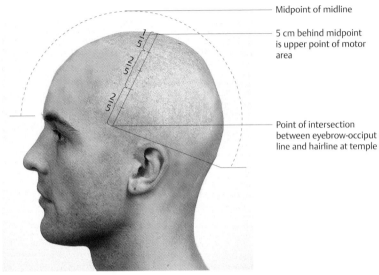

Midpoint of midline

5 cm behind midpoint is upper point of motor area

Point of intersection between eyebrow-occiput line and hairline at temple

A Scalp acupuncture.

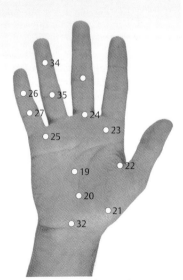

B Hand acupuncture. Palmar surface.

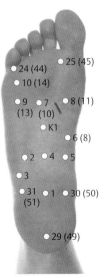

C Foot acupuncture.

Ear Acupuncture

Auricular or ear acupuncture is a widely used acupuncture microsystem. While its origins are essentially European it is now an integral part of Chinese acupuncture. It is also used around the world in supporting individuals experiencing substance abuse issues and post-traumatic stress.

Points on the ear, particularly on the tragus, are standard channel points. Although there is some evidence of the use of the auricle diagnostically and for limited applications of acupuncture and moxibustion, ear acupuncture cannot be said to have been part of classical Chinese acupuncture (Huang 1996).

In 1951, Dr. Paul Nogier, a French physician, encountered patients who had been treated for sciatica by burning (cautery) specific areas of the ear. These patients described relief from their symptoms (Nogier 1981, 1983). Nogier was intrigued and began what turned into a lifelong engagement with the therapeutic possibilities of stimulating the ear to treat medical conditions. He used a number of stimuli including acupuncture, which was well known in French medical circles due to the work of Soulié de Morant (1939 onwards). Nogier's critical insight was to describe a pattern of reflex areas that corresponded with an inverted homunculus of "little man" (**A**) that could be mapped onto the human ear.

Subsequent to its 1957 publication in Germany, his work was translated into Chinese and published in 1958. Based on earlier publications by Nogier and his work in China, the Beijing Academy of TCM published its version of an auricular acupuncture chart in 1977, blending Nogier's model with Chinese additions. From this point, auricular therapy can be said to be an important aspect of Chinese acupuncture.

Because of its roots, auricular acupuncture is typically used as a reflex system where areas on the ear are stimulated to address clinical problems in affected areas and organs. However, channel treatment paradigms can be incorporated by stimulating associated organ zones.

As a clinical example, recall our diabetic, chronic low back and knee pain patient, *John*, who has signs of kidney *yang* vacuity (see also Case Study pp. 198–199). Points would be selected on the ear and needled bilaterally. The areas associated with the lumbar vertebrae and knees would be examined for color changes, and gently probed to select areas for acupuncture. The kidney, heart, liver, endocrine, pancreas, and adrenal regions would also be needled. It is often the case that specific auricular points are selected and treated concurrently with standard channel points according to the diagnosis.

Ear acupuncture is used as an adjunct to group and behavioral therapies in supporting patients who are addressing substance abuse issues. Typically, what is known as the National Acupuncture Detoxification Association (NADA) protocol, ear points, *shen men*, liver, kidney, lung, and sympathetic, are needled bilaterally on a daily basis for a period of several weeks (**B**).

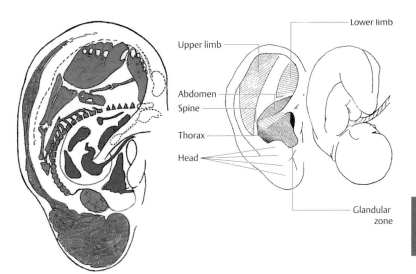

Upper limb

Abdomen

Spine

Thorax

Head

Lower limb

Glandular zone

A The auricle and the corresponding fetal image (© Raphael Nogier, reprinted by kind permission).

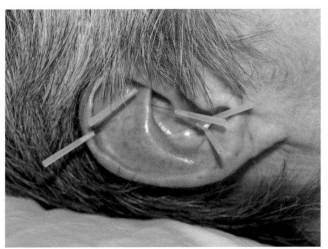

B Auricular acupuncture is typically done with 15mm needles that are placed at specific locations in the ear. Here the acupuncture points for the spirit *(shen men)*, the sympathetic nervous system, kidney, liver, and lung are needled to reduce stress and support physiological function.

➡ *Case Study John:*
69-year-old Male
with Chronic Low Back and
Knee Pain for 12 Years

Chronic low back and knee pain that developed gradually with no initial injury.

Description

Constant, low-level, fixed aching that is worse with exertion and fatigue and better with warmth and rest. It begins at the level of the second lumbar vertebrae and spreads over the left side of the back. There is one spot about 10 cm lateral to the spine, at the level of L4 that is particularly tender to palpation. The knee pain is in the anterior medial aspect of both knees. The knees are cold to the touch. *John* is overweight and has been diagnosed with diabetes, for which he takes insulin. He has difficulty controlling his glucose levels, and due to the diabetes, there is numbness in the toes and he gets toe blisters that take months to heal. *John*'s face is pale and he has large, puffy white bags under his eyes. His pulse is 62 bpm, deep and slippery. The tongue is swollen and pale with toothmarks and a thick white fur.

Diagnosis

Kidney *yang* vacuity and dampness causing low back and knee pain.

Treatment Principle and Method

Warm and invigorate kidney *yang*, transform damp and stop pain. Our most effective warming technique is moxibustion. Thus, we need to use moxibustion to warm the kidneys and the affected areas.

Prescription

To begin, we consider selecting points from the affected channels, including the urinary bladder, which traverses the back and travels the toes, the governing vessel, which travels up the spine, the spleen channel, which is important for transforming damp and traverses the knees, and the kidney channel to address the root condition and which also traverses the knees. The prescription that we will examine includes: BL-23, BL-52, GV-4, BL-32, a "That's It!" point on the back, BL-40, BL-60, SP-9, SI-3, and Ear Lower Back. This prescription has ten points (10 needles, GV-4 is not bilateral), moves the *qi* of the greater *yang*, and opens the governing vessel to stop pain. It treats the root through boosting the kidney *yang* and draining damp and it warms the *yang* with the use of moxibustion. It is balanced, addresses the root and the tip, and has local, adjacent, and distal points. Its overall function matches the treatment method and it is of an appropriate size (see **A**). *John*'s back pain is chronic and is due to a vacuity of the kidneys, therefore it is unlikely that it will completely resolve. With regular treatment, he should be able to remain active and to keep the pain level relatively mild.

➡ Case Study

Point Name and Number	Relevant Point Categories and Locations	Point Actions in the Prescription	Technique/Notes
BL-23 *Shen shu* 肾输 Kidney Transport	Local point Back transport point of the kidney Lies on the affected channel (BL)	Supports the movement of the channel *qi* Provides local relief Supplements the kidney and boosts essence Treats tip and root	Perpendicular insertion Supplementing technique Moxibustion to disperse cold and damp from the channel
BL-52 *Zhi shi* 志室 Will Chamber	Local Point Lies on the affected channel (BL)	Supports the movement of the channel *qi* Provides local relief Supplements the kidney and boosts essence Treats tip and root	Perpendicular insertion Supplementing technique Moxibustion to disperse cold and damp from the channel
GV-4 *Ming men* 命门 Life Gate	Local point Lies on the affected channel (GV)	Banks the origin and supplements the kidney Supports the movement of the channel *qi* Provides local relief Treats tip and root	Perpendicular insertion Supplementing technique Moxibustion to disperse cold and damp from the channel
BL-32 *Ci liao* 次廖 Second Bone Hole	Adjacent point	Opens the sacroiliac joint Supports the movement of the channel *qi* Provides local relief Treats the tip	Perpendicular insertion Neutral technique
"That's It" point	Local point at tender spot	Supports the movement of the channel *qi* Provides local relief Treats the tip	Perpendicular insertion Draining technique
BL-40 *Wei zhong* 委中 Bend Middle	Distal point Command point of the lower back Local point for knee pain	Supports the movement of the channel *qi* Provides local relief Treats the tip	Perpendicular insertion Strong draining stimulation
BL-60 *Kun lun* 昆仑 Kunlun Mountain	Distal point	Soothes the sinews and transforms damp Strengthens the lumbus and kidney Treats tip and root	Needle perpendicular through to KI-3 (*tai xi* 太溪 Great Ravine) thereby accessing the source point of the kidney
SP-9 *Yin ling quan* 阴陵泉 *Yin* Mound Spring	Distal point Sea point of the spleen	Transforms damp Provides local relief to the knee Treats tip and root	Perpendicular insertion Draining technique
SI-3 *Hou xi* 后溪 Back Ravine	Distal point on the arm Confluent point of the governing vessel	Balances the prescription upper and lower SI channel is hand greater *yang*; BL channel is foot greater *yang* SI points can move *qi* in the BL channel	Perpendicular insertion Neutral technique
Ear Lower Back	Microsystem point	Treats pain in the lower back	Draining technique

A Point selection for Case Study John.

→ *Case Study Alice:*
   23-year-old Female with Severe
   Dysmenorrhea for Eight Years

Every month, on day 27, she gets a bad headache, located at her temples. The first two days of menstruation are extremely painful. About one week prior to menstruation, she experiences breast tenderness, a feeling of tightness in her chest, and extremely labile emotions. The tongue is slightly purple and has stasis macules on the sides with a normal, thin white fur. The pulse is 72 bpm, stringlike, rough and forceful.

Diagnosis

Qi and blood stagnation in the liver and gallbladder channels causing menstrual pain.

Treatment Principle and Method

Move *qi* and blood in the liver and gallbladder channels to stop head pain and prevent painful menstruation. Here, we must consider that treatment will change depending upon where *Alice* is in her menstrual cycle. The focus remains on moving the *qi* and blood to stop pain, but this is mediated by whether she is about to begin menstruating or has just completed menstruating. For the sake of simplicity, let us assume that *Alice* is on day 27 of her cycle. She is experiencing pre-menstrual tension and has a headache.

Channel Involvement

The liver is responsible for moving *qi* and blood in the body, and it controls menstruation. When it fails to do its job correctly, *qi* and blood stagnation can result. The liver channel traverses the external genitalia, the lower abdomen, and the ribs, and travels up to the head. It is internally/externally associated with the gallbladder, which covers the sides of the head and the temples, traverses the ribs, and crosses the lower abdomen on its way to the toes. The penetrating vessel is also closely associated with menstruation and the spleen manages the blood as it moves through the vessels, thus points associated with these channels are chosen.

Prescription

The points chosen are: LI-4, LR-3, PC-6, SP-4, CV-17, BL-17, SP-8, GB-34, *tai yang*, Infant's Palace, Ear Liver, Ear Uterus, and Ear Endocrine. Although slightly large, if we needle LI-4/LR-3 contralaterally and PC-6/SP-4 contralaterally on the opposite sides, we will reduce the number of needles to 21. In this prescription we have chosen local, adjacent, and distal points and we have treated the root (the *qi* and blood stagnation) and the tip (the pain). The prescription is balanced upper and lower, left to right, and *yin* to *yang*. It is focused on relieving the headache and menstrual pain so that when *Alice*'s period arrives in the next 1–2 days, she should not experience as much pain as she usually does. *Alice*'s condition will not be fully relieved after one treatment. She will need to continue treatment for 3–5 months (see **A**).

➡ **Case Study**

Point Name and Number	Relevant Point Categories and Locations	Point Actions in the Prescription
LI-4 *He gu* 合谷 Union Valley	Distal point Command point of the face and mouth	Relieves pain and quiets the spirit: headache, pre-menstrual tension Together with LR-3, this point strongly moves *qi* Treats the headache Treats tip and root
LR-3 *Tai chong* 太冲 Supreme Surge	Distal point Source point of the liver Earth point	Soothes the liver and rectifies *qi*: liver *qi* stagnation Together with LI-4, this point strongly moves the *qi* As the earth point it keeps the liver from over-controlling the spleen Treats tip and root
SP-4 *Gong sun* 公孙 Yellow Emperor	Distal point Confluent point of the penetrating vessel	Regulates the sea of blood and harmonizes the penetrating vessel for menstrual pain Supports the spleen and stomach Treats root
PC-6 *Nei guan* 内关 Inner Pass	Distal point Confluent point of the *yin* linking vessel, paired with the penetrating vessel	Clears heat and eliminates vexation to reduce premenstrual tension On the hand reverting *yin* channel, connected to the liver foot reverting *yin* channel it opens the chest and soothes the liver Treats root
CV-17 *Shan zhong* 膻中 Chest Center	Adjacent point Influential point of *qi*	Regulates *qi* in the body Calms the spirit Treats tip and root
BL-17 *Ge shu* 膈俞 Diaphragm Transport	Adjacent point Influential point of blood	Rectifies vacuity and detriment to nourish and supplement the blood as well as move the blood Treats root
SP-8 *Di ji* 地机 Earth's Crux	Distal point Cleft point of the spleen	Harmonizes the spleen and rectifies the blood Harmonizes the womb Treats pain in the uterus and lower burner Treats tip
GB-34 *Yang ling quan* 阳陵泉 *Yang* Mound Spring	Distal point *Yang* channel point on the lower body to balance *yin* and *yang*	Moves *qi* in the liver and gallbladder Treats root
Infant's Palace *Zi gong* 子宫	Local point Extra point to treat the uterus and ovaries	Moves *qi* in the lower burner and relieves pain Treats tip
Tai yang	Local point Extra point located on the temple	Clears the head for lateral headaches Treats tip
Ear Liver	Microsystem point	Soothes the liver
Ear Uterus	Microsystem point	Regulates the uterus
Ear Endocrine	Microsystem point	Regulates the endocrine system

A Point selection for Case Study Alice.

➜ Case Study Jeremy: 45-year-old Male with an Acute Cold

Jeremy has been receiving acupuncture for treatment of fatigue due to overwork. On this visit he arrives with an acute cold. His symptoms include a sore throat, a sensation of heat that easily transforms into cold after sweating. His nose is stuffy, but it is difficult to expel any phlegm. When there is visible phlegm, it is slightly yellow. His body is sore, his eyes red, and he is fatigued. His tongue has not changed from its previous presentation, which is slightly pale, swollen, and tooth-marked, but his pulse is slightly rapid (82 bpm) and floating at the lung position.

Diagnosis

External invasion of wind–heat causing common cold.

Treatment Principle and Method

Resolve the exterior by effusing sweat, release toxins, and protect the lung.

Channel Involvement

As discussed earlier, when an evil invades the body, it first encounters the cutaneous and/or the sinew channels. When the evil is at this level of the body, the defense *qi* rises to the surface to battle with the evil *qi*. This is what causes the sensation of cold and heat that transforms into each other, as well as the floating pulse. The tongue has not changed because the evil has not been present long enough. Our job at this visit is to expel the evil from the exterior and prevent it from moving further into the interior, to the regular channels or the organs.

Prescription

Based on the presentation, our point prescription includes: LU-1, BL-13, GB-20, LI-4, KI-7, LU-5, LI-11, TB-5, and ST-36. We will also bleed LI-1/LU-11 and perform cupping on the upper back. Because this is an acute condition, the needles will only remain in for about 15 minutes. After removing the needles, LU-11 (*shao shang*/Lesser *Shang* 少商) and LI-1 (*shang yang* 商阳), the well points of the lung and large intestine channels are pricked to release a few drops of blood. As the well points, these are heat-clearing points. Bleeding will release heat quickly and relieve the sore throat almost immediately. Finally, we turn the patient over and apply cups to the upper chest. This will help release the evil from the exterior, and stop cough and transform phlegm. *Jeremy* should feel immediate relief from many of his symptoms and with a day or two of rest, feel healthy again. While we all eventually recover from colds, it is important to treat colds by resolving the exterior and dispelling the evil so that the evil does not lodge in the exterior or travel interiorly and cause further problems (see **A**).

→ **Case Study**

Point Name and Number	Relevant Point Categories and Locations	Point Actions in the Prescription	Technique/ Notes
LU-1 *Zhong fu* 中府 Central Treasury	Local point Alarm point of the lung channel	Clears and diffuses the upper burner and courses lung qi Used in combination with BL-13 (alarm and transport combination)	Oblique insertion
BL-13 *Fei shu* 肺输 Lung Transport	Local point Back transport point of the lung	With LU-1, diffuses the lung *qi* and boosts and protects the lung	Oblique insertion
GB-20 *Feng chi* 风池 Wind Pool	Adjacent	Courses wind and clears heat, and clears the head and opens the orifices	Oblique insertion
LI-4 *He gu* 合谷 Union Valley	Distal point Source point of the large intestine	Courses wind and resolves the exterior Clears and discharges lung heat Regulate sweat pores	Strong stimulation until sweat effuses
KI-7 *Fu liu* 付溜 Recover Flow	Distal river point of the kidney channel	Regulate sweat pores	Strong stimulation until sweat effuses
LU-5 *Chi ze* 尺泽 Cubit Marsh	Uniting point of the lung channel	Clears heat from the lung and stops cough	Perpendicular insertion
LI-11 *Qu chi* 曲池 Pool at the Bend	Uniting point of the large intestine channel	Resolves the exterior and courses evil heat	Perpendicular insertion
TB-5 *Wai guan* 外关 Outer Pass	Confluent point of the *yang* linking vessel	Dissipates wind and resolves the exterior, especially in cases of wind–heat	Perpendicular insertion
ST-6 *Zu san li* 足三里 Leg Three *Li*	Supports the correct and banks up the origin Dispels pathogens and prevents disease	Boost the right *qi* Prevents the evil from damaging the right *qi* and also helps the right *qi* to dispel the evil before it can move any further interior	Perpendicular insertion

A Point selection for Case Study Jeremy.

5

Tui Na

Michael McCarthy and Kevin V. Ergil

Introduction

Chinese therapeutic bodywork or massage is typically referred to as *tui na* (推拿), literally meaning "pushing and grasping," or *anmo* (按摩), literally meaning "pressing and rubbing." They are terms that are often used interchangeably though they are essentially distinguished by the harder and more forceful deep tissue movements and manipulations of the Chinese therapeutic bodywork referred to as *tui na* and the more gentle stroking and kneading movements referred to as *anmo*. In general, the term *tui na* refers to all aspects of Chinese therapeutic bodywork. *Tui na* encompasses a very broad collection of therapeutic methods, including massage, manual stimulation of acupuncture points, and manipulations of bones, joints, and soft tissue. Chinese medicine theory, and particularly acupuncture and channel theory, form the conceptual basis for most aspects of *tui na* therapeutics. There are also many points of intersection with the traditional practice of "bone righting" (*zheng gu*), or "bone setting," the traditional orthopedics of TCM, and with the use of topical or external therapies, since these are often used for treatment in conjunction with *tui na*. The language of contemporary orthopedics and physiatry also inform the practice since *tui na* can be involved with the correction of sprains, dislocations, and other musculoskeletal problems.

Tui na is applied to specific areas of the body, and the techniques can be quite forceful and intense. *Tui na* is applied routinely for orthopedic and neurological conditions (**A**). It would be a mistake, however, to view Chinese massage as concerned only with the musculoskeletal system since its therapeutic techniques are applied to acupuncture points and channels to influence the viscera and bowels towards the end of correcting internal disorders. *Tui na* is used in conditions that might not be thought of as susceptible to treatment through manipulation, such as asthma, dysmenorrhea, chronic gastritis, and others (**B**).

These methods have been practiced at least as long as moxibustion, if not longer, and like acupuncture, massage has a rich history in Chinese medical practice. Given the practical implications of the skills associated with Chinese massage it is not surprising that it has a strong relationship with martial arts traditions in China where massage and bone-setting techniques are used in first aid and rehabilitation. As with all aspects of Chinese medicine, regional styles and family lineages of practice abound, and this is particularly true in the case of massage given its association with martial arts traditions.

The first modern massage training class was created in Shanghai in 1956 (Wang et al. 1990, p.16), coincident with the national project of professionalizing and institutionalizing the education and practice of acupuncture and Chinese medicine in China. While massage is an important part of the professional practice of Chinese medicine, there are also many practice traditions outside of institutional settings.

Medical
– internal medicine
– orthopedics & physical medicine
– neurology
– gynecology
– pediatrics
Health promotion/wellness
Self-care
Athletic training

A Applications of *tui na*.

Orthopedics	Acute lumbar sprain, cervical spondolyopathy, semi-dislocation of sacroiliac joint, sprains of wrist and ankle joint, stiff neck
Internal Medicine	Abdominal pain, asthma, Bell's palsy, chronic gastritis, common cold, constipation, diarrhea, duodenal ulcer, dysmenorrheal, epigastric pain, epilepsy, gastric ulcer, gastroptosis, headache, hiccough, insomnia, mastitis, myopia, primary hypertension, ribside pain, sunstroke, vertigo, vomiting,
Pediatrics	Abdominal pain, asthma, common cold, constipation, cough, diarrhea, enuresis, fever, food stagnation, vomiting

B Conditions treated with *tui na*.

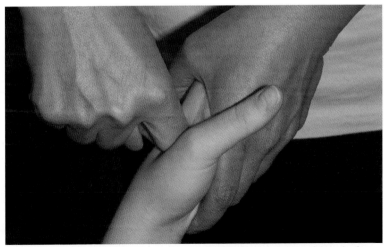

C Pointing *(dian fa)* is applied to the acupuncture point LI-4 using the joint of the index finger. This application relieves head and face pain, treats pain generally, and is used to support digestion.

Physical Preparation of the Practitioner

Tui na training is a component of acupuncture training programs because, despite its distinctiveness as a technique, its practice can be seen as an extension of the acupuncture paradigm. *Tui na* can range from being a minor component of a traditional medical education to being an area of full clinical specialization. While *tui na* can be used as an adjunct to acupuncture treatment, for example, to increase the range of motion of a joint, or instead of acupuncture when needles are uncomfortable or inappropriate, such as pediatric applications, it can also be used independently for many conditions. In the same way, acupuncture can be used as an adjunct to *tui na*.

A distinct aspect of *tui na* is its physicality. Clinically, this emerges in the extensive training of the hands that is necessary for clinical practice. The practitioner's hands are trained to accomplish focused and precise movements that can be applied to various areas of the body. Techniques such as pushing, rolling, kneading, rubbing, and grasping are practiced repetitively until they become second nature to the practitioner. Students practice on a small bag of rice until their hands have developed the necessary strength and dexterity.

Tui na is an active and demanding therapeutic activity and its practitioners typically undertake exercises to increase their stamina and flexibility, cultivate their *qi*, and improve the dexterity and strength of their hands.

Whilst all of these attributes are valued in the practice of acupuncture, especially hand strength and *qi* cultivation, the strenuous and repetitive movements of *tui na*, as well as the need to support and move patients, makes stamina and strength critical in its practice.

"*Lian gong*," literally meaning "practice skill," refers to the training practices that are used to prepare the practitioner of *tui na*. Exercises, which are also found within the martial arts traditions and physically active *qi gong* traditions, are used by students and practitioners to strengthen their bodies and cultivate their *qi*. Practices such as sinew transforming exercises (*yi jin jing*), the Shaolin internal cultivation practices (*shao lin nei gong*) and others, supply the exercises that are used. These exercises coordinate breath, attention, stance, and movement to build the combination of strength and flexibility to support both practice and training (**A**).

After learning and becoming adept at the physical exercises, hand training is the next step. Chinese massage employs a wide range of movements and manipulations that require mastery in application, dexterity, repetitive relaxed and repetitive fluid movement, and often, rapid or forceful movement. Prior to clinical practice, rice-filled practice bags about the size of a child's bean bag (15 cm by 30 cm) are used to practice many of the hand techniques. Students may be told to practice on a bag of rice until the rice grains themselves are reduced to powder (**B**).

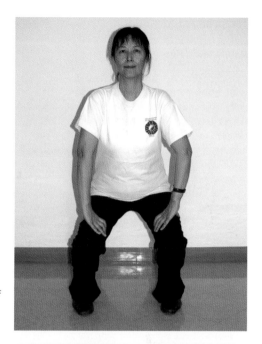

A Practitioner demonstrating the "horse stance." This is one of the many postures that is used to cultivate the practitioner's *qi* and stamina for *tui na* practice.

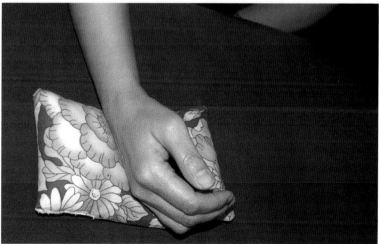

B *Tui Na* **hand movements require diligent practice.** Here a student practices "rolling" on a practice pad filled with grains of rice.

Therapeutic Techniques

Hand Movements

Pushing (*tui*) (**A**) can be carried out with many parts of the practitioner's body. The thumb, the palm, the exposed joints of a fist, or an elbow can be used to push along a muscle generally along the pathway of the channels. The choice between thumb and elbow depends on the area to be treated, the size of the patient, the disorder to be treated, and other factors. This method promotes the movement of *qi* by removing impediments or blockages of *qi* in the channels, thus stopping pain.

Grasping (*na*) (**B**) involves holding a muscle or tendon between the thumb and forefinger or all of the fingers, then slightly lifting and releasing the tissue. This movement is repeated with varying degrees of force, but always with a rhythmic and fluid movement. Grasping can be used on the nape of the neck, the shoulders, the trunk, anterior and posterior, and over the four limbs. Its application is used to treat external evils that may have entered the surface, to clear impediments from the channels, and to relax muscle or other tissue contraction or spasm. Together the names of these two techniques give the eponymous term *tui na*.

An fa, the pressing method (**C**), uses the thumb or palm to exert a focused steady pressure on an acupuncture point or area of the body. This steady pressure can be used to allow the muscles to progressively relax or to provide needed stimulus to a specific acupuncture point. This can range from light pressure to quite heavy pressure depending on the location being treated.

Mo fa, the round-rubbing method (**D**) uses the tips of the fingers or the palm heel of the hands to provide a gentle, or forceful stimulus to various parts of the body. It disperses congested *qi* and blood, producing the effect of rectifying the *qi* and quickening the blood. The method can be used in the area of CV-17 on the sternum to open the *qi* of the chest and reduce feelings of anxiety, or on the abdomen to normalize digestive function. Together, pressing and round-rubbing give us the term *anmo*, the other name for Chinese massage.

Dian fa, the pointing or dotting method (**E**), can be used to provide a very forceful stimulus to a small area. The tip of the index finger or middle finger, the joint of the thumb, or the second interphalangeal joint of the second or third finger can be used. The joint is protruded and its hard surface is pressed into the body. The technique is used to treat soreness, pain, or to eliminate wind.

Rou fa, the kneading method (**F**) is where the practitioner uses gentle pressure with the finger tips, thenar eminence, or palm, and pressing with a slight circular or kneading motion. Unlike a rubbing method the hand does not travel across the surface of the body; unlike a hitting method the hand does not leave the surface of the body, and unlike pressing there is no forceful pressing.

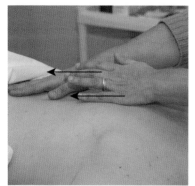

A Pushing.

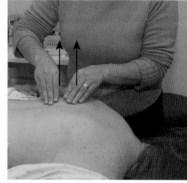

B Grasping.

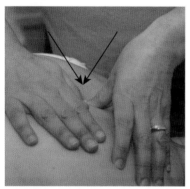

C Pressing.

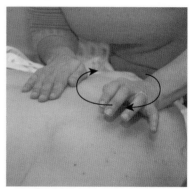

D Round rubbing.

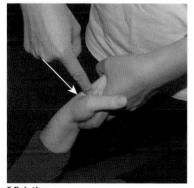

E Pointing.

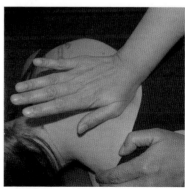

F Kneading.

Yi zhi chan tui fa (枝禅推法), the one-digit meditative pushing method, involves holding the hand in a loose fist with the thumb pointed downwards and pressing into the area to be treated and then gently and rhythmically moving the forearm back and forth, causing the thumb to oscillate. The movement involves relaxed and coordinated movement of the upper arm, lower arm, hand, and thumb. Once the optimal posture and hand positions have been achieved by the practitioner, then the movement is practiced extensively so that it can be applied effortlessly, often in a sequence with other movements. The technique itself has a wide variety of applications. Because it is used to provide moderate, but deep stimulation to acupuncture points, often producing sensations of *qi* moving along channel pathways, it can be very useful in helping to correct visceral function and bowel function depending on the points chosen for stimulation.

Gun fa (滚法), the rolling method, is a hard maneuver for beginners to grasp; it involves the steady rhythmic rolling of the ulnar edge of the hand (the minor thenar eminence) by alternately flexing and extending the forearm at the elbow while keeping the wrist loose. Gaining the ability to deliver fluid and forceful stimulus without jerkiness or fatigue requires substantial practice. The technique is used on areas of the body with large muscles such as the trapezius in the shoulder, the erector spinae muscles of the back, and the large muscle groups of the limbs. It is not used on the head, the face, the chest, or the abdominal areas. The method is useful for treating wind, or wind–cold, warming the channels, for quickening the blood to remove stasis, and for a variety of musculoskeletal and neurological conditions.

Hand movements can be combined in a variety of ways. They may be applied successively, as in pointing or pressing specific acupuncture points followed by kneading and pressing, or they can be applied in quick alternation, or simultaneously to different areas of the body.

Manipulation

Techniques (**A**) such as the back-carrying method, the rotation method, the twisting method, the grasping method (**B**) and the pulling-extending method, are manipulations that are used to restore a range of movement to a joint or to correct the alignment of the joint itself. Back carrying is used to hyperextend the patient's back to release the lumbar vertebrae. Rotation involves inducing passive movement around the affected joint, for instance the shoulder or hip, to increase range of movement, increase circulation, and free adhesions. Twisting can be applied to adjust the relationship of cervical, thoracic, and lumbar vertebrae.

Name	Chinese	Method
an fa	按法	pressing method
ba shen fa	拔伸法	pulling-extending method
ban fa	板法	twisting method
bei fa	背法	back-carrying method
ca fa	擦法	scrubbing method
cuo fa	搓法	foulage method
dian fa	点法	pointing method
dou fa	抖法	shaking method
gun fa	滚法	rolling method
ji fa	击法	tapping method
ma fa	抹法	wiping method
mo fa	摩法	round-rubbing method
na fa	拿法	grasping method
nian fa	捻法	twirling method
nie fa	捏法	pinching method
pai fa	拍法	patting method
rou fa	揉法	kneading method
tan fa	弹法	flicking method
tui fa	推法	pushing method
yao fa	摇法	rotating method
yi zhi chan tui fa	一枝禅推法	one-digit meditation pushing method
zhen fa	振法	vibrating method

A Therapeutic techniques.

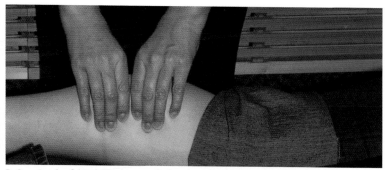

B Grasping *(na fa)* is shown here applied to the calf. This application addresses calf pain and tension and pain in the lower back.

Clinical Applications of Tui Na

Alice, the 23-year-old woman with dysmenorrhea, is familiar to us from earlier chapters. Her diagnosis is *qi* and blood stagnation in the liver and gallbladder channel causing menstrual pain. *Tui na* therapy would involve kneading, a gentle and slow circular pressure applied without rubbing, using the fingers in this case to provide a focused stimulus. Kneading is applied to CV-3 and CV-4, two points on the controlling vessel below the navel that are used to regulate the menses. Kneading is applied to the points SP-8 and SP-10 as well, both of which are used to treat painful menses. SP-8 lies on the inner side of the leg below the knee, and is primarily used for dysmenorrhea. SP-10 has an action of regulating the menses and quickening the blood. Finally, the fingers can be used to knead the sacral foramen, which is found at BL-32 to help relieve pain and discomfort. *Qi* stagnation is addressed by applying pointing and vibrating techniques (without force) to the Sea of *Qi* (CV-17) located on the sternum at the level of the nipples. This approach is used to help mobilize *qi* throughout the body.

Supplementary treatment can be given at other points as well. In some cases, a liquid medium prepared from herbs such as *Gao Ben* (ligusticum root/ Chinese lovage root) and *Dang Gui* (*tang kuai*/Angelica sinensis), which act to quicken the blood and relieve menstrual pain, can be used during the manipulation so that the effects of the herbs can be transmitted directly to the affected channels (Sun 1990, p.224). The areas chosen to treat this condition with massage have some similarities to locations for acupuncture treatment, but also with some quite significant differences.

The application of *tui na* to impotence is first approached through pattern differentiation. In the case of insufficiency of the "life gate fire" (or kidney *yang* vacuity), there are signs of dizziness, fatigue, weakness, and soreness of the lower back and knees, a pale face and tongue, and a deep and fine pulse. These are familiar signs of cold and vacuity affecting regions associated with the kidney. Treatment involves two approaches to stimulation. First, a range of stimulating hand techniques are applied over areas of the body associated with the kidney and larger areas associated with the channel pathways. Techniques such as pushing, pinching, grasping, pressing, and kneading are used along the path of the urinary bladder, the *yang* organ of the kidney, which traverses the back (**A**). Scrubbing and rolling the lower back, which is closely associated with the kidney can also be indicated. The "cinnabar field" (*dan tian*) below the umbilicus relates to reproductive function and the health of the kidney in both men and women. A vibrating technique with the palms can be used to improve its function. Treatment can also be applied to additional acupuncture points such as GV-4, BL-31 to BL-34 found on the lumbus, sacrum, and legs (ibid., p.190).

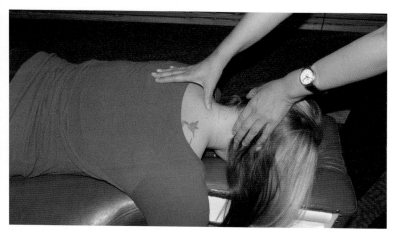

A Patient receiving *tui na* on the back. A patient receives pushing or *tui* along the upper portion of the urinary bladder channel. This technique improves the flow of *qi* and blood in the affected region and is used to relieve muscular tension and spasm, to release external evils, and to affect other regions of the body traversed by the internal and external pathways of the channel.

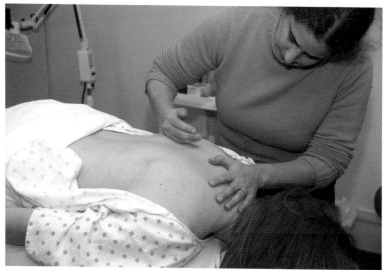

B Rolling involves a smooth continuous movement that can be seen to produce a dynamic pressure along the tissue where it is applied. Here it is used to remove stagnation and stasis from the area of the trapezius muscle and the sinew channels associated with the region.

Pediatrics

Pediatric applications (**A**) of *tui na* massage are now quite common. In fact, it is becoming something of a specialty in itself. Whilst acupuncture can be used on children with good effect there is no question that a needle-free approach is much more appealing to young children. The ability of *tui na* to regulate and move *qi* and blood, and to disperse evils without the use of potentially frightening invasive techniques makes this form of therapy very useful for children. Because children's bodies are still developing, it is considered that their channels and organs respond readily and rapidly to gentler therapies and simple manipulations.

While pediatric massage derives from traditional channel theory and point selection, coupled with standard *tui na* techniques, these are specifically adapted to the physiology and physical structure of children. Techniques are typically more gentle and limited. Specific regions are identified as particularly appropriate to pediatric patients.

Conditions such as cough, asthma, nausea and vomiting, abdominal pain, food stagnation, diarrhea or constipation, bedwetting, near-sightedness (myopia), and night terrors as they appear in children are among the conditions considered to be suitable for treatment with *tui na*.

For example, the treatment of abdominal pain in a child would involve a basic strategy of rubbing the abdomen with the palm of the hand and gently kneading the umbilicus and grasping the area lateral to and below the umbilicus. Channel points related to the spleen and stomach on the urinary bladder are pressed, and ST-36 on the leg below the knee is pressed and kneaded to normalize stomach function, reduce pain, and cause the descent of *qi*. Depending on the precise cause of the abdominal pain, pattern differentiation is used to guide the selection of other areas for stimulation.

Self-massage

The practice of self-help methods is an intrinsic part of *tui na* therapy especially with its close association with *tai ji* and *qi gong*. So self-massage with movement and meditative breathing exercises can be used in the development and maintenance of health, in the treatment of disease, and in rehabilitation (**B**). Therefore, with *tui na* as part of the practice of Chinese medicine, patients can be taught to carry out simple exercises in between visits to supplement the effects of acupuncture, *tui na*, or herbal treatment.

Qi gong and *tui na* work very well together and while they are related by the paradigm of channels and *qi*, *tui na* self-treatment focuses on directed physical stimulus where *qi gong* uses breath and mental activity to coordinate the movement of *qi*. However, a number of *qi gong* or self-massage techniques incorporate both elements, coupling breath control, posture, the intentional movement of *qi*, and direct physical stimulation of acupuncture points and channels, which can be very effective in improving the *qi* dynamic.

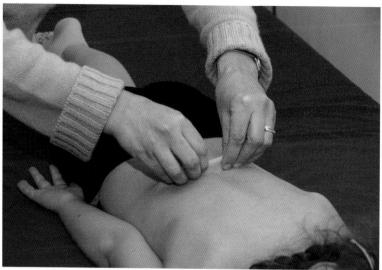

A Pediatric *tui na*. The pinching method is applied to the back to stimulate the transport points on the urinary bladder channel.

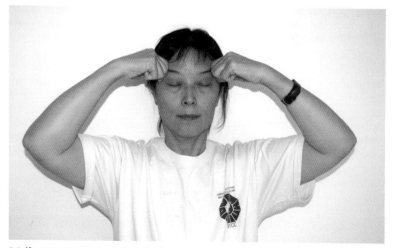

B Self-massage. A simple method of self-massage for stress reduction involves gentle stimulation of areas of the head, patting the vertex, pressing and kneading acupuncture points on the occipital area and on the forehead, and then pressing and kneading the points HT-7 on the wrist, SP-6 on the ankle, and KI-1 on the sole of the foot. Massaging the head opens the channels and collaterals and the stimulus to the distal points calms the spirit and causes *qi* to descend.

Bone Righting

"Bone righting" (*zheng gu*) or "bone setting," involves the reduction of fractures and the correction of dislocations with manipulation. While the techniques and resources of modern orthopedics, especially imaging, are routinely applied in the integrated Chinese medical settings, there are many aspects of traditional bone righting that are unique, distinctive, and clinically important. Conditions such as a fracture of the radius or ulna can be set using conventional or traditional methods and supported by imaging if necessary. However, these and other fractures can benefit from the traditional methods of local strapping. These lightweight methods of stabilizing a fracture immobilize the fracture using light splints and slings. Unlike a full cast, this permits the *tui na* practitioner to access points in the area of injury to stimulate the healing response. It also allows the patient to engage in limited exercise and movement, thus potentially reducing the muscular atrophy associated with casting. Because the interruption of the flow of *qi* and blood is considered detrimental to local tissue and the health of the body, methods that preserve maximum mobility and allow the free movement of *qi* and blood are highly valued.

For instance, an acute ankle sprain, without dislocation or fracture, is managed with a range of gentle pressing techniques applied to local and distal points. This treatment will reduce swelling and pain and, combined with kneading and pushing of the affected area will reduce swelling and improve local circulation (**A**). Acupuncture may also be used. Because of the marked effects of acupuncture and *tui na* in reducing swelling, ice is often avoided in the management of this type of injury because it can cause local stasis of *qi* and blood. In the late stages of an ankle sprain, massage may be used to disperse bruising, increase the rate at which function is restored, and where necessary break up adhesions.

Topical Preparations

Topical preparations play a significant role in Chinese massage. Preparations such as liniments, ointments, oils, and washes may be used in their own right or as a therapeutic medium in combination with massage. Poultices are used in traumatic injury. Depending on the condition, and the needs of the patient, soaks, plasters, poultices, and liniments are used. Often internal herbal formulas are used as well.

In the case of an injury such as the sprained ankle discussed above, the early treatment involves clearing the heat of inflammation while quickening blood to avoid blood stasis. Appropriate poultices offer a useful alternative to icing since they can address local inflammation while quickening the blood (**B**). As the injury heals, poultices and liniments that warm and quicken the blood are used to promote healing and eliminate stagnant blood.

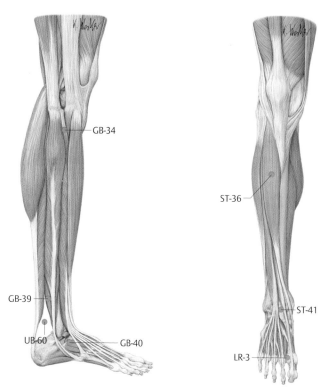

A Diagram of the ankle showing points to be pressed and kneaded, using finger techniques, for ankle sprain. (From THIEME Atlas of Anatomy, General Anatomy and Musculoskeletal System, © Thieme 2005, Illustration by Karl Wesker.)

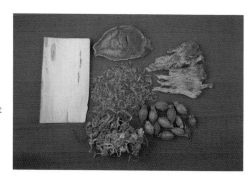

B Poultice ingredients to be ground and mixed with tea and applied at the early stages of sprain. The ingredients shown (from the top clockwise) are rhubarb *(da huang)*, scutellaria root *(huang qin)*, gardenia fruit *(zhi zi)*, dandelion *(pu gong ying)*, phellodendron bark *(huang bai)*, and (in the center) carthamus *(hong hua)*.

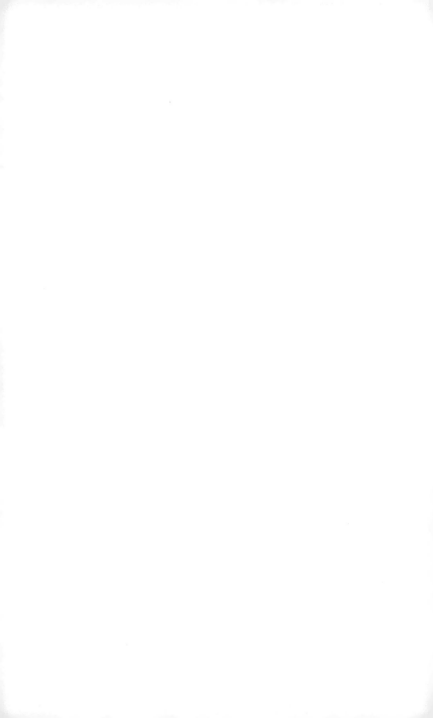

6

Traditional Chinese Pharmacotherapy

Simon Becker

The traditional pharmacotherapy of China is referred to in the West as "Chinese Herbal Medicine (CHM)." From the Chinese point of view, it is Chinese medicine. It is the primary therapeutic method among important, but secondary, practices such as acupuncture and *tui na*. Chinese medicine uses a wide variety of plant, animal, and mineral materials. Although it is common in the West to write about "Chinese herbs," the strict interpretation of "herbs" does not include animal or mineral materials, or even all plant parts. The Chinese themselves refer to *yao* (药) or drugs when they discuss the contents of the traditional materia medica and specify *cao yao* (草药) or plant drugs when discussing drugs of plant origin. Traditional Chinese pharmacotherapy or "herbal" medicine consists of the use of these medicinal agents singly, or, more often, in combination, in the context of the diagnostic and therapeutic theories of Chinese medicine. Where the term "herb" appears in this chapter it is in the broader sense of any substance in the materia medica.

This chapter discusses the historical development of the knowledge base of Chinese pharmacotherapy, the organization of individual substances in relation to traditional theory, and then examines the use of these medicinals in formulas. Where applicable, the clinical cases presented earlier will be used to illustrate the application of formulas.

Historical Overview

The earliest records of Chinese pharmacotherapy date to the late Zhou dynasty through the Han dynasty (see pp. 3, 12). The oldest extant work, *Formulas for 52 Diseases (Wu Shi Er Bing Fang)*, was found recently in the Ma Wang tombs (see also p. 28–29). In addition to therapeutic techniques such as moxa, stone therapy, cupping, and spells, it lists 170 medicinal formulas with 247 different ingredients. The formulas and treatments are arranged according to different illnesses. Another collection of formulas was found in West and Northwest China early in the 20th century. On 92 bamboo slabs, 30 formulas consisting of 100 different medicinals were discussed. These texts list complex formulas containing from five to 15 different substances and discuss delivery methods, such as powders, pills, drops, and even suppositories, and the use of vehicles such as honey, lard, milk, and camel cheese (Unschuld 1986, p. 16). Neither of the two works engages basic medicinal theory or single medicinal substances. The first work to do that, *The Divine Husbandman's Materia Medica (Shen Nong Ben Cao)* was written in the late Han dynasty (p. 29).

From antiquity to the 19th century, over 2605 titles devoted to medical theory, formulas, and medicinals have been written (**A**). A short discussion of the most outstanding and important of these works provides a brief illustration of the development of Chinese pharmacotherapy over the past two millennia.

30 formulas and 100 medicinals on 92 bamboo slabs

Wu Shi Er Bing Fang
(Formulas for 52 Diseases)

Shang Han Za Bing Lun
(Treatise On Cold Damage and Miscellaneous Diseases)
including *Shang Han Lun* (On Cold Damage) and *Jing Gui Yao Lue* (Essential Prescriptions of the Golden Coffer)

Shen Nong Ben Cao
(The Divine Husbandman's Materia Medica)

Ben Cao Jing Ji Zhu
(Collective Notes to the Classic of Materia Medica)

Qian Jin Fang
(Thousand Gold Pieces Prescriptions)

Xin Xiu Ben Cao
(Newly revised Materia Medica)

Tai Ping Hui Min He Ji Ju Fang
(Imperial Grace Formulary of the Taiping Era)

Pi Wei Lun
(Discussion of Spleen and Stomach)

Dan Xi Xin Fa
(The Heart Method of Zhu Dan Xi)

Ben Cao Gang Mu
(Comprehensive Herbal Foundation)

Zhong Yao Da Ci Dian
(Great Dictionary of Chinese Medicinals)

Zhong Hua Ben Cao
(Chinese Materia Medica)

Timeline: -200, 0, 200, 500, 1200, 1600, 2000

A Important works in Chinese pharmacotherapy.

The Divine Husbandman's Materia Medica is the *locus classicus* of Chinese pharmacotherapy. It is attributed to Shen Nong, one of the three legendary emperors who is said to have tasted plants and thus encountered their medicinal effectiveness and identified potential toxicities (p. 4–5).

The Divine Husbandman's Materia Medica discusses the basic theory of herbal medicine including: the five flavors and the temperatures; the different ranks in formula combinations and different methods of preparations such as pills, powders, water decoctions, wines, and pastes. Even the correct time to take medicines is specified:

> "In case of illness located above the diaphragm, the medications should be taken after meals. For illnesses situated below the diaphragm, medications should be taken before meals. If the illness is located in the four limbs or in the blood vessels, the medications ought to be taken in the morning on an empty stomach. If the illness is in the bones, the medication should be taken at night after eating." (Yang 1998, p. ix)

The Divine Husbandman's Materia Medica discusses a total of 365 substances divided into three classes: an upper class, a middle class, and a lower class (**A**). Upper class medicinals are:

> "non-toxic medicinals that are able to nurture life and therefore bestow longevity … middle class medicinals are able to cultivate personality or modify temperament … [they] may be toxic [and] their formula

requires care. [Lower] class medicinals specifically treat disease. These substances, due to toxicity and other factors, cannot be taken in large amounts or for prolonged periods of time (Yang 1998 p. ix)."

The Divine Husbandman's Materia Medica includes medicinals from the plant, animal, and mineral kingdoms, a few coming from as far as Vietnam and Korea. For each medicinal entry, the identification, taste, temperature, functions and indications, secondary names, as well as the specific or general name of origin, are discussed (**B**).

Besides the mythical Shen Nong, two other authors must be mentioned in an overview of Chinese Pharmacotherapy. The first, Tao Hong Jing, born in 456, expanded *The Divine Husbandman's Materia Medica*. In a format that would become common and of great importance for the preservation of old classics, Tao Hong Jing added his commentaries in a different color to the original work. For most entries, he added the region of origin, appearance, characteristics, preparation, and storage. In Tao Hong Jing's commented version, information such as the antimalarial function of Artemesia capillaris (*yin chen hao*), or the idea that ephedra (*ma huang*) should be harvested at the beginning of fall were included. Also very important for the development of Chinese Pharmacotherapy was the fact that his *Collective Notes to the Classic of Materia Medica (Ben Cao Jing Ji Zhu)*, contained an index. This made Tao's work a practical and useful work for physicians.

Class	Characteristics	Preface	Actual Number
Upper class	Non-toxic; able to nurture life and bestow longevity	120	141
Middle class	Able to cultivate personality or modify temperament; may be toxic; use of these medicinals requires care	120	111
Lower class	Specifically treat diseases; at least slightly toxic Cannot be taken in large amounts or for prolonged periods of time without developing negative side-effects	125	103

A The three classes of substance as described in *The Divine Husbandman's Materia Medica*.
According to its preface, the number of substances in each category should be 120 upper class, 120 middle class, and 125 lower class. According to Unschuld (1986, p. 21) the actual number of substances is 141 upper class, 111 middle class, and 103 lower class.

Category of Discussion	Example from the Entry of *Tang Kuei (Dang Gui)*
Substance	*Dang gui* (Angelicae sinensis Rx)
Flavor	Sweet
Nature	Warm
Functions and indications	It is non-toxic, treating mainly cough and counterflow *qi* ascent, warm malaria with fever persisting within the skin, leaking causing infertility in females, various malign sores, and incised wounds It can be [constantly] taken after being cooked
Secondary names	*Gan gui* (dry Angelicae sinensis Rx)
Specific or general name of origin	It grows in rivers and valleys

B Information presented in *The Divine Husbandman's Materia Medica* on *dang gui*
(adapted from Yang 1998, p. 39).

Li Shi Zhen (1518–93) (see p.40) wrote the *Comprehensive Herbal Foundation (Ben Cao Gang Mu)*, posthumously published in 1596. This text presents detailed information on a total of 1892 substances, with illustrations provided for 1160 substances. Li Shi Zhen established 10 criteria for each substance: 1) information on earlier false classifications; 2) secondary names with their sources; 3) collected quotes from earlier authors explaining the origin (**A**), occurrence, appearance, time of collection, medicinally useful parts, and similarities with other drugs; 4) preparatory information; 5) doubtful issues; 6) correction of mistakes; 7) properties of the medicinals; 8) main indications; 9) explanations of the effects of the drug; and 10) formulas in which the drug is used, the preparation and dosage of these formulas.

The *Comprehensive Herbal Foundation* is considered the greatest work on materia medica in the history of Chinese medicine:

"The value of this enormous achievement … written by one person, goes far beyond the scope of a pharmaceutical-medical drug work, and, in fact, constitutes an extensive encyclopedia of knowledge concerning nature and the technology required for the medicinal use of nature." (Unschuld 1986, p.145)

Since its publication in 1596, it has been translated into 60 languages. (**B**)

The writing of Zhang Zhong Jing (pp.30–31), one of the most revered Chinese medical scholars, is an important early text on herbal formulation. This was edited into two volumes: *On Cold Damage (Shang Han Lun)* and *Essential Prescriptions of the Golden Coffer (Jin Gui Yao Lue)*. Both contain formulas that are still widely used today. For example, *Chinese Herbal Medicine: Formulas and Strategies* by Bensky and Barolet (1990) lists 604 formulas. Over 20% of all of the formulas in this modern collection of clinical formulas from the past two millennia derive from these two texts.

The Tang dynasty formulary collections by Sun Si Miao (see pp.36, 300), *Thousand Gold Pieces Prescriptions (Qian Jin Yao Fang)* (and its companion, *Supplement to Thousand Gold Pieces Prescriptions/Qian Jin Yi Fang)* are rich sources of formulas, as is the Song dynasty work *Imperial Grace Formulary of the Taiping Era (Tai Ping Hui Min He Ji Ju Fang)*. The latter was compiled after the Emperor Tai Zong ordered the collection of all effective secret formulas. The resulting work contained over 16,000 formulas.

Two physician-scholars of the Jin/Yuan period developed formulas that are frequently used in modern practice (see p.40): Li Dong Yuan, proponent of the School of Supplementing the Spleen and Stomach and author of *Discussion of the Spleen and Stomach (Pi Wei Lun)*, and Zhu Dan Xi, proponent of the School of *Yin* Nourishment and author of *(The Heart Method of Zhu Dan Xi) Dan Xi Xin Fa* .

Important formulas have been contributed by the School of Warm Diseases (*Wen Bing Xue*), which developed during the Qing dynasty (1644–1911) (see p.42). The School of Warm Diseases was a response to the *On Cold Damage* theories developed by Zhang Zhong Jing 1700 years earlier in the Han dynasty.

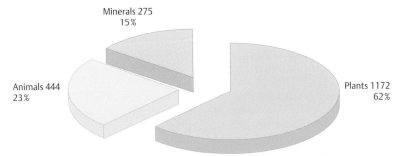

Minerals 275
15%

Animals 444
23%

Plants 1172
62%

A Origin of medicinal substances in the *Ben Cao Gang Mu*.

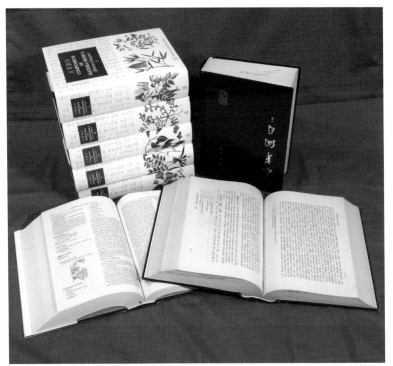

B The *Ben Cao Gang Mu* was written by Li Shi Zhen and published in the late 16th century.
It describes nearly 2000 medicinal substances in great detail, including exact drawings.
This monumental work has been translated into 60 languages. The picture shows a Chinese
two-volume print and an English six-volume translation.

Pharmacopoeias

An official pharmacopoeia is "a book or treatise describing the drugs, preparations, etc., used in medicine; especially, one issued by official authority and considered as standard" (*Merriam Webster's Collegiate Dictionary*). Although it has been suggested that the *Newly Revised Materia Medica (Xin Xiu Ben Cao)* from the Tang dynasty (618–907) was the first such pharmacopoeia in the world, most experts do not consider it a true pharmacopoeia. Although it was a government-sponsored work, it was simply one of many pharmaceutical works and had no legal or binding character.

It was not until 1930 that the first official Chinese pharmacopoeia, the Chinese Republic's (ROC) *Dictionary of Medicinals (Zhong Hua Yao Dian)* was published. The first edition contained 676 medicinal agents. Interestingly, almost no traditional substances were discussed. Rather, this first pharmacopoeia was not much more than a translation of parts of European pharmacopoeias into Chinese. After the establishment of the People's Republic of China (PRC) in 1949, a "new" pharmacopoeia was published in 1953. It contained 531 monographs. Similar to the ROC's pharmacopoeia, most substances were not traditional medicinals but chemical constituents, or preparations made from them, such as tincture Nucis Vomicis or Extractum Belladonnae (p. 42–43).

It was the second edition of the PRC pharmacopoeia that finally published monographs of substances traditionally used in China. Published in 1963,[*] the two-volume work included 446 descriptions of traditional Chinese drugs and 197 prepared formulas in Volume I and 667 descriptions of Western drugs in Volume II. In the most recently released 2005 edition of the official PRC pharmacopoeia, Volume I contains 551 traditional Chinese medicinal substances and 564 prepared medicines. Volume II is devoted to Western medicines.

More closely following in the tradition of Li Shi Zhen's *Comprehensive Herbal Foundation* is the *Great Dictionary of Chinese Medicinals (Zhong Yao Da Ci Dian)* (**A**), published in 1977, and its successor the *Chinese Materia Medica (Zhong Hua Ben Cao)*, which catalogues over 9000 substances. In contrast to the science-oriented pharmacopoeias, these works "represent so far the most advanced synthesis of traditional pragmatic *ben cao* [materia medica] knowledge and modern science" (Unschuld 1986, p. 287). However, this large number of substances are by no means all used frequently. Many of them are local plants that are largely unknown, even in other areas of China let alone the larger world.

A Chinese medicine practitioner, in China or in the West, typically works within the domain described by the 2005 PRC pharmacopoeia and may use from 150 to 500 different substances, depending on the nature of their practice.

---

[*]   According to Unschuld (1986), the publication date of the second pharmacopoeia was 1977. According to my research, in 1977 the third edition of the PRC pharmacopoeia was published. It contained 882 single substances, 270 prepared formulas, and 773 Western medicines.

Category	Comment
Main name	The main Chinese name serves as the title of the entry
Other names	Various other names are discussed, including the source of other names
Species information	Description of the employed species
Cultivation	Information on the cultivation of the plant
Harvest	Information on the best time to harvest for medicinal purposes
Dried herb description	Monographical description of the characteristics of the dry substance
Chemical constituents	A list of the common chemical constituents
Pharmacology	Research findings on various pharmacological functions
Toxicity	Information about the toxicity of the medicinal
Processing	Description of the different forms of processing
Characteristics and channel entry	The most common and generally accepted characteristics and channel entry are listed first, followed by a list of other classifications according to major medicinal works of the past
Functions and indications	A list of the main functions and respective indications is followed by statements on function from various ancient sources
Method of application and dosage	Statement as to the common method of application (decoction, powder, pill, and so on) and the dosage
Contraindications	A list of the contraindications including statements as to its contraindications from important ancient medical books
Selected combinations	A list of common combinations and formulas sorted according to indications with reference to the source of the combination
Clinical application reports	Summary presentations of clinical research reports for different indications
Selected scholar opinions on clinical application	A list of discussion of the medicinal in various ancient medical books
Notes	Various other notes regarding the medicinal

A Common categories in a monograph from the *Great Dictionary of Chinese Medicinals.*
(Zhong Yao Da Ci Dian).

Medicinal Substances

Chinese medicinal substances are of plant, mineral, and animal origin, although most are plants. Often, different parts of a plant are used in different ways. For example, the twigs (*sang zhi*), the fruits (*sang shen*), the leaves (*sang ye*), and the root bark (*sang bai pi*) of the mulberry tree (**A**) are all used, each with traditional usages. Another example is the tangerine. The outermost peel (*ju hong*), the peel (*chen pi*), the white vein-like net within the skin (*ju luo*), and the seeds (*ju zi*) are all used, albeit in this case, all have similar functions. Different stages of plant development may be used as different medicinals: the unripe bitter orange (*zhi shi*) is a much stronger *qi*-moving substance than the ripe bitter orange (*zhi ke*). Different plant parts may have opposite functions. A prominent example is the ephedra plant. The more popular herb part of ephedra (*ma huang*) is a strong stimulant and diaphoretic. The root (*ma huang gen*) is an astringent that treats spontaneous or night sweating.

Examples of medicinal substances derived from the animal kingdom are the earthworm (*di long*), scorpion (*quan xie*), sick silkworm (*jiang can*), deer horn *(lu jiao)*, and centipede (*wu gong*). Animal shells such as the oyster shell and the abalone shell are also used. Mineral substances include gypsum, amethyst, hematite, and magnetite.

Identification of Medicinal Substances

Identification of medicinals, particularly plants, can be complex. Many different species of the same plant grow in different parts of China. A different species may grow and be used in the North rather than in the South. To address this, and to set an all-China standard, the Chinese government released its first official Chinese pharmacopoeia including Chinese herbs in 1963. In it, exact species for each Chinese name are identified.

To think that only one species is listed per Chinese substance name is incorrect. Two or three species may be "correct" for one Chinese name. This is because all fulfill the requirements established by the pharmacopoeia commission: for a species to be included, there must be historical records of its use, it must be available on the market, and phytochemical and clinical studies must prove its effectiveness for some of its indications. The 2005 edition of the Chinese pharmacopoeia lists 551 single medicinals. Each edition adds or deletes medicinals or increases specifications. In the 2005 edition, most aristolochia species have been removed due to their toxicity, and entries with several species were divided. In the 2000 edition, two species are correct for pueraria (*ge gen*): Pueraria lobata and Pueraria thomsonii. These are chemically quite different and likely to have different actions, thus, they were split into two entries in the 2005 edition.

The identification of Chinese medicinals is a complicated issue. The official Chinese pharmacopoeia is becoming a reliable worldwide standard that may serve as an instrument for jurisdictional regulation.

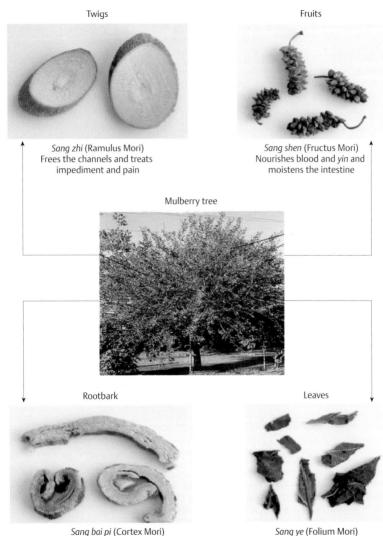

Twigs

Fruits

Sang zhi (Ramulus Mori)
Frees the channels and treats
impediment and pain

Sang shen (Fructus Mori)
Nourishes blood and *yin* and
moistens the intestine

Mulberry tree

Rootbark

Leaves

Sang bai pi (Cortex Mori)
Clears lung heat and stops cough

Sang ye (Folium Mori)
Resolves the surface and clears
wind–heat; clears the eyes

**A From the mulberry tree, the leaves, twigs, fruit as well as the root bark are used
medicinally.** They all have different medicinal functions.

Why is a Chinese Herb Chinese?

Is it because these plants only grow or appear in China? Or is it because they were first discovered there? Neither is correct. Many substances came from outside of China. Early materia medica depict "round-eyed barbarians" bringing substances to the Chinese people. Examples of such foreign substances are olibanum (frankincense) resin (*ru xiang*), myrrh resin (*mo yao*), and camphor (*zhang nao*). What is true of most "Chinese herbs" is that they are classified according to the theoretical foundations of Chinese medicine, including their flavor, their temperature and their channel of entry. Out of this system of classification grow the functions and indications of the substances based on Chinese medicine theory.

Medicinal Properties

Flavor

There are five flavors, two *yang* and three *yin*. The *yang* flavors are acrid and sweet; the *yin* arc bitter, sour, and salty. An herb can also be bland, which is an absence of the five flavors. Each flavor has different properties that influence the substance's therapeutic action. Acridity is active, moving and dispersing; sweetness is supplementing, harmonizing, and moistening; bitterness dries and drains; sourness astringes, secures, and keeps fluids from leaking; saltiness drains downward and softens hard masses; bland percolates dampness and disinhibits urination. Substances may have more than one flavor (**A**).

Medicinal formulas must be balanced in terms of flavor. If a patient suffers from internal accumulation of dampness secondary to a spleen *qi* vacuity, herbs would be selected from three categories: bland to percolate dampness and disinhibit urination; bitter to dry dampness; and sweet to supplement the spleen. Sweet medicinals need to be combined with acrid ones to move and disperse and with aromatic ones to open and penetrate. Acrid medicinals need to be combined with sweet and nourishing medicinals so that the active acridity does not over-disperse *qi* and fluids.

Nature

All medicinals are ascribed a nature: cold, cool, neutral, warm, or hot. Cool and cold medicinals treat heat diseases. Warm and hot medicinals treat cold diseases. Diseases that present without distinct signs of heat or cold require a neutral formula (**B**). If a patient presents with high fever, strong sweating, and big thirst, this is repletion *yang* and gypsum (*shi gao*), one of the coldest medicinals, might be prescribed. However, because the middle burner likes warmth and dislikes cold, cold medicinals damage spleen *yang* and lead to diarrhea, lack of appetite, and fullness and bloating. If cold medicinals are prescribed, they are usually combined with herbs to protect the middle burner. The most common of these "protecting medicinals" is licorice root (*gan cao*). Hence, in the formula for high fever, gypsum is combined with, among other herbs, licorice.

Flavor		Properties
Sweet	→	Supplementing, harmonizing, moistening
Sour	→	Astringing, securing
Bitter	→	Drying, draining
Acrid	→	Active, moving, dispersing
Salty	→	Draining downward, softening hard masses
Bland	→	Percolating dampness, disinhibiting urination

A Flavor of Medicinals. The flavor or taste of Chinese medicinals is used to understand their fundamental actions. Above are shown the basic associations of the six flavors. It should be noted that the bland flavor is considered to be produced by the absence of the other flavors.

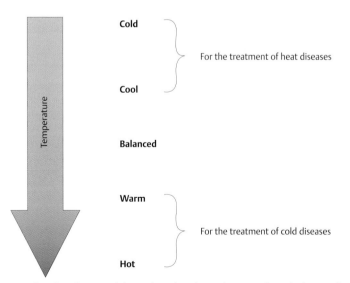

B *Qi* of Medicinals. It is said that each medicinal agent has a specific *qi* which generally is characterized as the nature or temperature of the substance. The notion of temperature refers to the impact of the agent on the body's internal environment, whether it is cooling, warming, or balanced.

Warm and hot substances are used in cold conditions. For example, cold limbs, aversion to cold, watery diarrhea and a pale facial complexion indicate that a patient's spleen and kidney *yang* has been damaged. Warm and hot medicinals like dried ginger (*gan jiang*) and aconite (*Fu zi*) might be prescribed. Because hot medicinals are drying, they may damage *yin* and blood. Hence, they are often combined with cool or even cold, moistening medicinals such as white peony root (*bai shao*) or unprepared rehmannia root (*sheng di huang*) to protect *yin* and blood from being damaged by the hot medicinals. Clinically, patients rarely present with a purely hot or a purely cold condition. A person with phlegm heat in the upper burner for which cool and cold medicinals are required may also present with weak spleen *qi* for which warm medicinals are required. Or a patient with cold in the middle burner, which requires warm and hot medicinals, may also suffer from liver depression with *qi* stagnation generating heat. The warm and hot medicinals treating the middle burner may in this instance promote the transformative heat. Hence, cool and cold medicinals also need to be added.

Channel Entry

Each medicinal also enters one or several channels. The concept of channel entry associates the action of the substance with specific channels and or-gans (**A**). For example, slightly warm and sweet astragalus root (*huang qi*) enters the lung and spleen channels and it supplements and boosts *qi* especially of these organs. Angelica dahurica root (*bai zhi*) is an acrid and warm medicinal that strongly resolves the exterior and unblocks the nose. Because of its strong exterior *qi*-dispersing action, it moves *qi* in the superficial layers and treats all kinds of pain. Angelica dahurica root enters the lung channel to resolve the exterior and it enters the stomach channel, which runs down the front of the face. Therefore, it is a good medicinal to treat all kinds of pain on the front of the face, particularly if from sinus congestion. It is added to most if not all formulas to treat frontal headaches, sinusitis, or toothaches.

Toxicity

From the earliest records describing the systematic use of medicinals in China, the toxicity of specific agents has been noted. The *Comprehensive Herbal Foundation* (*Ben Cao Gang Mu*) by Li Shi Zhen described a number of toxic medicinals including veratrum root (*li lu*), prepared aconite accessory root (*fu zi*), aconite main tuber (*wu tou*), and aspidium (*guan zhong*). Many other substances such as centipede (*Wu gong*) and croton seed (*ba dou*) are well understood as toxic substances throughout the centuries in various texts.

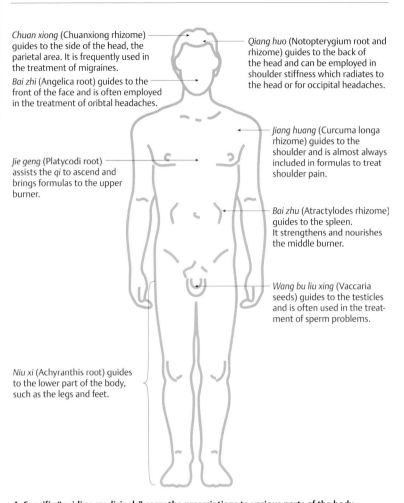

Chuan xiong (Chuanxiong rhizome) guides to the side of the head, the parietal area. It is frequently used in the treatment of migraines.

Bai zhi (Angelica root) guides to the front of the face and is often employed in the treatment of oribtal headaches.

Qiang huo (Notopterygium root and rhizome) guides to the back of the head and can be employed in shoulder stiffness which radiates to the head or for occipital headaches.

Jie geng (Platycodi root) assists the *qi* to ascend and brings formulas to the upper burner.

Jiang huang (Curcuma longa rhizome) guides to the shoulder and is almost always included in formulas to treat shoulder pain.

Bai zhu (Atractylodes rhizome) guides to the spleen. It strengthens and nourishes the middle burner.

Wang bu liu xing (Vaccaria seeds) guides to the testicles and is often used in the treatment of sperm problems.

Niu xi (Achyranthis root) guides to the lower part of the body, such as the legs and feet.

A Specific "guiding medicinals" carry the prescriptions to various parts of the body.

This tradition has continued to modern times. Toxicity is one of the properties described in all materia medica. Many traditionally toxic medicinals are also considered toxic by modern standards. For example, scorpion was traditionally considered to be toxic and its recommended dosage is very low. Modern research confirms the toxicity of scorpion. Sometimes, the traditional toxicities cannot be confirmed by modern research, as in the case of curculigo (*xian mao*), traditionally a toxic substance not suitable for long-term use. Research has not yet confirmed this toxicity. In many instances, an herb's toxicity is an aspect of its usefulness as a medicine; this is particularly true in the case of aconite (*cao wu*), which must be processed to render it safe for therapeutic use (**A**, **B**, **C**).

Processing of Medicinals

Almost all medicinal substances undergo some degree of processing before being used clinically. Minimally, substances are cleaned, dried, and cut or milled. Special processing techniques are used to enhance desirable properties of a substance, reduce its toxicity, or change its flavor or nature. These methods are collectively referred to as "processing of medicinals" (*pao zhi*), literally "blast frying and mix frying." For example, the very popular blood-nourishing root of the Polygonum multiflorum plant (*he shou wu*) has to be cooked for over 24 hours in a soup prepared of black beans. Only after this preparation does it lose its stool-loosening properties and becomes useful to supplement the blood.

Processing is often used to change the flavor, nature, or other properties of a medicinal so that an aspect of its action is altered. An example is licorice root (*gan cao*). The cut and dried root is used to mildly supplement *qi* and to clear heat from the lungs. If fried in honey to produce the distinct medicinal honey mix-fried licorice (*zhi gan cao*) it more strongly strengthens the spleen and the middle burner due to its sweeter flavor and warmer nature.

The substance used to prepare medicinals may modify medicinal properties. While honey is sweet and strengthens the middle burner, vinegar is sour and astringes and wine is active and moves. Frying schisandra berries (*wu wei zi*) in vinegar strengthens their astringent property; frying cyperus root (*xiang fu*) with vinegar focuses more strongly on the liver, and soaking tang kuei (*dang gui*) in rice wine strengthens its ability to quicken the blood. Processing can also be done without adding another substance. For example, charring substances strengthens their hemostatic properties.

Detoxification of substances such as aconite (**A**, **B**, **C**) is accomplished by the use of heat, salt, vinegar, and/or sulfur depending on the exact nature of the final product desired.

The preparation of a medicinal can strongly reduce its toxicity. The toxic as well as the analgesic and anti-inflammatory effects of the root and lateral root of aconite stem from the diester diterpenoid alkaloids aconitine and its analogues. More exactly, the toxic-active sites of these compounds are the two ester groups at C14 and C8. Hydrolisis of the esters, accomplished by such processing methods as boiling, steaming or treating with dilute acid or alkali for a few hours, results in detoxification of the alkaloids by losing the acetyl group at C8, forming benzoylaconine. This compound is 100–1000 times less toxic than the original aconitines. Further hydrolysis loses the benzoyl group at C14, forming non-toxic aconine. What is special about aconine is that it retains its analgesic and anti-inflammatory functions but loses its heart toxicity (Zhu, p. 18).

A Aconite detoxification.

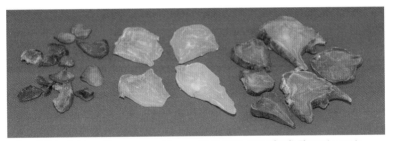

B From left to right are three prepared forms of Aconitum carmichaeli. The main root is processed with water, by soaking then boiling with licorice and soybeans, and sun drying to make *zhi chuan wu*. The lateral root is shown here in two prepared forms *bai fu pian* and *hei fu pian*. Both are prepared with water and salt, the white *(bai)* aconite slices are then steamed with sulfur.

C Traditional aconite production plant in Sichuan, China. Here, the aconite is being dried after having been soaked in a special salt bath.

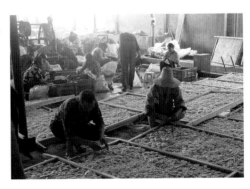

Medicinal Categories

By combining all three classification systems (flavor, nature, and channel entry), the specific functions and actions of individual substances result. A warm and acrid medicinal treats cold diseases and resolves wind from the exterior. Hence, it resolves wind–cold from the exterior. A cold and bitter medicinal treats heat diseases and is drying; hence, it treats damp-heat disorders. If that same medicinal also enters the urinary bladder, kidney, and large intestine channels, it will treat damp heat in the lower burner. In the practice of Chinese medicine, substances are combined to balance the flavor and nature of a formula to make it suit the picture of disharmony.

In most modern materia medica, Chinese medicinals are categorized according to their functions, which correspond closely to the treatment methods discussed in Chapter 2. Typically, 18 major categories are distinguished (**A**). Medicinals in a category all share at least one major function, that of the category. Often they will have similar flavors and natures and they may even enter similar channels. Within a category, medicinals are distinguished by their differences. For example, cimicifuga (*sheng ma*) and chrysanthemum (*ju hua*) are both acrid and slightly cold, belong to the exterior wind-resolving category and treat wind–heat symptoms. Cimicifuga also ascends clear *yang* and chrysanthemum clears ascendant liver–fire. Both enter the lung channel to resolve exterior conditions. Cimicifuga enters the stomach channel and clears toxic heat from the mouth whereas chrysanthemum enters the liver channel and clears heat and fire from the eyes. So, even though these medicinals are in the same primary category, they have very different secondary functions. Frequently, medicinals are clinically employed for their secondary or tertiary functions. For example, even though slightly cold, acrid, and bitter bupleurum root (*chai hu*) is in the same exterior-resolving category as cimicifuga and chrysanthemum clinically, it is much more commonly prescribed to resolve liver depression *qi* stagnation.

The following pages provide an overview of medicinal categories and their subcategories and introduce representative medicinals.

Category	Subcategory
1 Exterior-resolving medicinals	Acrid warm medicinals resolving wind–cold
	Acrid cool medicinals resolving wind–heat
2 Heat-clearing medicinals	Repletion heat-clearing medicinals
	Blood-cooling medicinals
	Damp-heat-clearing medicinals
	Toxin-resolving medicinals
3 Precipitating medicinals	Offensive-precipitating medicinals
	Moist-precipitating medicinals
	Water-expelling medicinals
4 Dampness-percolating medicinals	Warm, neutral, and cool medicinals
5 Wind–damp-dispelling medicinals	Warm, neutral, and cool medicinals
6 Phlegm-transforming and cough- and panting-suppressing medicinals	Cold medicinals to transform hot phlegm
	Warm medicinals to transform cold phlegm
	Suppress cough and calm panting medicinals
7 Aromatic dampness-transforming medicinals	
8 Food-dispersing medicinals	
9 *Qi*-rectifying medicinals	
10 Blood-rectifying medicinals	Blood-stanching medicinals
	Blood-quickening medicinals
11 Interior-warming medicinals	
12 Supplementing medicinals	*Qi*-supplementing medicinals
	Blood-nourishing medicinals
	Yin-enriching medicinals
	Yang-fortifying medicinals
13 Securing and astringing medicinals	
14 Spirit-quieting medicinals	Blood-nourishing and spirit-quieting medicinals
	Heavy settling and spirit-quieting medicinals
15 Orifice-opening medicinals	
16 Liver-calming and wind-extinguishing medicinals	
17 Worm-expelling medicinals	
18 External use medicinals	

A An overview of 18 medicinal categories.

Exterior-resolving Medicinals

Medicinal substances in this category are used if exterior evils such as wind–cold or wind–heat assail the exterior (see p. 88). Acrid medicinals are needed to disperse and diffuse the wind evil from the exterior. In the case of wind–cold, acrid, warm medicinals disperse the wind–cold; in the case of wind–heat, acrid cool medicinals disperse and cool the wind–heat. The acrid flavor, common to all substances in this category, expels the wind evil. Most of these substances enter the lung channel, which controls the defense *qi* that circulates in the body's exterior. In the early stage of invasion, the evil is just underneath the skin or in the exterior layers of the muscles. The strategy is to effuse the evil outward through the skin to the exterior by promoting sweating. Many of the medicinals in this category thus cause sweating or outthrust rashes. They are active, moving *yang* medicinals that move *qi* up and out. Many are flowers and leaves, light substances floating to the exterior and top of the body.

Ephedra (*ma huang*) (**A**), an acrid, slightly bitter, and very warm medicinal that enters the lung and urinary bladder channels, is representative. It strongly promotes sweating and thus disperses wind–cold evils from the exterior. Furthermore, ephedra has a lung *qi*-dispersing and descending function and is indicated in the treatment of obstruction of lung *qi*. Cinnamon twig (*gui zhi*) (**B**) is sweet, warm, and acrid. It resolves the surface and enters the lung and is often combined with ephedra to treat wind–cold.

A representative acrid, cool medicinal is mint (*bo he*) (**C**). By way of its light and dispersing taste, it enters the exterior and resolves wind–heat from the surface, thereby relieving such symptoms as sore throat, fever with simultaneous aversion to wind, and headache. Its cooling and dispersing property make it particularly effective to resolve throat pain, especially throat pain caused by exterior wind–heat. Furthermore, its acrid flavor and aromatic smell help to open the nose, which is blocked secondary to lung *qi* congestion. Similar to many wind–heat-dispersing medicinals, it also has the ability to "resolve the muscle layer," which means to disperse evils lodged in the muscles, such as heat rashes.

Heat-clearing Medicinals

The heat-clearing category is the largest in the materia medica. It contains medicinals that clear many different manifestations of heat: repletion heat, damp heat, blood heat, summer heat, and toxic heat. Almost all of these medicinals are cool or cold in temperature. Many are also bitter. The combination of cool or cold and bitter makes many of them hard to digest because the bitter flavor and the cold temperature injure the spleen's *yang qi*.

A Ephedra *(ma huang)* is a typical representative of the acrid warm medicinal category. It has strong diaphoretic properties and thus effuses invading cold evils outward through the skin.

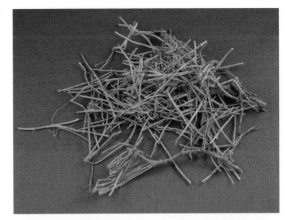

B Cinnamon twig is acrid and warm and thus resolves the exterior. It also promotes the transformation of fluids in the body and can be applied in the case of dampness accumulation in the middle burner.

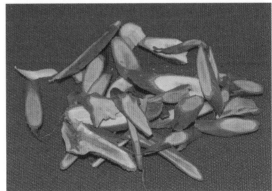

C Mint is a representative medicinal of the acrid cool medicinal category. It not only resolves wind–heat from the exterior by effusing it outward but it also pushes heat rashes out through the muscle layers, thus treating measles and other skin rashes.

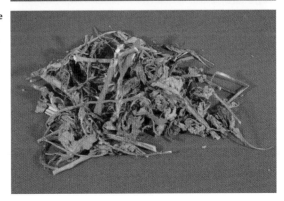

Medicinals that clear repletion heat or fire are the coldest substances in the materia medica. Because fire and heat rise upward in the body, many of these substances not only clear heat but also have a descending function. In contrast to acrid, cool medicinals that dispel heat from the exterior, fire-clearing substances clear heat from the interior, with different substances clearing heat from different aspects and organs. Substances in this category address symptoms such as high fever, irritability, red eyes, and thirst. Representatives of this category are: gypsum (*shi gao*), anemarrhena rhizome (*zhi mu*) and prunella spike (*xia ku cao*).

Blood-cooling medicinals clear heat that has penetrated to the construction and blood aspects. At this stage of disease, heat has penetrated deeply and damaged fluids and *yin*. Heat in the construction level leads to rashes; heat in the blood causes the blood to flow frenetically, leave the vessels, and cause bleeding. These medicinals staunch bleeding due to blood heat. Heat in the blood or construction is not the same as *yin* vacuity heat, although it is often accompanied by it. Hence, many blood heat-clearing medicinals also have *yin* vacuity heat-clearing properties. Representatives are water buffalo horn (*shui niu jiao*)*, unprepared rehmannia root (*sheng di huang*), and scrophularia root (*xuan shen*).

Medicinals that clear damp heat are cold and bitter. Their bitter flavor dries dampness; their cold nature clears heat. Many of the substances in this subcategory have antibacterial and anti-fungal properties. They are often used in infections with pronounced heat and dampness signs such as dysentery, urinary tract infections, eczema, and so on. The three most prominent representatives in this category are the "three yellows". All three substances have a yellow color and therefore the Chinese word for yellow (*huang*), in their name: scutellaria root (*huang qin*) (**A**), coptis root (*huang lian*) (**B**), and phellodendron bark (*huang bai*) (**C**). Each clears heat and dries dampness in one of the three burners.

Substances that clear heat and resolve toxins address inflammation produced by animal or insect venom or by an accumulation of heat evil. For example, a sore throat can be due to heat in the lungs, but if there is severe pain and inflammation then it is considered toxic heat. Medicinals that resolve toxins are often used where heat symptoms are pronounced or where pus and abscesses are present. For example, the most popular wind–heat formula, Lonicera and Forsythia Powder (*Yin Qiao San*), is named after two toxic heat-clearing medicinals: lonicera (honeysuckle) flower (*jin yin hua*) and forsythia fruit (*lian qiao*), thus blurring the line between heat and toxic heat. As the heat becomes stronger, more toxic heat substances may be added.

---

*   Originally, rhinoceros horn (*xi jiao*) was used, but now water buffalo horn is used instead due to the endangered status of rhinoceros.

A–C *Huang* **means yellow in Chinese; the "three yellows" are the prominent representatives of the damp–heat-clearing category.** Each one of them is attributed to a different burner: *huang qin* (scutellaria) to the upper burner, *huang lian* (coptis) to the middle burner, and *huang bai* (phellodendron) to the lower burner. They are among the most bitter medicinals in the Chinese pharmacopoeia and have strong antibiotic properties.

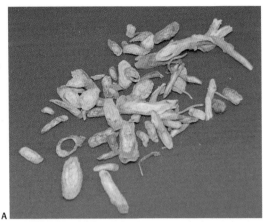

A

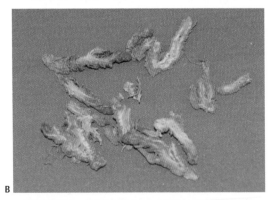

B

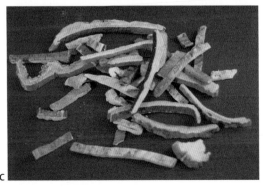

C

Precipitating Medicinals

Precipitation refers to helping the stools to move freely. Substances are categorized as offensive precipitants, moist precipitants, and water-expelling medicinals. Rhubarb (*da huang*) (**A**) is an offensive precipitant used for acute constipation. Rhubarb also has blood-moving, heat-clearing, and stop-bleeding properties for which it is frequently used. If used for its precipitating effect, rhubarb should be cooked for a short period of time (5–10 minutes). If used for its heat-clearing and blood-moving properties, it is cooked together with the other herbs for at least 20 minutes, to reduce its precipitating action.

If *qi* or blood vacuity has produced dryness in the intestines, causing chronic constipation, a moist precipitant such as hemp seed *(huo ma ren)* is selected. However, most seeds, even from other medicinal categories, have intestine-moistening properties.

Water-disinhibiting, dampness-percolating Medicinals

These medicinals promote urination and drain dampness. Some of the dampness-dispelling medicinals also clear heat that may be engendered if dampness blocks the free flow of *qi* transforms into heat.

Medicinals from this category are generally combined with spleen-supplementing and dampness-transforming medicinals or with heat-clearing and dampness-drying medicinals.

Poria (*fu ling*) (**B**) is sweet and neutral, and so can be used in hot or cold conditions. It has a slight supplementing function and is ideal for spleen vacuity with dampness accumulation. Talcum (*hua shi*) is a cold water-disinhibiting medicinal to treat damp heat in the urinary bladder, a condition that essentially corresponds to urinary tract infection.

Wind–damp-dispelling medicinals

These medicinals are specific for the treatment of wind–damp impediment (*bi*) conditions. Wind, damp, and cold are common causes of impediment, which manifests with pain in the joints, sinews, or bones, and heaviness or numbness of the limbs. These substances, typically acrid and aromatic, hot or cold, are combined with agents from other categories to address all aspects of impediment syndrome: water-disinhibiting and dampness-percolating medicinals, cold-dispersing medicinals, blood-quickening medicinals, or supplementing medicinals.

Angelica root (*du huo*) (**C**) treats wind–damp cold impediment in the lower back and legs. It is bitter, acrid, and warm, disperses dampness, dispels cold, and courses *qi* to dispel wind.

Vines are found among the wind–damp-dispelling medicinals as they enter the channels and network vessels, dispelling the dampness and wind impeding the free flow of *qi* and blood. Star jasmine stem (*luo shi teng*) is a bitter and slightly cold vine that enters and frees the network vessels and is especially useful in the treatment of wind–damp-heat or wind–dampness impediment in the extremities.

A Rhubarb root is not only a strong laxative, which is used in case of constipation due to heat, but it also activates blood and clears damp heat. Similar to the "three yellows" (see p. 243) it is of a yellow color, has a very bitter taste and strong antibiotic properties. It is often combined with two of the three yellows to produce an all-purpose heat-clearing external remedy by the name of "Three Yellow Powder" *(San Huang San)*.

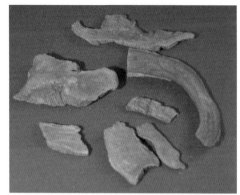

B Poria is quite bland in taste and neutral in temperature. It gently percolates dampness and supplements the spleen.

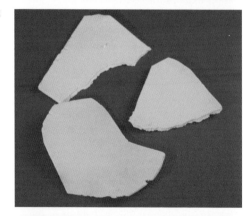

C Angelica root is bitter, acrid, and warm. Its bitterness dries dampness; its acridity moves *qi* and frees obstructed channels and network vessels; and its warmth dispels cold. Furthermore, it focuses on the lower back. Hence, it is an ideal medicinal to treat impediment due to wind–damp-cold in the lumbar area and lower extremities.

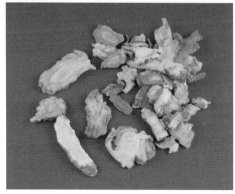

Phlegm-transforming, Cough-suppressing, Panting-calming Medicinals

Divided into cold medicinals that transform hot phlegm, warm medicinals that transform cold phlegm, and cough-suppressing medicinals, these substances primarily address respiratory tract conditions, but may be used to treat phlegm anywhere in the body (see pp. 92 and 132).

Arisaema root (*tian nan xing*) is warm and transforms cold phlegm. If it is pulverized and prepared with bitter and cold bile, it turns cool and is able to transform hot phlegm (Bile Cured/ *dan nan xing*).

Fritillaria bulb (*zhe bei mu*) (**A**) is bitter and cold and treats spitting and coughing of yellow phlegm. It can be compared with a bulb of the same family, Sichuan fritillaria bulb (*chuan bei mu*) (**B**), which is bitter, cold, and sweet, transforms hot phlegm and moistens and engenders *yin* fluids. While fritillaria bulb is best used early on during a cough, before fluids are damaged, Sichuan fritillaria bulb is used in later stages when the heat has dried up the phlegm and the *yin* fluids are injured.

Medicinals in the last subcategory are, based on their nature, used for hot or cold patterns of cough and for dry or damp coughs. Perilla seed (*zi su zi*) is acrid and warm and treats cold-type coughs with phlegm. Mulberry root bark (*sang bai pi*) is cold and sweet and treats hot, dry cough or cough due to *yin* vacuity, because the sweet taste nourishes *yin* and moistens fluids.

Aromatic Dampness-transforming Medicinals

These substances are all aromatic and acrid. Their aromatic nature opens and disperses the heaviness of dampness and awakens the spleen. Their acridity moves *qi* and penetrates dampness. They are mostly warm in temperature. They do not promote urination but rather disperse and penetrate dampness. They are indicated for symptoms of accumulated dampness such as fullness in the epigastrium and abdomen, loss of appetite, heaviness, or diarrhea. Amomum fruit (*sha ren*) (**C**) enters the spleen and stomach channels, is acrid, warm, and aromatic. Its acridity moves *qi*, its warmth activates the middle burner, and its aroma opens congestion.

Food-dispersing Medicinals

If the spleen and stomach are not able to move and transform food due to vacuity, to overeating, or to bad food, the food stagnates and blocks the normal flow of *qi* (see Ch. 7). Symptoms of food stagnation are belching, bad breath, diarrhea with a foul smell, bloating and fullness, and lack of appetite. Food-dispersing medicinals are used according to their specific characteristics. Rice and barley sprout (*gu ya* and *mai ya*) resolve food stagnation, have spleen and stomach fortifying properties, and are used where spleen vacuity is the root of the food stagnation. Crataegus fruit (Chinese hawthorn) (*shan zha*) disperses meaty and fatty foods, barley sprout disperses rice, wheat flour, and fruit.

A–B Two types of fritillaria bulbs with two different medicinal applications. While the bitter and cold fritillaria bulb **(A)** clears heat and resolves phlegm, the sweet, bitter, and cold Sichuan fritillaria bulb **(B)** also nourishes *yin* due to its sweetness. The former is used for acute coughs with copious yellow sputum; the latter for chronic coughs with dry, difficult-to-expectorate sputum.

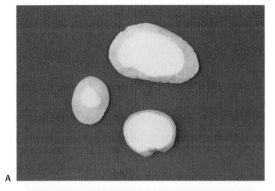

A

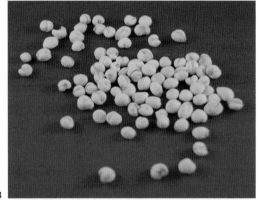

B

C The aromatic nature of amomum makes this a superior medicinal to penetrate turbid dampness blocking and obstructing the middle burner and to promote a healthy appetite. It is representative of the aromatic dampness-transforming medicinal category.

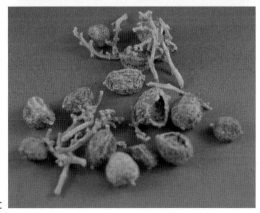

C

Qi-rectifying Medicinals

To rectify *qi* is to correct its counterflow or stagnant movement (see p. 132). Counterflow lung *qi* manifests as cough. Counterflow stomach *qi* presents with belching, nausea, and vomiting. Because cough-suppressing medicinals are classified with the phlegm-transforming substances, medicinals in this group mainly downbear counterflow stomach *qi*. Persimmon calyx (*shi di*) treats hiccough. Its neutral temperature permits use in counterflow stomach *qi* due to heat or cold.

Qi-moving medicinals focus primarily on the stomach and spleen, or the liver. Signs of *qi* stagnation include fullness, distension, and pain. *Qi*-rectifying medicinals frequently have an acrid flavor, which disperses *qi*. Tangerine peel (*chen pi*) (**A**) moves *qi* in the spleen and stomach. Its acrid and aromatic properties move depressed *qi*. Its warmth supports the spleen and stomach. Its bitterness dries dampness and phlegm. Cyperus root (*xiang fu*) enters the liver and gallbladder and moves liver *qi*. It is used in the treatment of gynecologial problems due to liver depression *qi* stagnation.

Blood-rectifying Medicinals

To rectify blood involves staunching bleeding, or quickening, transforming, or breaking static blood (see p. 132). Blood-staunching medicinals may be cool or warm. Sanguisorba root (*di yu*) is cold, bitter, and sour. It cools the blood, astringes, and stops bleeding. It treats rectal bleeding due to damp heat in the lower burner. Mugwort leaf (*ai ye*) is bitter, acrid, and warm. When charred, it enters the spleen, liver, and kidney channels and treats gynecological bleeding due to cold. Some of these substances simultaneously quicken blood and stop bleeding. Static blood blocks the vessels and causes blood to extravasate. When the congealed blood is moved, extravasation will stop. Notoginseng root (*san qi*) (**B**) treats injuries from contusions or falls. It stops bleeding and dissipates stasis to stop pain.

Fixed and stabbing pain is a clear sign of blood stasis. Blood-quickening agents are used where pain is due to blood stasis. In common with *qi*-rectifying medicinals, many blood-quickening medicinals are acrid, bitter, and warm. Acridity moves and disperses, bitterness frees and opens the channels, and warmth invigorates *yang qi*, thus supporting movement.

The blood-quickening medicinals vary in the areas on which they act and the strength of their stasis-dispersing effects. Chuanxiong rhizome (ligusticum) (*chuan xiong*) moves upward, and treats blood stasis in the head and chest. Cyathula root (*chuan niu xi*) descends and is used for blood stasis in the lower limbs. Salvia root (*dan shen*) is a mild quickening agent that both quickens and nourishes the blood. It is frequently used for blood stasis in the chest. Carthamus (*hong hua*) (**C**) and peach kernel (*tao ren*) are more forceful stasis-transforming agents often used to treat gynecological conditions.

A *Qi*-rectifying medicinals either move *qi* in the middle burner or in the liver or both. Tangerine peel is representative of the middle burner *qi*-moving substances. It also transforms phlegm and is an important ingredient in the basic phlegm-eliminating prescription Two Matured Ingredients Decoction.

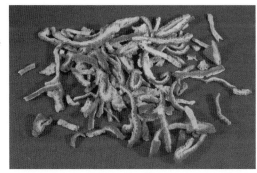

B Notoginseng root is a very special and rather expensive medicinal: it not only moves blood but it also stops bleeding. It is a superior medicinal for the treatment of cases that present with stasis and bleeding at the same time. Because of its price, it is usually not decocted but swallowed as a powder with the decoction.

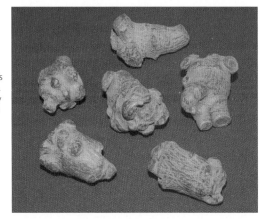

C Carthamus flower is a typical representative of the blood-quickening medicinal category. It can be applied for most types of blood stasis problems, externally as well as internally.

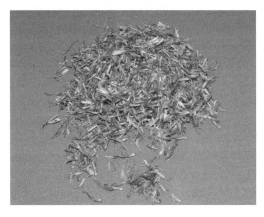

Interior-warming Medicinals

These are warm or hot and acrid substances that dispel cold and invigorate *yang*. They treat both replete and vacuous interior cold patterns. Heat warms cold; heat and acridity invigorate *yang*. Together these properties disperse interior accumulation of cold. They are used for repletion cold conditions, in which exterior cold enters the body and blocks *yang qi*, and to invigorate weak *yang* or rescue collapsed *yang*. *Yang* collapse describes a critical condition marked by very cold limbs and body, profuse and cold sweat, and a faint pulse. Representative of this category is aconite accessory root (*fu zi*) (**A**). Aconite is toxic, hot, and acrid, and it invigorates *yang* and the flow of *yang qi*. It is commonly prescribed in combination with *yang*-supplementing medicinals for the treatment of general *yang* vacuity patterns. In combination with wind–dampness-eliminating and blood-activating medicinals, it treats wind–cold-damp impediment pain by entering the channels and network vessels and powerfully freeing the flow of *yang*, *qi*, and blood. Dried ginger (*gan jiang*) (**B**), is rather static and primarily warms the *yang* of the middle burner and the lungs. The combination of dried ginger and aconite is one of the most powerful *yang*-warming combinations; one is active and warms the kidney and heart *yang*. The other is static and focuses on the *yang* of the spleen and lungs.

Supplementing Medicinals

The supplementing medicinals are divided into four subcategories, one for each of the four essential substances: *qi*, blood, *yin*, and *yang*. This category contains some of the most popular and widely known medicinals, including all of the different ginseng varieties, *tang kuei (dang gui)*, Cordyceps sinensis (*dong chong xia cao*) and cooked rehmannia root (*shu di huang*). These medicinals are indicated in vacuity when the body is weak and one or several of the basic substances are damaged.

Sweet is the *yang* flavor with supplementing properties. Most substances in the supplementing category are sweet. Their temperature depends on which substance they supplement: *qi*- and *yang*-supplementing medicinals are generally warm, whereas *yin*-supplementing medicinals are more commonly neutral or cool. Blood-supplementing medicinals may be warm, neutral, or cool.

Most of the *qi*-supplementing medicinals enter the spleen and/or stomach and focus on the middle burner. By supplementing these organs, *qi* in the entire body is fortified.

The best-known *qi*-supplementing medicinal is Panax ginseng (*ren shen*) (**C**). Sweet, slightly bitter and slightly warm, it enters the spleen and lung channels. It powerfully supplements *qi* of the middle burner and the original *qi*. Its original *qi*-supplementing function differentiates ginseng from other *qi*-supplementing medicinals that focus primarily on the spleen and stomach. Further, ginseng gently nourishes *yin* and quiets the spirit.

A–B Aconite and dried ginger are the most popular representatives of the interior-warming medicinal category. Both have intensely warm properties. Aconite is an active, moving medicinal and warms the true *yang* of the kidney, spleen, and heart, i.e., the entire body. In contrast, dried ginger is rather static and mainly warms the spleen and lungs. They are often combined in order to strongly warm the *yang* of the body.

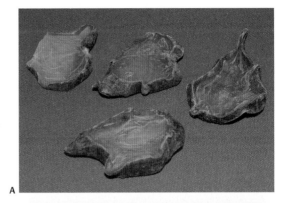

A

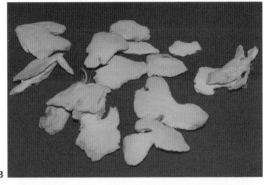

B

C Ginseng is probably the most popular Chinese medicinal in the world. It belongs to the *qi*-supplementing medicinal category. In contrast to the other *qi*-supplementing medicinals, it is unique in fortifying the original *qi*, i.e., the essential *qi* of the kidneys. Panax ginseng comes in two forms: white *(bai)* and red *(hong)*. If the root is steamed, it becomes red. This makes the nature of red ginseng warmer and thus more *yang* strengthening.

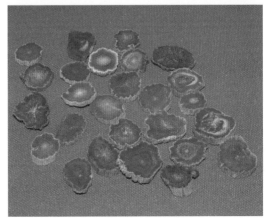

There are several ways in which ginseng is processed that change its nature and actions: white ginseng (*bai ren shen*) refers to the cultivated and then sun-dried root. This form is not as warm as other forms and so is suitable in a greater variety of conditions. When the fresh root is steamed and then sun-dried, it becomes red ginseng (*hong ren shen*), which is warmer than white ginseng and should not be used when heating is contraindicated. American ginseng (*xi yang shen*), is an entirely different species (Panacis quinquefolii) that is cool or cold, depending upon when it is harvested. American ginseng is in the *yin*-supplementing category because it enriches *yin* and supplements *qi*, and also clears vacuity heat.

The best-known of the blood-supplementing medicinals is *tang kuei (dang gui)* (**A**). *Tang kuei* nourishes blood and, by way of its acrid and warm properties, moves blood and unblocks *yang* and *qi*. It can be used to treat blood vacuity conditions such as delayed or scanty menses, and conditions in which blood is static and vacuous.

Many of the *yang*-supplementing substances not only powerfully invigorate and supplement *yang* but also nourish *yin*. In order to supplement *yang*, *yin* must also be enriched as the two are closely interconnected and when one is damaged, the other is directly affected. Kidney *yang* damage manifests with bodily cold including cold extremities, a pale and swollen tongue, a cold and sore low back, lack of energy and decreased sexual function. Two representatives of *yang*-invigorating and *yin*-nourishing properties are cuscuta seed (*tu si zi*) and cordyceps (*dong chong xia cao*) (**B**). Cuscuta is able to warm without drying and to secure desertion. It is also an important substance for use with threatened miscarriage due to kidney vacuity. Cordyceps supplements kidney *yang* and lung *yin* and is especially useful for vacuity-type panting or pulmonary tuberculosis.

Yin-supplementing medicinals are cool or cold, nourishing, and moistening. They primarily enrich the *yin* of the lung, the stomach, and the kidneys. For example, ophiopogon tuber (*mai men dong*) (**C**) enters the heart, lung, and stomach and nourishes the *yin* of these organs.

Due to their moistening characteristics and cool temperatures, many *yin*-supplementing medicinals are somewhat cloying and more difficult to digest. Therefore, they may damage the spleen and stomach and can lead to such symptoms as abdominal fullness, diarrhea, and lack of appetite. To prevent them from stagnating the *qi* of the spleen and stomach, *qi*-regulating medicinals like citrus peel are frequently added. Yang- and *qi*-supplementing substances on the other hand, can be too warming and drying and so may need to be modulated with cooling and moistening substances.

A Pressed slices of the *tang kuei* root. *Tang kuei* is the most popular blood-supplementing medicinal. It not only supplements blood but due to its acrid nature also gently moves blood. Hence, it is also said to be a blood-harmonizing medicinal.

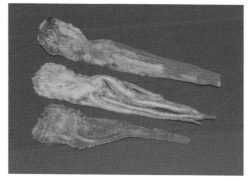

B Cordyceps, a popular representative of the *yang*-strengthening category, is called *dong chong xia cao* in Chinese. This translates as "winter insect summer herb." The name has its origin in the fact that this medicinal substance is composed of a fungus ("herb") growing on the larvae of a caterpillar ("insect"). It is one of the most precious substances in the Chinese materia medica and strongly supplements the body. Due to its high cost, it is never cooked in a decoction but rather taken with the decoction as a powder or pills.

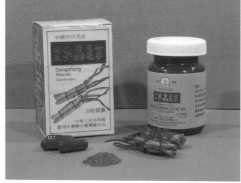

C Ophiopogon tuber belongs to the "upper *yin*-nourishing" medicinals. It nourishes the *yin* of the lungs and stomach in contrast to the "lower *yin*-nourishing" substances that nourish the *yin* of liver and kidneys. It not only nourishes *yin* but also has the ability to resolve phlegm in the lungs. It is therefore frequently used in the treatment of cough with dry phlegm.

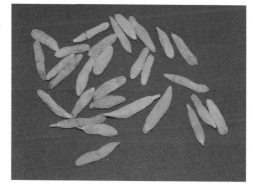

Securing and Astringing Medicinals

The securing and astringing function of these medicinals focuses on the lungs, the intestines, the bladder, the uterus, and the pores of the skin. They hold in bodily substances that have a tendency to leak out. They treat conditions such as diarrhea, urinary frequency, enuresis, and spontaneous or night sweating. All of these medicinals have an astringent property and many are sour, as the sour flavor astringes.

Rubus berry (*fu pen zi*) is sweet, astringent, and neutral and enters the kidney and liver channels. It supplements the liver and kidney, secures essence, and is used in the treatment of urinary incontinence or enuresis. Schisandra berry (*wu wei zi*) (**A**) is warm and sour and enters the lung and kidney channels. It constrains the lung and enriches the kidney to treat abnormal sweating or nocturnal emissions. Because these substances often have no supplementing action, securing and astringing medicinals are typically added to formulas that treat the root of the leakage, such as vacuity of kidney *yang* or spleen *qi*.

Not every leakage should be treated by astringing. "The thief should not be locked in the house" is a statement of fact in Chinese medicine. If a repletion evil such as damp heat causes leakage, for example, diarrhea, astringing medicinals should not be prescribed. The correct treatment is to clear damp heat from the lower burner.

Spirit-quieting Medicinals

The spirit resides in the heart and is nourished by blood. It can be unsettled either by heat disturbing it or by an insufficient amount of blood to nourish it. Spirit-quieting medicinals are divided into two subcategories: medicinals that settle fright and quiet the spirit and medicinals that nourish the heart and quiet the spirit. The former are mostly heavy minerals that subdue the *yang*. For example, dragon bone (*long gu*) (**B**) and oyster shell (*mu li*), are both heavy mineral substances with a settling effect. They quiet the spirit when the heart is disturbed by repletion evil. Most substances in this category also have additional functions such as constraining perspiration and securing essence.

The latter group quiets the heart and calms the spirit by nourishing the heart and blood. Prominent representatives are biota seed (*bai zi ren*) and spiny jujube kernel (*suan zao ren*) (**C**). While both nourish the heart and quiet the spirit, biota seed focuses on the heart and spiny jujube kernel focuses on the liver. For heart blood vacuity symptoms such as forgetfulness, loss of concentration, and palpitations, biota seed is appropriate. For liver blood vacuity spirit disquietude with such signs as irritability, palpitations, and pale tongue sides, spiny jujube kernel is the medicinal of choice.

A Schizandra berries are called *wu wei zi*, five flavor seeds. The berry combines all five flavors and is said to supplement all viscera. Its main flavor is sour and thus its main function is to astringe. Its sour flavor also makes it a fluid-generating medicinal. Because of this, it has been integrated into some mainstream beverages for its thirst-quenching abilities.

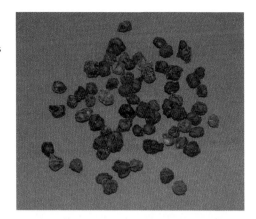

B So-called dragon bones, fossilized bones from large mammals, are heavy and settle the mind and spirit. Heavy mind-settling medicinals are mainly used in repletion patterns when the mind is disturbed by heat.

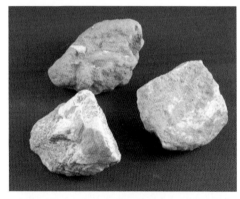

C The spiny jujube kernel belongs to the nourishing spirit-quieting medicinals. In contrast to the heavy settling substances, they nourish the blood, which in turn supports the spirit. Spiny jujube kernels have an affinity to the liver and particularly nourish liver blood.

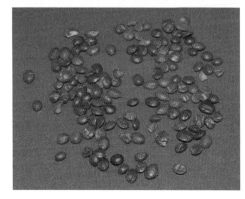

Orifice-opening Medicinals

The spirit communicates and interacts with the outside world through the clear orifices. If the orifices are obstructed by phlegm, interaction between the spirit and the world is obstructed and the patient may lose consciousness or become muddled. Orifice-opening medicinals, aromatic and acrid in nature, assist in opening the orifices to revive the patient or clarify thinking. These substances are not commonly used in the West, in part because these are not commonly seen indications in a Chinese medical practice, and in part because some of these substances are difficult to buy, very expensive and/or toxic. Examples are musk (*she xiang*), liquid styrax (*su he xiang*), benzoin (*an xi xiang*), cattle bezoar (*niu huang*) and borneol (*bing pian*). The only commonly administered substance is acorus root (*shi chang pu*) (**A**). Acorus is acrid and warm and enters the heart, liver, and spleen channels. It is often employed to penetrate phlegm and dampness accumulation. It is prescribed in combination with aromatic herbs to awaken the spleen. Acorus sharpens the mind as it clears away phlegm and dampness and so it is often employed to increase concentration or to treat conditions such as Attention Deficit Disorder.

Liver-calming, Wind-extinguishing Medicinals

Wind evil can be divided into two types: external and internal wind. External wind is treated with exterior-resolving medicinals. Interior wind may arise due to upflaming liver fire, ascendant hyperactivity of liver *yang* or liver *yin* or blood vacuity. Whether the cause of the wind is a repletion, mixed vacuity and repletion or vacuity pattern, liver wind stirring internally always has a relationship to the liver. As the medicinals in this category treat internal wind, almost all enter the liver channel and are cool or cold. Many of the substances in this category are of animal origin, for example, scorpion (*quan xie*) (**B**), centipede (*wu gong*), and earthworm (*di long*) (**C**). Because these animals not only extinguish wind but also enter and unblock the channels, they are also effective in the treatment of pain. Besides the animal substances, many medicinals in this category are of mineral origin. They weigh down ascending *yang* or clear upflaming fire. Examples are bitter and cold hematite (*dai zhe shi*) and salty and cold abalone shell (*shi jue ming*). One manifestation of internal wind is dizziness. In the treatment of dizziness, we might use substances in this category such as gastrodia root (*tian ma*). Gastrodia root's sweet and neutral properties make it ideal to treat repletion as well as vacuity patterns of dizziness.

Liver-calming, wind-extinguishing medicinals are frequently used in modern clinical practice. They are employed in the treatment of many patterns of hypertension, migraine headaches, tics and tremors, paralysis, and other such wind conditions.

A Acorus root is the only commonly administered medicinal from the orifice-opening category. It "opens" in different ways: in combination with aromatic medicinals, it "opens" the spleen; in the treatment of ear infections, it is applied to "open" and unblock the ear; and in combination with phlegm-transforming and brain stimulating medicinals, it "opens" the brain, i.e., sharpens the mind.

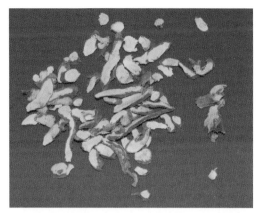

B Scorpion is toxic and potent. Besides extinguishing liver–wind, it is particularly useful for entering into the channels and network vessels and freeing these. Hence, it is a powerful pain-stopping medicinal frequently used for migraine headaches, arthritis, or neuralgias.

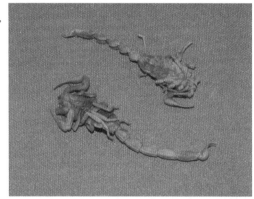

C Just as the earthworm crawls through the dirt, it enters the channels and network vessels and unblocks them. Like the scorpion but less potent, besides extinguishing wind, it also stops pain. Furthermore, earthworm is also employed in the treatment of asthma and coughs, as it can resolve spasms of the bronchi, also a type of internal wind.

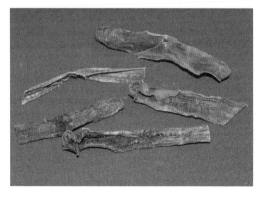

Worm-expelling Medicinals

This is a small category that in modern practice is not frequently used. The worms for which these medicinals are indicated, such as roundworms, tapeworms, and hookworms, are often more effectively expelled with biomedicine. However, the Chinese word for worm, *chong*, can be extended in meaning to also cover such intestinal parasites as candida. Following this idea, today, many worm-expelling medicinals are prescribed in patterns of candida or intestinal dysbiosis. An example from this category is melia bark (*ku lian pi*) (**A**), which not only kills worms but because of its bitter and cold properties also treats damp heat. It is ideal to treat vaginal candidiasis. However, like other medicinals from this category, it is toxic and should be prescribed with caution.

External Use Medicinals

Medicinals in the external application category have a wide spectrum of actions. Some are used for itching, others for promoting the healing process, others for burns or for bleeding. What they have in common is that they are typically only applied on local external areas and that most commonly they are applied in the form of powders, ointments, washes, steams, or soaks.

Most of the substances in this category should not be taken internally. Many are toxic and may lead to serious side-effects if ingested. A typical example is alum (*bai fan*) (**B**), which treats external dampness and toxicity and stops itching. It is applied, mostly as a powder, in the treatment of eczema, tinea, scabies, and vaginal itching. It also stops bleeding and can be applied externally in combination with other blood-stanching medicinals. It has the internal function to stop diarrhea, clear heat, and resolve phlegm, such as in the treatment of cough or delirium, however, internal administration of this medicinal should not exceed 3 g in decoction or 1 g in powder form and toxic side-effects such as nausea, dizziness, headache, and so on have been reported. Alum is a frequently used medicinal for external application but very rarely prescribed internally. Other substances still commonly listed in this category in modern materia medica are highly toxic and should be used with great caution, for example, mylabris (*ban mao*) (**C**) and toad venom (*chan su*), or not at all, for example, lead oxide (*qian dan*) (see also p. 218).

The 18 categories of medicinals described above all contain substances that have the general category function as well as individual functions. It is the individual functions that differentiate the substances in each category and help the practitioner to decide which substance is the most appropriate in a given condition. However, it is very unusual for Chinese medicinal substances to be used individually. Most often, several substances are combined to create a formula that will address the specific condition with which a patient might present.

A Bitter, cold, and slightly toxic, melia bark belongs to the worm-dispelling category but is frequently used in the treatment of damp heat vaginal fungal infections. Its "worm-killing" properties assist in killing off pathologic microorganisms such as candida.

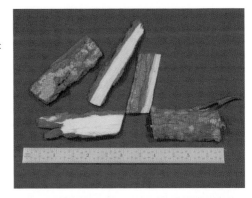

B Alum belongs to the external use medicinal category. Although it has an internal function, it is only rarely included in decoctions that are ingested. Its main application is externally for itching wet skin disorders.

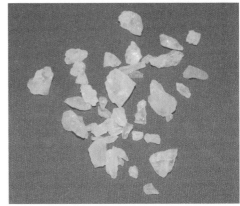

C Although mylabris, the Spanish fly, is still listed frequently in modern materia medica and treatment manuals, it is not a commonly used substance, and is avoided by most practitioners. Its use is restricted to exceptionally low doses and very specialized clinical applications (e.g. dermatology and oncology), that exploit its poisonous irritant properties. It is highly poisonous and a very strong irritant to the skin.

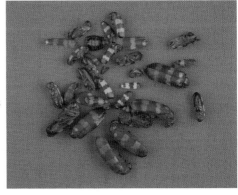

Chinese Medicinal Formulas

Chinese medicinals are rarely dispensed individually. Rather, they are dispensed as formulas consisting of anywhere from two to 20 or more medicinals. On average, a formula contains eight to 12 substances. Formulas are generally constructed on an individual basis for a single patient. One patient's formula may not be the same as another patient's formula with the same condition.

Throughout the history of Chinese medicine, thousands of formulas have been recorded and passed down. Today, these are recognized as classical formulas and form the basis of most modern formulas. For example, *On Cold Damage (Shang Han Lun)* recorded combinations that have become classical formulas and are some of the most commonly used formulas today. While collections of traditional formulas list tens of thousands of "classical" formulas, only a few hundred are commonly used. Modern formula textbooks list 250–300 different formulas. Some have very specific indications; others are broad in application. About 100 formulas are extremely commonly used. The other 150–200 are used for specific indications.

Formulas have actions that correspond to methods of treatment and indications that match specific symptoms and diseases. Depending on the disease pattern and the selected treatment method, several small, simple formulas may be combined to make a larger formula. Or a large formula may be modified by adding or removing medicinals so that it better fits the pattern. Classical formulas do not represent definite and unchangeable "medicines." Rather, they represent building blocks and serve as a guide in the selection of a strategy. As has been pointed out by famous doctors of the past, to use a formula does not mean to use its ingredients but to use its "ideas." "Ideas" refers to strategies of combining medicinals from different categories for various symptoms and patterns.

For example, medicinals from the dampness-eliminating category could be combined with medicinals to support the spleen *qi*. This is the case in Ginseng, Poria, and Ovate Atractylodes Decoction (*Shen Ling Bai Zhu San*) (**A**), a popular traditional formula that fortifies the spleen, eliminates dampness, and stops diarrhea. Besides the spleen-fortifying and dampness-eliminating medicinals, substances from the astringent category are added to stop diarrhea.

The ideas contained in such formulas can be quite complex. There are also many simple two-, three-, or four-substance formulas that are quite popular and frequently used as building blocks. For example, in the above-mentioned formula, the *qi*-supplementing portion is the four-medicinal *qi*-supplementing formula Four Gentlemen Decoction (*Si Jun Zi Tang*). Medicinals are added to eliminate dampness and to stop diarrhea. As such, Ginseng, Poria, and Ovate Atractylodes Decoction could also be considered a modification of Four Gentlemen Decoction.

Ginseng	Strengthens the spleen so that there is sufficient *qi* to transform dampness	
Ovate actractylodes	Supports ginseng in strengthening the spleen and transforms dampness	In combination, this constitutes the basic spleen *qi*-fortifying prescription Four Gentleman Decoction
Poria	Gently strengthens the spleen and percolates dampness, thus supporting ovate atractylodes and the other dampness-resolving medicinals	
Honey mix-fried licorice	Strengthens the spleen and harmonizes all the medicinals in the prescription	
Dioscoreae root	Strengthens the spleen and eliminates dampness; gently secures the intestines to stop diarrhea	
Coix seed	Eliminates dampness and gently fortifies the spleen	Combination focusing on dampness and diarrhea
Lotus fruit/seed	Astringent medicinal to stop diarrhea, which also supplements the spleen and eliminates dampness	
Lablab bean	Moderate, neutral medicinal to support the spleen and eliminate dampness	
Amomum fruit	Acrid and aromatic medicinal to penetrate dampness and activate the spleen to transform dampness	Assisting medicinals
Platycodon root	Upbearing medicinal to send the sinking spleen *qi* up to the lungs	

A Analysis of Ginseng, Poria, and Ovate Atractylodes Decoction.

Formula Structure

A Chinese medicinal formula is a composition of medicinals, organized hierarchically with a sovereign (*jun*), minister (*chen*), assistant (*zuo*) and courier (*shi*). Each performs a specific function in the formula.

The sovereign expresses the treatment method that will be applied to the disease pattern(s) or pathological process(es). For example, Agastache *Qi Righting Powder* (*Huo Xiang Zheng Qi San*) is indicated for external wind dampness assailing the middle burner with exterior signs, accompanied by nausea and vomiting. The sovereign is agastache (*huo xiang*), which addresses all three of the main pathologies: its aromatic property transforms dampness, its acridity dispels wind from the exterior, and it checks nausea and vomiting. A formula may have two or more sovereigns, each addressing aspects of the pathology. For example, if a patient suffers from dizziness due to phlegm and wind, Pinellia, Ovate Atractylodes and Gastrodia Decoction (*Ban Xia Bai Zhu Tian Ma Tang*) can be given. One sovereign, gastrodia (*tian ma*), extinguishes wind; the other, pinellia (*ban xia*), transforms phlegm.

The minister supports and complements the sovereign's functions and addresses secondary pathologies. In the *qi*-supplementing formula Four Gentlemen Decoction, the sovereign, ginseng, functions to strongly supplement *qi*. The minister, ovate atractylodes (*bai zhu*) aids in *qi* strengthening by fortifying the spleen, and its bitter,

warm nature addresses the secondary pathology of dampness. More than one substance may have the role of minister.

The assistant has three possible roles. The helpful assistant (*zuo zhu*), supports the chief or minister or addresses a minor aspect of pathology. The corrective assistant (*zuo zhi*) reduces the toxicity or moderates the harshness of the sovereign or minister ingredients. Honey-prepared licorice root and Chinese dates are frequently used corrective assistants. The opposing assistant (*zuo fan*) counteracts and opposes the sovereign ingredients' functions. This strategy is employed when opposing pathological events occur simultaneously. For example, in conditions presenting signs of both heat and cold, a bitter, cold sovereign might be opposed by a hot, acrid assistant. A formula can contain many assistant substances.

The courier has two roles. It may focus the action of a formula on a particular area or channel of the body. For example, for frontal headaches or sinus pain, Angelica dahurica root can lead the formula to the stomach channel. The courier may also harmonize all the ingredients and their actions. Licorice root is commonly used in this role. The dosage of the courier is generally small.

Not every formula contains medicinals in all roles. One sovereign and one minister together with a courier may suffice in simple cases. The overall structure and composition of formulas typically follows the classic rubric of the four roles (**A**, **B**).

Medicinal Role	Description of Function
Sovereign *Jun*/君	Performs the principal function in the formula and addresses the main aspect of the pathology. Often dosed higher than the other medicinals. May be one or more medicinals
Minister *Chen*/臣	Provides direct assistance to the sovereign and addresses possible secondary pathologies. Often dosed lower than the sovereign. May be one or more medicinals
Assistant *Zuo*/佐	Helpful assistants *(zuo zhu)* support the chief or minister or address a minor aspect of the pathology. Corrective assistants *(zuo zhi)* reduce the toxicity or moderate the harshness of the sovereign or minister ingredients. Opposing assistants *(zuo fan)* counteract and oppose the sovereign ingredients' functions. Dosage is similar to the minister. Often the majority of ingredients
Courier *Shi*/使	Focuses the action of a formula on a particular area or channel of the body and/or harmonizes all the ingredients and their actions. Often only one or two per prescription

A The structure of a formula.

Astragalus	Sovereign: strongly supplements the *qi* and ascends *yang qi*
Ginseng	Ministers: strengthen the middle burner
Ovate atractylodes	
Honey mix-fried licorice	
Tang kuei	Assistants: supplement the blood *(tang kuei)* and regulate the middle (tangerine peel), assuring that the supplementing medicinals can be digested
Tangerine peel	
Cimicifuga root	Couriers: guide upwards and raise the clear *yang qi*
Bupleurum root	

B Supplement the Center and Boost *Qi* Decoction (see also p. 265) is an imporant classical formula used to strengthen the *qi* of the spleen and stomach and to lift the clear *yang. The formula displays a complex organization with multiple ministers, assistants, and couriers.

Forms of Formula Administration

Medicinal formulas are delivered in a myriad of ways: decoctions, teas, powders, wines, tinctures, traditional and modern pills, dry and liquid extracts (**A**). Formulas are also applied topically, as liniments, ointments, sprays, baths, washes, plasters, and poultices.

Water Decoction

The most commonly used traditional form of administration is the decoction (*tang*), prepared by cooking the medicinals in water for 15 minutes to an hour, depending on the purpose. Again depending on the purpose, the herbs may be decocted a second time or discarded after one cooking. The resultant decoction is divided according to the physician's instruction and drunk two or three times per day.

The cooking time for an ingredient may vary according to its characteristics. Many minerals and toxic substances such as aconite, are decocted by themselves for 60 minutes before the other ingredients are added. Substances containing essential oils, such as mint leaves, are added just before the decoction is finished cooking. Expensive and valuable medicinals may be decocted separately or ground into powder, a small amount of which is swallowed with the strained decoction. A separately decocted herb is ginseng; a medicinal taken as powder is notoginseng root.

Formulas prepared by water decoction or dried extracts are often modified according to the specific needs of the patient. Typical aspects of patient presentation that can influence the adjustment of formulas include age, gender, weight, and underlying issues of constitution and pathology. Formulas may be adjusted by increasing or decreasing the dose of specific medicinals, as well as by removing or adding substances to address specific clinical issues.

Dried Extracts

Dried extracts of formulas or individual substances adapt traditional techniques of decoction and concentration to the production of dry concentrates using contemporary technologies. These products have gained increasing popularity due to their ease of use. Dried extracts permit the combination of standard formulas with extracts of individual herbs, which allows for formula modification and individualization.

Prepared Medicines

Prepared Chinese medicines have existed in China for centuries. Physicians, monasteries, and pharmacies sold medicines for specific indications, and many of these preparations became quite famous. Many of the "classic" guiding formulas discussed below are available in prepared form. This eliminates the possibility of their modification, but their convenience sometimes outweighs this drawback. The modern name *zhong cheng yao*, Chinese prepared medicines, appeared with the beginning of the modern pharmaceutical industry, and the market for Chinese prepared medicines is now quite large.

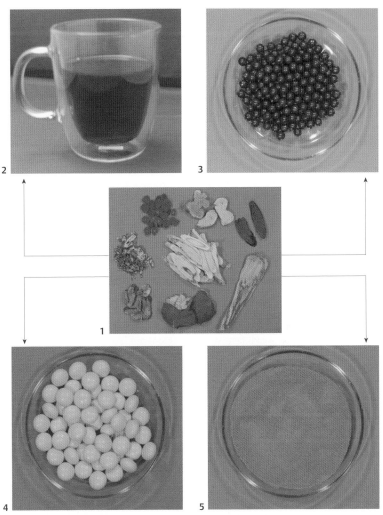

A Different forms of delivery for the classic *qi*-boosting and *yang*-rising prescription Supplement the Center and Boost *Qi* Decoction. The crude herbs (1) are cooked together into a *tang* (2), and herbal soup or decoction. This is the original and moste potent form of administration of Chinese medicines. Modern teapills (3) involve contemporary production methods, but retain the appearance of the traditional product. Ground medicines and extracts are surrounded by an enteric coating (4). Granulated preparations of spray dried herbal decoctions (5) are readily soluble in water. These more modern forms of delivery are convenient and taste better.

The early Chinese prepared medicines, called teapills, were small (2–3 mm in diameter) black pellets. Teapills are made from highly concentrated decoctions of individual ingredients that are blended with specifically selected powdered substances, made into pills and polished or coated. Chinese prepared products are also available in other forms, including tablets, syrups, coated pills, capsules, powders, and so on.

Chinese prepared products are typically based on traditional Chinese medicine theory. However, today, their composition may also be based on modern biomedical research. For example, Double Yellow and Lonicera (*Shuang Huang Lian*) tablet is composed of lonicera flower, forsythia fruit, and scutellaria. All of these substances have antiviral and antibacterial properties. The indications listed for this product include: wind–heat with such signs as common cold, cough, and sore throat. Although it can be applied according to Chinese medicine, the formula design is based on biomedical research.

Medicinal wines are another traditional form of administration. They are prepared by soaking a combination of herbs in an alcoholic beverage such as rice wine or vodka for several weeks to a year, and then drinking the result in small doses as required. Wines are mostly used as supplementing formulas or anti-rheumatics.

Medicinal Formula Categories

Just as the individual medicinal substances are organized into different categories of actions, formulas are grouped into categories according to their primary functions. These categories are based on the methods of treatment discussed earlier. These categories are further divided into subcategories, which express the treatment method embodied by the formula more precisely. The use of subcategories provides a precise delineation of the clinical application of a formula. Considered as a whole, categories and subcategories can provide over 60 distinct divisions for formulas.

While many of the categories used to organize formulas are the same as those used to organize the single substances, others are different. There can be variation between the precise delineation and number of categories and subcategories used to organize formulas. The list provided here (**A**) describes 18 categories of formulations primarily for internal use; schemes with 20 or more categories can be found depending on how the categories are divided and what types of formulas are included. Other schemes might include ejection formulas as a primary category, or describe formulas for external use. This chapter does not discuss topical preparations at all although topical preparations are discussed briefly in the chapter on *tui na*.

The following discussion of formulas addresses representative formulas in the context of their clinical applications.

Formula Category	Action
1 Exterior-resolving	Dispels exterior evils, that is, wind–heat and wind–cold from the surface of the body
2 Heat-clearing	Clears all types of heat from all aspects of the body
3 Precipitant	Frees the stool in constipation from various causes
4 Harmonizing	Harmonizes the channels, organs, and substances
5 Dryness-moistening	Resolves external and moistens internal dryness
6 Dampness-dispelling	Disperses dampness accumulation due to internal or external causes
7 Interior-warming	Disperses cold and warms the interior in replete or vacuity cold patterns
8 Supplementing	Supplements *qi*, blood, *yin*, and *yang* of the viscera and bowels
9 *Qi*-rectifying	Restores the free flow of *qi* when it is stagnant or counterflow
10 Blood-quickening	Quickens the blood and transforms stasis to promote free movement of blood
11 Blood-stanching	Stops bleeding due to a variety of causes including trauma
12 Securing and astringing	Stops diarrhea, cough, and other leakages where vacuity is both cause and consequence of the leakage
13 Spirit-quieting	Settles and quiets the spirit or nourishes and calms the spirit
14 Wind-dispelling	Extinguishes or settles wind in the interior or channels
15 Orifice-opening	Removes obstructions to the orifices to restore mental clarity or consciousness
16 Phlegm-transforming	Resolves phlegm from various different sites in the body: middle burner, lungs, nodulations, and so on
17 Dispersing formulas	Disperses stagnant food blocking the middle burner
18 Worm-expelling	Kills or eliminates various types of worms

A The 18 primary formula categories.

Exterior-resolving Formulas

Formulas in the exterior-resolving category treat external invasion where the evil remains on the surface of the body. The category includes formulas for the very early stages of wind invasion, for wind–heat and for wind–cold, for pain due to wind invading the head and neck, for wind invading a weak and vacuous body where supplementing medicinals are combined with exterior-resolving ones, and for a combination of interior repletion with exterior wind invasion.

Ephedra Decoction (*Ma Huang Tang*) was first described by Zhang Zhong Jing (p. 30) around 220 CE. It is a famous formula used to treat a patient attacked by a wind–cold evil or who, using the pattern identification system described in *On Cold Damage*, has a greater *yang* stage pattern. The presentation includes fever and chills, no sweating, muscle aches, and possibly cough. The pulse is tight and moderate and the tongue normal.

Ephedra is the sovereign, dispelling wind and cold from the surface of the body and coursing the lung *qi*; cinnamon twig (*gui zhi*), is the minister, reinforcing the warming and exterior-resolving effects of ephedra; apricot kernel (*xing ren*) is the assistant, reinforcing ephedra's action of coursing the lung *qi* to stop cough; and honey-fried licorice is the courier, harmonizing the action of the ingredients, boosting the *qi*, and moistening the lungs. The ingredients are decocted in water and the resulting liquid is taken warm to induce sweating, a sign that the *qi* of the surface of the body that had been impeded by the cold evil is free to move and dispel the evil. After drinking the tea, a bowl of rice is eaten to boost the *qi*. Once sweat arrives no further doses of the tea are taken. The sweating signals the resolution of the exterior.

Lonicera and Forsythia Powder (*Yin Qiao San*) is a very popular exterior-resolving formula indicated if wind–heat invades the body and causes sore throat, fever, aversion to wind, headache, and slight body aches. Although this is an exterior-resolving formula, its two sovereign medicinals, lonicera flower and forsythia fruit belong to the clear heat, resolve toxin category. The other main ingredients come from the exterior-resolving category. This highlights the fact that formulas are not simply a mix of medicinals from a single category, rather, they are composed of medicinals from various categories. What is important is the overall function of the formula, which in this case resolves exterior wind–heat.

This formula would be very applicable to *Jeremy*'s clinical presentation (see Chapter 3, p. 101 for details). *Jeremy* presents with an attack of wind–heat in the early stages, against a backdrop of *qi* vacuity. While it might be advisable to include some herbs to support *Jeremy*'s *qi*, perhaps American ginseng, most clinicians would provide this medicine in prepared form and recommend that *Jeremy* use it for 2–3 days until the symptoms subsided (**A**).

→ **Case Study**

Jeremy, 45-year-old man with an acute cold with a sore throat, sweating, and slightly yellow phlegm (also see Chapter 3 Diagnosis and Jeremy's case study in Chapter 4 Acupuncture)
Formula: Lonicera and Forsythia Powder

Medicinal and Dosage	Category and Role	Actions
Lonicera (9–15 g)	Heat-clearing, toxin-resolving Sovereigns	Clear heat and resolve toxins to treat early onset external invasion of wind–heat. An herb pair with these two are essential for wind–heat patterns. They help to clear the heat, stop the sore throat, and resolve the condition
Forsythia (9–15 g)		
Fermented soybean (9–12 g)	Wind–heat-dissipating Ministers	These two ministers help the sovereign pair to resolve the exterior and dispel the evil by promoting sweating
Mint (3–5 g)		
Arctium (9–12 g)	Wind–heat-dissipating Minister	These two ministers focus on diffusing the lung *qi*, transforming phlegm, and stopping cough. Together they support the sovereigns to clear heat, with a focus on the throat
Platycodon (3–6 g)	Phlegm-transforming Minister	
Schizonepeta (6–9 g)	Wind–cold-dissipating Assistant	Although in the category of wind–cold-dissipating medicinals, schizonepeta enhances the formula's ability to resolve the exterior
Fresh phragmites (15–30 g)	Heat-clearing, drain fire Assistant	These three assistants all engender liquids to stop thirst and prevent damage to *yin* from the heat Raw licorice also helps the platycodon and arctium to stop the sore throat
Lophaterum leaf (3–6 g)	Heat-clearing, drain fire Assistant	
Raw licorice (3–6 g)	*Qi*-supplementing, harmonizing Assistant + courier	

Frequently given in pill form, this formula will help Jeremy to get rid of his cold because it resolves the exterior, clears heat, and resolves toxins. Although the cold would likely go away anyway, it is important to make sure the evil is expelled so that is does not go deeper and cause other problems. Jeremy would only take the formula for a few days, so the damage to his spleen from the cold medicinals would be minimal.

A Application of the formula Lonicera and Forsythia Powder to *Jeremy's* treatment.

Heat-clearing Formulas

An expression of the treatment method "clearing," this category contains formulas to clear *qi* aspect heat, to clear construction (*ying*) and to cool the blood (*xue*). These therapeutic approaches address the patterns of febrile disease identified by the four aspects patterns of the School of Warm Diseases (see pp. 42 and 130).

The category includes formulas to clear heat and resolve toxins. Toxic heat presents with such symptoms as high fever, irritability, carbuncles, deep-rooted boils, incoherent speech, a forceful pulse, and a red tongue with a thick and yellow tongue fur. This symptom complex, indicating fire toxins, can be treated with Coptis Toxin-resolving Decoction (*Huang Lian Jie Du Tang*), a small and powerful representative from the clear heat and resolve toxin category (**A**).

In addition, there are formulas that clear heat from the organs. In many of these formulas the organ is represented by a reference to its five-phase color: Drain the White Powder (*Xie Bai San*) clears lung heat, Abduct the Red Powder (*Dao Chi San*) clears heart heat, Drain the Yellow Powder (*Xie Huang San*) clears heat from the spleen, and Drain the Blue-green Pill (*Xie Qing Wan*) clears liver heat.

A representative of the "clear organ heat" subcategory is Gentian Liver-draining Decoction (*Long Dan Xie Gan Tang*). This is the primary formula to clear liver fire and damp heat in the liver channel. This function is completed by the sovereign herb, bitter and cold gentiana root (*long dan cao*). It is supported by bitter and cold, urination-promoting minister and assistant medicinals. The formula also contains two corrective assistants to protect *yin* and blood from the bitter and cold medicinals as well as from the burning and drying of the liver fire.

Precipitant Formulas

If heat damages the fluids, drying the intestines and leading to repletion heat constipation, it is necessary to clear heat and precipitate the bowels. Major Qi-coordinating Decoction (*Da Cheng Qi Tang*), addressing greater *yang* organ heat, is used. Its main ingredients, rhubarb and mirabilitum (*mang xiao*) clear heat, move the bowels, and soften hardness. They are supported by the *qi*-rectifying and distension-resolving medicinals immature aurantium fruit (*zhi shi*) and magnolia bark (*hou po*).

If the stool does not move due to dryness, moist precipitant formulas are used. Hemp Seed Pill (*Ma Zi Ren Wan*), consisting of various seeds that all have a bowel-moistening function can be used.

If cold accumulates in the intestine, blocking the free flow of *qi* and *yang*, presenting with gripping cold abdominal pain with constipation, Rhubarb and Aconite Decoction (*Da Huang Fu Zi Tang*) is used. In this formula, hot medicinals that dispel cold (aconite accessory root) are combined with precipitating medicinals (rhubarb) to warm the interior and move the bowels (**B**).

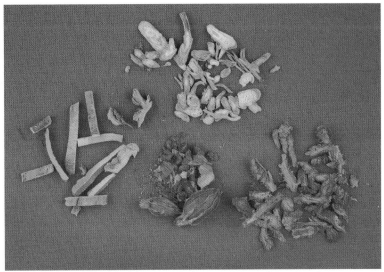

A Coptis Toxin Resolving Decoction is a potent heat-toxin (or toxic heat) resolving prescription. It is a combination of four bitter and cold medicinals from the damp-heat clearing category. Pronounced damp heat quickly leads to what is considered toxic heat in Chinese medicine. Among the four medicinals in this prescription are the "three yellows" which each clears damp heat from one of the three burners, thus clearing damp heat from the entire body. The fourth ingredient, red gardenia fruits, clears damp heat from all three burners.

Heat-clearing Formulas	Precipitant Formulas
Clear *qi* aspect heat	Cold precipitation
Clear construction and cool the blood	Moist precipitation
Clear both *qi* and construction	Warm precipitation
Clear heat and resolve toxins	Expel water
Clear organ heat	Simultaneous supplementation and attack
Clear vacuity heat	
Clear heat and resolve summer heat	

B Actions of heat-clearing and precipitant formulas.

Harmonizing Formulas

Harmonization refers to adjusting an imbalance between two separate, often opposing, pathological events. Often, medicinals from opposing categories are combined in harmonizing formulas. There are three groups of harmonizing formulas: 1) formulas that harmonize the lesser *yang* where disease evils are trapped between the exterior and interior; 2) formulas that harmonize wood and earth when the liver overwhelms the spleen or stomach and disrupts proper digestive functioning; and 3) formulas that harmonize the stomach and intestines, when cold and heat combine and block the middle burner (**B**).

Representative of this category is Minor Bupleurum Decoction (*Xiao Chai Hu Tang*) (**A**). Originally designed by Zhang Zhong Jing to treat the lesser *yang* channel presentation in which an externally invading cold evil lodges between the interior and exterior, it combines medicinals that clear internal heat with medicinals that resolve external heat. The combination of acrid, bitter, and slightly cold bupleurum root (*chai hu*) with bitter and very cold scutellaria root (*huang qin*) has become a standard combination to clear and resolve heat in the liver. Minor Bupleurum Decoction includes assistants to supplement the spleen and fortify the *qi*, and assistants to transform phlegm and regulate stomach *qi*. It is indicated for much more than the general presentation of a lesser *yang* pattern with alternating fever and chills, dry throat, nausea and vomiting, dizziness, sensa-

tion of fullness in the chest and hypochondriac region and a string-like pulse. It may also used for childhood conditions such as otitis media because it elegantly addresses the common pediatric pathologies of heat, dampness, and spleen vacuity. Similarly, it is one of the primary formulas to treat hepatitis, which often presents with a complex pattern involving heat, *qi* stagnation, dampness, and vacuity.

Dryness-moistening Formulas

If dryness evil invades the body, acrid exterior-resolving medicinals are combined to dispel the exterior evil through the surface. For example, Apricot Kernel and Perilla Leaf Powder (*Xing Su San*), contains no moistening medicinals but instead acrid exterior-resolving herbs. Similarly, the classical formula for heat dryness, Mulberry Leaf and Apricot Kernel Decoction (*Sang Xing Tang*), is governed by acrid and cool exterior resolving herbs and contains only two moistening medicinals.

If internal dryness develops, then moistening formulas are used. Because the lung is particularly sensitive to dryness, many of the formulas in this category moisten the lungs and nourish lung *yin*. For example, Lily Bulb Metal-securing Decoction (*Bai He Gu Jin Tang*), nourishes *yin*, moistens the lungs, transforms phlegm and stops coughing, and is indicated for lung dryness and lung *yin* vacuity signs such as coughing with blood-streaked sputum, dry mouth and throat, heat in the five hearts, and a red tongue with thin or peeling fur (**B**).

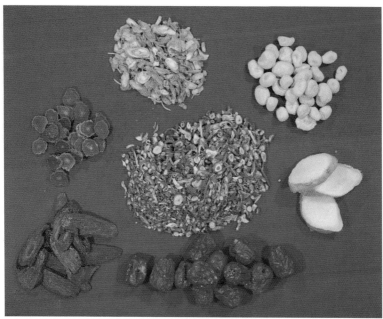

A Minor Bupleurum Decoction is the most representative prescription for resolving *Shaoyang* **Channel Patterns.** Due to its combination of heat-clearing, phlegm-resolving, and *qi*-supplementing medicinals, it is an ideal prescription to treat children. As such, it is the most popular prescription for many childhood illnesses.

Harmonizing Formulas

Harmonize lesser *yang*

Harmonize liver and stomach

Harmonize stomach and intestines

Dryness-moistening Formulas

Moisten dryness by light diffusion

Enrich *yin* and moisten dryness

B Action of harmonizing and dryness-moistening formulas.

Dampness-dispelling Formulas

Formulas in the dampness-dispelling category address damp accumulation, however, the manner of doing this varies according to the presentation. Poria Five Powder (*Wu Ling San*) (**A**, **B**) is a formula that "disinhibits water and percolates dampness." It combines three bland and neutral or slightly cool substances that disinhibit urine with atractylodes macrocephala rhizome and cinnamon twig, which support the spleen's transformative action. Poria Five Powder is indicated for general dampness accumulation signs such as edema, generalized sensation of heaviness, diarrhea, and urinary difficulty.

The sovereign medicinals in formulas that "dry dampness and harmonize the stomach" are from the aromatic, transform damp category. Dampness evil enters as wind–cold–dampness assailing the spleen or manifest when wind–cold assails a person with spleen damp. The result is fever and chills, headache, a sensation of fullness and oppression in the chest, pain in the epigastrium and abdomen, nausea and vomiting, and diarrhea. Agastache *Qi* Righting Powder treats this by combining aromatic dampness-penetrating medicinals with exterior-resolving and *qi*-rectifying substances.

Eight Rectification Powder (*Ba Zheng San*), which combines bitter and cold medicinals from the dampness-draining category with bitter and cold medicinals from the heat-clearing category, belongs to the subcategory of formulas that "clear heat and dispel dampness." It clears heat, drains fire, disinhibits urine, and frees painful uri-nation. It is indicated if damp heat lodges in the urinary bladder, manifesting as urinary tract infections.

Formulas that warm and dispel water damp are used when dampness combines with cold to form cold dampness. True Warrior Decoction (*Zhen Wu Tang*) combines acrid and hot aconite root with dampness-transforming and urination-promoting ovate atractylodes and poria. It warms *yang* and disinhibits urine and is indicated if damaged and vacuous *yang* fails to transform water, which then accumulates in the body.

Formulas that dispel wind and overcome dampness are used to treat impediment patterns. The sovereign and minister ingredients are from the dampness-dispelling category, such as Angelica root (*du huo*) and gentiana root (*long dan cao*). Medicinals from other categories are used to address wind–dampness lodged in the joints. For example, in Angelica pubescens and Mistletoe Decoction (*Du Huo Ji Sheng Tang*), medicinals that supplement the liver and kidney are added, thus treating wind–damp-cold with kidney and liver vacuity. In Cinnamon Twig, White Peony, and Anemarrhena Decoction (*Gui Zhi Shao Yao Zhi Mu Tang*), a formula indicated for early stage wind–dampness in the superficial layers of the joints, ephedra is added to disperse the wind. Because dampness always combines with wind when invading the joints, every formula in this subcategory contains wind-dispelling medicinals, most commonly saposhnikovia root (*fang feng*) (**C**).

Medicinal and Role	Category	Actions
Alisma Sovereign	Water-disinhibiting Dampness-percolating	Disinhibits urination and dispels dampness
Poria Minister	Water-disinhibiting Dampness-percolating	Disinhibits urination, dispels dampness, and gently fortifies the spleen
Polyporus Minister	Water-disinhibiting Dampness-percolating	Disinhibits urination and dispels dampness
Ovate atractylodes Assistant	Supplements *qi*	Fortifies the spleen and dries dampness
Cinnamon twig Assistant	Wind–cold-dissipating	Warms the spleen, supports *qi* transformation, and thereby transforms dampness

A Analysis of Poria Five Powder.

B Poria Five Powder is the basic prescription to fortify the spleen and promote urination, thus eliminating dampness. It combines dampness-eliminating medicinals such as poria and polyporous with warm water-transforming cinnamon twig and dampness-transforming ovate atractylodes, thus making use of three separate ways in which pathological water and dampness is eliminated from the body.

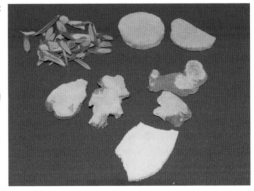

C Actions of dampness-dispelling formulas.

Dampness-dispelling Formulas

Disinhibit water and percolate dampness

Dry dampness and harmonize the stomach

Clear heat and dispel dampness

Warm and transform water damp

Dispel wind and overcome dampness

Interior-warming Formulas

Interior cold has its origin either in repletion cold or in vacuity cold. Repletion cold occurs when external cold invades the body and either passes through the greater *yang* channel and moves to the interior or directly invades the interior. Vacuity cold arises when the *yang qi* of an organ, usually the heart, the spleen, or the kidney, becomes vacuous and so the *yang* is unable to warm the body or particular areas of the body, especially the limbs. The formulas in this category can be divided into three groups: formulas that warm the channels and dissipate cold, formulas that warm the center and dispel cold and formulas that return *yang* and stem counterflow (**B**).

If *yang qi* is depleted, it does not warm the extremities, which become icy cold. Acrid and hot medicinals that enter the channels and network vessels and invigorate the flow of *yang qi* as well as disperse cold are indicated. *Tangkuei* Counterflow Cold Decoction (*Dang Gui Si Ni Tang*) combines such medicinals with blood-supplementing substances and is the main formula for cold hands and feet secondary to blood vacuity and *yang* debility.

The second group of formulas warm the center and dispel cold. They act to warm the *yang* of the middle burner. Center Rectifying Pill (*Li Zhong Wan*) or its hotter modification, Aconite Center Rectifying Pill (*Fu Zi Li Zhong Wan*) (**A**),

are representative formulas. Center Rectifying Pill warms the middle burner and fortifies spleen *qi*. It contains dried ginger, which acts to warm the spleen and stomach. The formula is indicated for spleen *yang* vacuity manifesting as diarrhea with watery stool, nausea and vomiting, lack of appetite, abdominal pain, a pale tongue with white fur, and a deep and forceless pulse. When cold signs are more severe, the addition of prepared aconite produces the formula Aconite Center Rectifying Pill.

Finally, there are several small, powerful formulas to return the *yang* and stem counterflow. These formulas treat *yang* desertion, a dangerous state where *yang* is exhausted to the point where it leaves the body. The two representatives both include acrid and hot aconite accessory root. Ginseng and Aconite Decoction (*Shen Fu Tang*) contains only aconite accessory root and ginseng root. This formula is meant to be used in acute conditions where there is a severe vacuity of original *qi*. It should not be used long term. After the acute state is resolved, the patient should be appropriately treated based on their condition. Counterflow Cold Decoction (*Si Ni Tang*) focuses more strongly on invigorating *yang* and combines aconite accessory root with dried ginger root and honey mix-fried licorice root. This formula may be used for a longer time in order to rectify a severe condition (**B**).

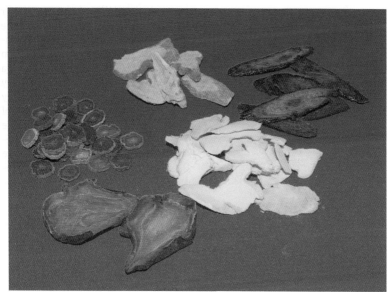

A Aconite Center Rectifying Pill consists of five medicinal substances from three different categories. These are the *qi*-supplementing medicinals such as panax ginseng and ovate atractylodes; urination-promoting medicinal poria; and hot true *yang*-rectifying aconite accessory root. It thus strongly supplements the *yang* fire in the middle burner and is indicated for vacuity cold of the spleen.

Interior-warming Formulas

Warm the channels and dissipate cold

Warm the center and dispel cold

Return *yang* and stem counterflow

B Actions of interior-warming formulas.

Supplementing Formulas

As with the supplementing medicinals, these formulas are divided into four sub-categories, each focused on one of the four main substances: *qi*, blood, *yin*, and *yang*. This very large category contains some of the most basic and frequently used formulas. For each of the four sub-categories, one representative can be considered the "prototype" for supplementation of the respective substance. Often, these formulas are used as the base for a myriad of other formulas.

Four Gentleman Decoction (*Si Jun Zi Tang*) (**A**) is the classic formula to fortify the spleen and supplement *qi*. Each of its four herbs focuses on a slightly different aspect of *qi* vacuity. Ginseng root, the sovereign, powerfully fortifies *qi*, ovate atractylodes, the minister, fortifies the spleen to support the sovereign and, through its bitter taste, dries dampness. Poria, the assistant, slightly supplements the spleen and drains dampness. Honey mix-fried licorice root, the courier, harmonizes all the medicinals and aids in gently supporting the middle. This formula is the base for many *qi*-supplementing formulas (see p. 261).

Four Agents Decoction (*Si Wu Tang*) (**B**) is the primary blood-supplementing formula. It combines three blood-supplementing medicinals (*tang kuei*, prepared rehmannia root, and white peony root) with a blood- and *qi*-moving medicinal (ligusticum/*chuan xiong*), to supplement and gently move blood. It is the base of many blood-supplementing formulas.

When these two formulas are combined, they become a basic eight-herb

formula to supplement *qi* and nourish blood, Eight Gem Decoction (*Ba Zhen Tang*) (**C**), which is also the base of many *qi*- and blood-supplementing formulas.

Whereas the basic *qi*- and blood-supplementing formulas share a similar structure, the basic *yin*- and *yang*-enriching formulas share almost the same ingredients. The eight-ingredient *yang*-supplementing formula Golden Coffer Kidney Qi Pill (*Jin Gui Shen Qi Wan*) was written by Zhang Zhong Jing as a part of the *Essential Prescriptions of the Golden Coffer (Jin Gui Yao Lue)*. It contains three groups of substances. The first consists of processed aconite accessory root and cinnamon bark to warm the interior and invigorate *yang*.[*] The second consists of three *yin*-supplementing medicinals: prepared rehmannia root, cornus fruit, and dioscorea root (*shan yao*). This group is complemented by the third group, three moving and dampness-eliminating medicinals: alisma (*ze xie*), moutan (*mu dan pi*), and poria. The six medicinals in the second and third sets can be grouped to form three pairs that match a supplementing medicinal with a moving medicinal: cooked rehmannia and alisma treat the kidneys, cornus fruit and moutan treat the liver, and dioscorea and poria treat the spleen. The three active, moving medicinals ensure that the sticky, slimy qualities of the *yin*-enriching medicinals do not cause stagnation.

---

[*]   Traditionally the formula contained cinnamon twig, but most clinicians feel that cinnamon bark is a more *yang*-invigorating substance.

A–C Four Gentlemen Decoction (A) is the basic four-herb *qi*-supplementing prescription. Four Agents Decoction **(B)** is the basic four-herb blood-supplementing prescription. The combination of these two four-herb combinations for *qi* and blood supplementation leads to the basic eight-herb *qi*- and blood-supplementing formula Eight Gem Decoction **(C)**.

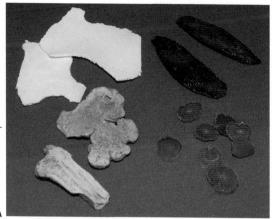

A

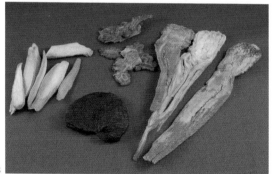

B

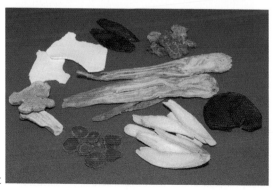

C

Nearly 1000 years after Zhang Zhong Jing, Qian Yi, in his *Formulary of Pediatric Patterns (Xiao Er Yao Zheng Zhi Jue)*, modified the Golden Coffer Kidney *Qi* Pill to create the Six Ingredient Rehmannia Pill (*Liu Wei Di Huang Wan*). In this formula, the two *yang*-supplementing substances (aconite accessory root and cinnamon bark) are removed to create a simple *yin*-nourishing formula. In modern usage, Six Ingredient Rehmannia Pill has become the standard *yin*-nourishing formula.

Yin and *yang* are interrelated. There must be sufficient *yang* to produce *yin* and sufficient *yin* to provide the basis for engendering *yang*. The Golden Coffer Kidney *Qi* Pill relies on the principle that if *yin* is fortified and strong, a small but powerful group of *yang*-invigorating medicinals is sufficient to supplement and warm the *yang*. Hence, this formula is indicated in the treatment of kidney *yang* vacuity, presenting with low back pain with a cold feeling, weak and aching lower extremities, generalized cold, a deep and forceless pulse, and a pale tongue. Often this pattern is accompanied by signs of dampness because the *yang* is unable to move the fluids, and underneath the dampness by signs of *yin* vacuity, which are harder to discern.

If we return to *John*, our 69-year-old male with chronic low back and knee pain, we can understand the action of the Golden Coffer Kidney *Qi* Pill and Six Ingredient Rehmannia Pill (**A**). *John*'s diagnosis was kidney *yang* vacuity and dampness causing low back pain (see Chapter 3, pp. 101, 150–151 and Chapter 4, pp. 198–199). In *John*'s case, the vacuity of kidney *yang* is unable to warm the fluids and steam them back up to the lungs. Additionally, the warming action of the kidney is insufficient to warm the spleen *yang*, creating problems with the movement of fluids in the body and with the production of *qi*. The lack of steaming and fluid movement creates an accumulation of dampness. When this type of pathological damp appears, it is important not to simply drain the damp or there will be damage to the physiological fluids. When there is repletion of pathological damp, this may indicate that elsewhere in the body there is vacuity of physiological fluids. Thus, a formula like the Golden Coffer Kidney *Qi* Pill will invigorate the *yang*, drain the fluids, and protect the *yin* from damage.

Because *John*'s case is quite complicated, modifications would be made to his formula. Modifications might include adding astragalus root to fortify the spleen *qi* and a blood-quickening medicinal such as spatholobus root and vine (*ji xue teng*) to relieve pain. Other *yang*-supplementing medicinals such as dipsacus root (*xu duan*) or eucommia bark (*du zhong*) might also be added both for the *yang* and to relieve pain. Additionally one might add amomum fruit (*sha ren*) to help the spleen digest the decoction.

→ **Case Study**

John, 69-year-old male with chronic low back and knee pain for 12 years.
Formula: Golden Coffer Kidney *Qi* Pill.

Substance and Dosage	Category and Role	Actions
Processed aconite root (3 g)	Interior Warming Minister	Dissipates cold and eliminates dampness by warming the kidney and spleen *yang*. Dispels cold from the channels and frees the blood vessels. Specifically used for dampness and pain due to cold-damp impediment. In *John's* case it will help to relieve his back and knee pain and to eliminate the damp accumulation
Cinnamon bark (3 g)	Interior Warming Minister	Supplements original *yang*, eliminates accumulated cold and frees the blood vessels. It will help to relieve the back and knee pain by dispelling cold and warming the kidney *yang*
Prepared rehmannia root (24 g)	Blood-supplementing Sovereign	Nourishes blood and enriches *yin*. It will protect *John's yin* fluids from damage by the hot and drying cinnamon bark and processed aconite accessory root and build *yang* by enriching *yin*
Alisma (9 g)	Dampness-dispelling Assistant	Disinhibits water and percolates dampness. It will help to drain pathologic fluids through the urine while helping the kidney to process fluids, allowing physiologic fluids to return to where they belong and draining pathologic fluids
Cornus fruit (12 g)	Secure and astringe Minister	Supplements the liver and kidney *yin* and astringes essential *qi*. Balances the formula to prevent excessive loss of fluid through urination
Moutan (9 g)	Heat-clearing, blood-cooling Assistant	Clears heat, cools blood, harmonizes the blood and disperses stasis. This will help to protect the *yin* and prevent the development of pathological heat. Additionally, it will help the aconite and cinnamon bark to move the blood and stop pain
Dioscorea root (12 g)	*Qi*-supplementing Minister	Fortifies the spleen, secures the kidney, and boosts essence. Works with cornus fruit to prevent excessive loss of essential *qi* through the urine and fortifies the spleen to help with the movement of fluids
Poria (9 g)	Dampness-dispelling Assistant	Disinhibits water and percolates dampness, and boosts the spleen. Together with alisma it drains pathological fluids. Together with dioscorea root it fortifies the spleen to aid in the movement of fluids

This formula will 1) warm and invigorate *John's* kidney and spleen *yang* to move the pathological fluids and so that the home of the kidney, the lower back, will be warm, allowing *qi* and blood to flow smoothly and reducing pain; 2) protect the kidney *yin* from damage; 3) fortify the spleen qi to manage the movement of fluids through the body; 4) drain pathological fluids from the body to eliminate dampness

A Application of the formula Golden Coffer Kidney *Qi* Pill to *John's* treatment.

Qi-rectifying Formulas

Most of the sovereign and minister ingredients in these formulas stem from the *qi*-rectifying medicinal category. The category is broken into two subcategories: the subcategory of *qi*-moving formulas treat *qi* that is blocked and inhibited in its free flow, requiring acrid, *qi*-moving medicinals to free the *qi* flow; the subcategory of formula that downbears counterflow and check vomiting treats *qi* that flows counter to its intended direction, requiring medicinals to treat counterflow *qi* signs such as cough or nausea and vomiting (**A**).

Stagnant *qi* engenders pain, thus *qi*-moving formulas all stop pain. *Qi* is the motive force of the body. If *qi* stagnates, then blood, fluids, and food may stagnate and, over time, transform into heat. Zhu Dan Xi, one of four great medical scholars of the Jin/Yuan dynasty (see pp. 40, 226), established the theory of the six depressions and created the prototypical formula Depression Overcoming Pill (*Yue Ju Wan*), which treats five of the six depressions. It includes one medicinal for each depression: cyperus root (*xiang fu*) for *qi* depression; ligusticum (*chuan xiong*) for blood stasis; gardenia fruit (*zhi zi*) for fire depression; atractylodes root (*cang zhu*) for dampness depression; and medicated leaven (*shen qu*) for food depression (**B, C**). Although Depression Overcoming Formula is not a very commonly used formula due to lack of specificity, it is a starting point for the treatment of all kinds of depression.

Other *qi*-regulating formulas deal specifically with localized *qi* stagnation. Pinellia and Magnolia Bark Decoction (*Ban Xia Hou Po Tang*) treats stagnation of *qi* and phlegm in the throat. Trichosanthis, Chinese Chive, and White Liquor Decoction (*Gua Lou Xie Bai Bai Jiu Tang*) treats stagnation of *yang* and *qi* in the chest, manifesting with chest impediment symptoms including pain. *Tian Tai* Lindera Powder (*Tian Tai Wu Yao San*) treats stagnation of *qi* and cold in the liver channel, manifesting with severe lower abdominal pain radiating to the testicles.

The formulas to downbear counterflow can be divided into the stomach *qi*-downbearing group to treat hiccough, burping, nausea and vomiting, and the lung *qi*-downbearing category to stop cough. Perilla Fruit *Qi* Downbearing Decoction (*Su Zi Jiang Qi Tang*) and Panting Stabilizing Decoction (*Ding Chuan Tang*) are both formulas of the latter category and stop panting and coughing by sending counterflow lung *qi* downward. Perilla Fruit *Qi* Downbearing Decoction contains warm medicinals such as perilla fruit (*su zi*), *tang kuei*, and magnolia cortex and treats coughing and panting due to cold phlegm blocking the lungs. Panting Stabilizing Decoction contains cool and cold medicinals such as scutellaria and Mulberry Bark (*sang bai pi*) and is indicated in the treatment of coughing and panting due to phlegm heat blocking the lungs.

A Action of *qi*-rectifying formulas.

Qi-rectifying Formulas

Move *qi*

Downbear counterflow and check vomiting

Medicinal and Role	Category	Actions
Cyperus Sovereign	*Qi*-rectifying	Courses *qi* and resolves *qi* depression
Ligusticum Minister	Blood-rectifying	Quickens blood and transforms blood stasis
Gardenia Minister and assistant	Heat-clearing	Clears heat and resolves heat depression
Atractylodes Minister and assistant	Dampness dispelling	Transforms and dries dampness and resolves dampness depression
Medicated leaven Minister and assistant	Food-dispersing	Transforms stagnant food and resolves food depression

B Depression Overcoming Formula.

C *Yue Ju Wan* means "Depression Overcoming Formula." Depression here refers to a stagnation or accumulation. This traditional prescription contains five ingredients, one for each type of depression (clockwise, beginning in the top left-hand corner, middle last): medicated leaven for food stagnation; ligusticum for blood stasis; atractylodes root for dampness; gardenia fruit for heat accumulation; and cyperus root for *qi* stagnation.

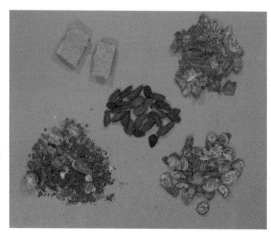

Blood-quickening Formulas

Formulas that dispel stasis and quicken blood address pain and dysfunction caused by static blood. A formula that is prescribed for many types of blood stasis is Peach Kernel and Carthamus Four Agents Decoction (*Tao Hong Si Wu Tang*), which is a modification of Four Agents Decoction (*Si Wu Tang*) (see p. 278). By adding peach kernel and carthamus flower, the formula both quickens and nourishes the blood.

Formulas in this category often deal with blood stasis due to a specific cause or in a specific place. House of Blood Stasis Expelling Decoction (*Xue Fu Zhu Yu Tang*) expands upon the idea of Peach Kernel and Carthamus Four Agents Decoction by adding *qi*-rectifying and chest-opening medicinals. Originally formulated for blood stasis in the chest, today it is used as a base formula for all types of blood stasis. Sudden Smile Powder (*Shi Xiao San*) is composed of two medicinals: typha pollen (*pu huang*) and flying squirrel droppings (*wu ling zhi*). Both strongly quicken the blood and stop bleeding. This is an important formula for blood stasis menstrual pain.

Alice, who suffers from severe dysmenorrhea due to *qi* and blood stasis (see above and, Chapter 3, pp. 101, 152–153) and Chapter 4, pp. 200–201) could be treated with a combination of Peach Kernel and Carthamus Four Agents Decoction and Sudden Smile Powder. She was seen at Day 27 of her cycle, presenting with severe headache and anticipating severe pain during the first two days of her cycle. The eight agents in this formula, with appropriate specific modifications would be very suitable for her condition (**A**).

Salvia Beverage (*Dan Shen Yin*) contains salvia root (*dan shen*), the main medicinal for blood stasis in the chest as its sovereign. Salvia Beverage primarily treats blood stasis chest impediment. If stasis is due to cold congelation, medicinals to warm and disperse cold are added to the stasis-transforming and blood-quickening medicinals. Warm the Menses Decoction (*Wen Jing Tang*) warms the menses and treats cold menstrual pain. In it, warm evodia fruit (*wu zhu yu*) and cinnamon twig are combined with ligusticum and moutan bark. If traumatic injury leads to swelling and pain, formulas from this category can be selected (see p. 235).

Blood-stanching Formulas

Bleeding can be due to hot blood frenetically stirring outside of the vessels, to vacuous *qi* not holding blood in the vessels, to stasis blocking the vessels and causing blood to extravasate into the surrounding tissue and to traumatic injury severing the blood vessels.

These formulas are specific to stopping bleeding and deal with a specific type of bleeding. Cephalanoplos Drink (*Xiao Ji Yin Zi*) treats blood in the urine, Sophora Flower Powder (*Huai Hua San*) treats blood in the stool, Blood Cough Formula (*Ke Xue Fang*) treats coughing of blood and Heat-clearing Uterine Bleeding Decoction (*Qing Re Zhi Beng Tang*) stops excessive menstrual bleeding.

→ Case Study

Alice, 23-year-old female with severe dysmenorrhea for 8 years. Presenting on Day 27 of cycle with a very bad headache and anticipating severe menstrual pain.
Formula: Peach Kernel and Carthamus Four Agents Decoction and Sudden Smile Powder

Medicinal and Dosage	Category and Role	Actions
Tang kuei (6 g)	Blood-supplementing Sovereign	Supplements and harmonizes the blood, regulates menstruation and relieves pain. One of the most important substances for supplementing blood and regulating menstruation to stop pain
Cooked rehmannia root (6 g)	Blood-supplementing Minister	Enriches *yin* and supplements blood. One of the most important ways to supplement the blood is via the *yin*, thus this minister supports the supplementing aspect of *tang kuei*
White peony root (6 g)	Blood-supplementing Assistant	Nourishes the blood and emolliates the liver, moderates the center and relieves pain. Another very important substance for menstrual pain, peony root assists *tang kuei* in supplementing and it stops pain
Ligusticum root (3 g)	Blood-quickening Courier	Moves *qi* and relieves depression and quickens the blood and stops pain. This courier focuses Four Agents Decoction on movement of the *qi* and blood. It is especially good for headaches and menstrual pain
Peach kernel (6 g)	Blood-quickening Assistant	Breaks the blood and moves stasis. An extremely strong blood-quickening substance that, when added to Four Agents Decoction, works with carthamus to move blood and relieve menstrual pain
Carthamus (3 g)	Blood-quickening Assistant	Quickens the blood and frees menstruation, eliminates stasis and relieves pain. The herb pair of peach kernel and carthamus is the most commonly used pair for treating menstrual pain
Typha pollen (9–12 g)	Blood-quickening	Quickens the blood and disperses stasis. The first substance in Sudden Smile Powder, a formula that focuses on the treatment of pain due to blood stasis in the lower burner
Flying squirrel droppings (9–12 g)	Blood-quickening	Moves the blood and relieves pain. The second substance in Sudden Smile Powder. These two substances are remarkably effective for stopping pain due to blood stasis

This formula contains the basic blood-supplementing formula Four Agents Decoction with the addition of peach kernel and carthamus. Because the blood vacuity signs are not prominent here, the amount of prepared rehmannia root might be slightly reduced. The other substances all move the blood and stop pain. After the menses are completed, Sudden Smile Powder would be removed and the dosages of prepared rehmannia root and *tang kuei* increased to build blood while continuing to move it, albeit more gently

A Application of Peach Kernel and Carthamus Four Agents Decoction and Sudden Smile Powder to *Alice's* treatment.

Securing and Astringing Formulas

The securing and astringing formulas are a diverse group of formulas that secure that which leaks from the body due to insecurity or lack of holding. This group of formulas can be divided into four subcategories: securing and astringing the exterior and the lungs; securing and astringing intestinal leakage; securing and astringing the kidneys; and securing and astringing the womb.

A representative lung-securing formula is Jade Wind-barrier Powder (*Yu Ping Feng San*) (**A, B**). This small, elegant formula combines acrid exterior-resolving medicinals to treat assailing wind with *qi*-boosting and spleen-fortifying medicinals. A key ingredient in this formula is astragalus root (*huang qi*), which powerfully boosts *qi* and secures the exterior. This formula is indicated when the defensive *qi* is "insecure" and external evils attack the body frequently, manifesting as recurrent colds.

Representative of the intestine-astringing subcategory is the Four Spirits Pill (*Si Shen Wan*). The Four Spirits Pill is indicated for severe diarrhea. Although the cause of the diarrhea is an advanced *yang* depletion of the kidneys and spleen, the treatment principle is to warm the spleen and kidney *yang* and astringe and secure to stop the diarrhea. The formula combines *yang*-warming psoralea fruit (*bu gu zhi*) and acrid and hot, cold-dispersing evodia fruit (*wu zhu yu*) with the warm, intestine-securing myristica seed (nut-meg) (*rou dou kou*) and schisandra berry (*wu wei zi*).

Kidney *qi* controls the lower orifice. Spontaneous seminal emissions as well as enuresis or incontinence are signs of weakened kidney *qi*. In addition to fortifying kidney *qi*, it is sometimes necessary to use stabilizing and securing medicinals to stop leakage. For example, the formula Stream Reducing Pill (*Suo Quan Wan*) combines three astringing medicinals to stop urinary frequency and two medicinals to warm the kidney and dispel cold. Stream Reducing Pill is indicated in patients complaining of frequent, clear, prolonged urination and/or enuresis accompanied by kidney *yang* vacuity signs.

Womb-securing formulas astringe discharge from the uterus, including vaginal bleeding or vaginal discharge. Again, this subcategory has to be used in combination with other formula categories because the focus is primarily on stopping leakage without treating the root problem. For example, Thoroughfare Securing Decoction (*Gu Chong Tang*) primarily stops uterine bleeding due to spleen *qi* not securing. This condition can also be treated by boosting *qi* and fortifying the spleen. However, supplementation would focus only on the root and would not act quickly enough to stop the bleeding. Besides containing *qi*-boosting and spleen-fortifying medicinals, Thoroughfare Securing Decoction also contains astringing medicinals to stop bleeding, such as cornus fruit, dragon bone, oyster shell, and sepia bone (*hai piao xiao*) (**C**).

Medicinal and Role	Category	Actions
Astragalus Sovereign	*Qi*-supplementing	Secures the exterior, fortifies the spleen, and supplements defense *qi*
Ovate atractylodes Minister	*Qi*-supplementing	Fortifies the spleen, supplements the *qi*, and transforms dampness
Saposhnikovia root Assistant	Exterior-resolving	Resolves exterior wind

A Jade Wind-barrier Powder.

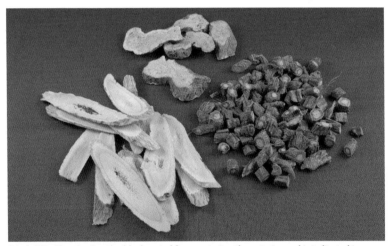

B Jade Wind-barrier Powder blocks wind from entering the exterior and is indicated in people who easily catch cold. In Chinese medicine, this symptom indicates poor defensive *qi* guarding the exterior of the body. In this prescription, astragalus and ovate macrocephalae strengthen the *qi* by supplementing the middle. Acrid and slightly warm saposhnikovia root courses wind and protects the exterior.

C Actions of securing and astringing formulas.

Secure and Astringing Formulas

Constrain sweat and secure the exterior (constrain lung and suppress cough)

Astringe the intestines and stem desertion

Astringe essence and check seminal emission and enuresis

Secure and astringe the womb

Spirit-quieting Formulas

There are three causes for a disquieted spirit: lack of nourishment of the spirit (heart blood or heart *yin* vacuity), heat disturbing the spirit (heart fire or *yin* vacuity), and obstruction of the spirit (blood stasis and phlegm blockage). This category contains formulas to nourish and quiet the spirit and to clear heat and quiet the spirit. Blockage of the spirit is addressed in the phlegm and blood stasis categories.

Celestial Emperor's Heart Supplementing Elixir (*Tian Wang Bu Xin Dan*) nourishes heart *yin* and blood and calms the spirit. It is a complex formula with almost 15 ingredients. Clinically, it is very effective in quieting the spirit secondary to lack of nourishment of the heart by *yin* and blood.

The second subcategory consists of settling and clearing formulas. Heat is downborne with heavy medicinals like magnetite (*ci shi*) and dragon bone and cleared with bitter and cold medicinals like coptis. Many of the formulas in this category traditionally contain cinnabar (*zhu sha*), a toxic medicinal that is no longer used.

Wind-dispelling Formulas

Wind-dispelling formulas address wind in the skin and channels and internal wind. Wind in the skin manifests primarily as itching. For widespread skin itching with weeping red rashes, Wind-dispersing Powder (*Xiao Feng San*) is indicated. This formula is composed of three groups of medicinals: wind-resolving medicinals serving as sovereigns and resolving exterior wind to stop itching, dampness-eliminating and urination-promoting medicinals serving as ministers, and heat-clearing medicinals serving as ministers.

Wind in the channels refers to external wind attacking the channels and blocking the flow of *qi*, leading to paralysis or nerve pain. Wind invading the channels describes acute and localized paralysis attacks such as Bell's Palsy as well as nerve pain such as trigeminal neuralgia and peripheral neuritis. A representative formula is Pull Aright Powder also known as Lead to Symmetry Powder (*Qian Zheng San*), which treats sudden facial paralysis with deviated eyes and mouth.

Internal wind is closely linked with the liver. If liver fire is strong, extreme heat can lead to wind. A clinical example is a child with high fever who develops cramping, which can be treated with Antelope Horn and Uncaria Decoction (*Ling Jiao Gou Teng Tang*)*, a formula combining cool and cold wind-extinguishing medicinals with liver fire-clearing and *yin*- and blood-nourishing substances.

Internal wind may also arise due to ascendant liver *yang* secondary to liver *yin* vacuity. In this case Gastrodia and Uncaria Beverage (*Tian Ma Gou Teng Yin*) (**A, B**) is chosen. This formula consists of wind-settling medicinals, heat-clearing medicinals, blood-quickening medicinals, and *yin*-nourishing medicinals (**C**).

---

*   Due to the endangered status of antelopes, their horns are no longer used. They are substituted with Cornu caprae (*shan yang jiao*), goat horn.

Medicinal and Role	Category	Actions
Gastrodia Sovereign	Liver-calming, wind-extinguishing	Extinguishes internal wind and quiets the liver
Uncaria Sovereign	Liver-calming, wind-extinguishing	Extinguishes internal wind and quiets the liver
Abalone shell Minister	Liver-calming, wind-extinguishing	Quiets the liver and heavily settles rising *yang*
Cyathula root Minister	Wind–damp dispelling	Moves blood downward and quickens blood
Gardenia Assistant	Heat-clearing	Clears heat from the liver
Scutellaria Assistant	Heat-clearing	Clears heat from the liver
Leonuris Assistant	Blood-rectifying	Quickens blood and disinhibits urination
Eucommia Assistant	*Yang-*supplementing	Supplements and nourishes the kidneys
Mistletoe Assistant	Wind-damp dispelling	Supplements and nourishes the liver and kidneys
Flowery knotweed stem Assistant	Blood-supplementing	Quiets the spirit and quickens the blood
Poria root Assistant	Spirit-quieting	Quiets the spirit and disinhibits urination

A Gastrodia and Uncaria Beverage.

B Gastrodia and Uncaria Beverage is a rather large and complex formula combining medicinals from six different medicinal categories. The sovereign and minister medicinals ensure that uprising *yang* is guided downward and wind is extinguished. The many assistant medicinals clear heat, calm the spirit, and nourish the kidney. Biomedically speaking, given that the Chinese medicine pattern is correct, this is a very effective formula in the treatment of migraine headaches.

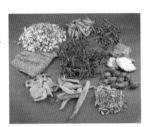

Spirit-quieting Formulas	Wind-dispelling Formulas
Nourish the heart and quiet the spirit	Course and dispel external wind
Quiet the spirit with heavy settlers	Calm and extinguish external wind
Other spirit-quieting formulas	Dispel wind and resolve tetany

C Actions of spirit-quieting and wind–dispelling formulas.

Orifice-opening Formulas

Orifices can be blocked by heat toxins sinking into the pericardium or by cold and phlegm congesting and confounding the heart. The common clinical manifestation for all types of blocked orifices is loss of consciousness or loss of clarity of mind. All the formulas in this category are emergency formulas and are generally prepared as powders or pills that can be ingested immediately. These formulas are all strong acting and often contain toxic ingredients, therefore they are not commonly used. The standard formula for *yang* block is Peaceful Palace Bovine Bezoar Pill (*An Gong Niu Huang Wan*). It clears heat, resolves toxicity, transforms phlegm, opens the orifices, and quiets the spirit. It is indicated if heat toxins sink into the pericardium and the patient presents with high fever, irritability, restlessness, delirium, and impaired consciousness. Among its over 10 ingredients are such powerful and toxic medicinals as cow bezoar (*niu huang*), musk (*she xiang*), realgar (*xiong huang*), borneol (*bing pian*), and cinnabar (*zhu sha*). If prescribed at all, these formulas should only be employed during acute attacks. For the sequela, appropriate formulas are selected from other categories (**C**).

Phlegm-transforming Formulas

This large category contains formulas to deal with various types of phlegm. The main subcategories are phlegm-transforming and heat-clearing formulas for hot phlegm in the lungs or the stomach; phlegm transforming and moistening formulas, for dry phlegm in the aftermath of hot phlegm in the lungs, when heat has dried up the fluids; phlegm-transforming and nodule-dissipating and -softening formulas for all types of nodulations; warming and transforming cold phlegm formulas for cold phlegm in the lungs or the middle burner; and phlegm-transforming and wind-extinguishing formulas for wind phlegm complex patterns (**C**).

The basic phlegm-transforming formula, Two Matured Ingredients Decoction (*Er Chen Tang*) (**A**, **B**), is contained in many of the other phlegm formulas and is very important. Two Matured Ingredients Decoction dries dampness, transforms phlegm, regulates *qi*, and harmonizes the middle burner. With appropriate modifications, it is indicated for the treatment of any type of phlegm.

Two Matured Ingredients Decoction contains four primary ingredients: its sovereign medicinals are acrid and warm pinellia and acrid, bitter, warm, and aromatic citrus peel. These two medicinals harmonize the middle and transform phlegm. The minister ingredient is poria, which assists citrus peel in rectifying and fortifying the spleen and addresses dampness. The courier medicinal is honey mix-fried licorice root, which supplements the spleen and harmonizes the other ingredients. Sometimes, fresh ginger and mume fruit *(wu mei)* are added as assistants. Fresh ginger supports pinellia in regulating the middle; sour and astringent mume controls the dispersing qualities of the sovereign medicinals (**A**, **B**).

Medicinal and Role	Category	Actions
Pinellia Sovereign	Phlegm-transforming	Dries dampness and transforms phlegm; harmonizes the stomach, downbears counterflow *qi*, and stops vomiting
Poria Minister	Dampness-dispelling	Fortifies the spleen, disinhibits urination, and dispels dampness
Tangerine peel Minister	*Qi*-rectifying	Regulates *qi* in the middle burner, dispels dampness, and transforms phlegm
Fresh ginger Assistant	Exterior-resolving	Harmonizes the stomach and downbears counterflow *qi*; transforms rheum; reduces the toxicity of pinellia
Mume fruit Assistant	Securing and astringing	Astringes the lungs and the fluids and protects lung *qi* and fluids from the drying and dissipating medicinals
Honey mix-fried licorice root Courier	*Qi*-supplementing	Harmonizes all the medicinals in the prescription; harmonizes and supplements the middle burner; moistens the lungs and stops coughing

A Two Matured Ingredients Decoction.

B Two Matured Ingredients Decoction is the basic prescription for transforming phlegm. Because its temperature is not very warm, it can readily be modified to also treat hot phlegm. It contains four main ingredients (pinellia, tangerine peel, poria, and honey mix-fried licorice) and thus also belongs to the group of the small but basic and important four-ingredient prescriptions like *Si Wu Tang* or *Si Jun Zi Tang*.

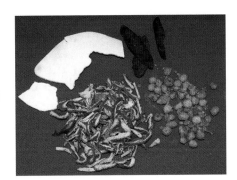

Orifice-opening Formulas	Phlegm-dispelling Formulas
Expel cold and open orifices	Dry dampness and transform phlegm
Transform phlegm and open orifices	Clear heat and transform phlegm
	Moisten the lung and transform phlegm
	Disperse goiter, scrofula, and phlegm
	Warm the lung and transform phlegm rheum
	Control wind and transform phlegm

C Actions of orifice-opening and phlegm-transforming formulas.

Formulas to moisten and transform phlegm are indicated if heat has dried up phlegm, leading to dry phlegm. For example, Fritillaria and Trichosanthes Powder (*Bei Mu Gua Lou San*) moistens the lungs, clears heat, regulates *qi*, and transforms phlegm. It is indicated in the treatment of cough with difficult to expectorate, sticky, and viscous phlegm. Often, this appears in the aftermath of acute phlegm heat coughs. This formula combines medicinals to moisten the lungs and transform phlegm, such as fritillaria (*chuan bei mu*) and trichosanthis fruit (*gua lou*) and root (*tian hua fen*) with acrid and bitter phlegm-drying and -transforming medicinals like citrus peel.

Dispersing Formulas

The food stagnation-dispersing category is represented by one especially popular formula: the Harmony Preserving Pill (*bao he wan*). In this formula, the sovereign and minister ingredients, crataegus fruit, medicated leaven, and radish seed (*lai fu zi*) stem from the food stagnation-dispersing category of medicinals. Because retained food blocks the spleen's function and leads to accumulation of phlegm and dampness, one group of assistants combines to form Two Matured Ingredients Decoction. Also, stagnant food blocks the free flow of *qi* and transforms into heat. To prevent such heat transformation, forsythia is added as an additional assistant. Thus, this formula consists of three groups of medicinals: the sovereign and ministers address the main problem by resolving food stagnation; the assistant medicinals address secondary complications by regulating the middle and transforming phlegm and dampness and by clearing transformative heat. In combination, the Harmony Preserving Pill treats acute food retention with such symptoms as epigastric and abdominal fullness, distension and pain, rotten-smelling belching, sour regurgitation, nausea and vomiting, dislike of food and foul-smelling diarrhea (**A**, **B**).

Worm-expelling Formulas

The formulas in this category were originally devised for the treatment of tapeworms, pinworms, ringworms, and other parasites. Although they are no longer commonly used for these indications, the parasite-expelling formula category contains at least one very important and still frequently used formula: Mume Pill (*Wu Mei Wan*).

Mume Pill warms and cools, supplements and clears, and disperses and astringes. Bitter, cold coptis and phellodendron root are combined with hot, acrid aconite, asarum (*xi xin*) and Sichuan pepper (*chuan jiao*) and with warm, *qi*-supplementing ginseng and *tang kuei*. Mume Pill is a very interesting example of how medicinals from opposing categories are combined to complement each other. Looking beyond its traditional functions, this formula supplements *qi* and blood, fortifies and warms the middle and also clears heat and eliminates dampness.

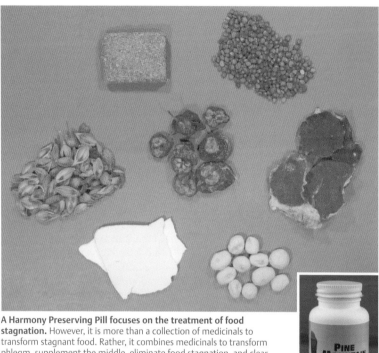

A Harmony Preserving Pill focuses on the treatment of food stagnation. However, it is more than a collection of medicinals to transform stagnant food. Rather, it combines medicinals to transform phlegm, supplement the middle, eliminate food stagnation, and clear heat. Thus, *Bao He Wan* is an effective medicinal for acute overeating with such symptoms as bloating, fullness, abdominal pain, belching, nausea, and vomiting, as well as foul-smelling diarrhea.

B Actions of dispersing formulas.

Dispersing Formulas

Disperse food and abduct stagnation

Disperse goiter, scrofula, and phlegm nodes

Disperse concretions, conglomerations, accumulations and gatherings

The Safety of Chinese Medicinals

"Chinese medicines are all natural substances that have been used for hundreds of years." This assertion sometimes leads to the erroneous conclusion that Chinese medicine is inherently safe and non-toxic. This is wrong. Although Chinese medicine is a relatively safe and side-effect-free medicine if used correctly, it contains many strong-acting and a few toxic substances. One of the big problems is that side-effects or toxic effects of Chinese medicines have not been recorded systematically over their long period of use. Hence, relying on its safety simply because of long-term use is not safe in all instances. For example, modern research has shown beyond doubt that aristolochic acid is nephrotoxic and can lead to acute kidney failure. How many patients have died over the past 1000 years from aristolochic-acid-induced nephropathy is uncertain. Arguing that aristolochia species herbs like *guang fang ji* or *guan mu tong* are safe because they have a long history of use is therefore not valid.

However, simply isolating medicinal ingredients and evaluating their toxic potential is equally incorrect. Chinese medicinals are prescribed as whole substances and often combinations with other substances. This certainly influences the toxicity of individual substances. Hence, evaluation of the toxicity of Chinese medicine must take these facts into consideration. Unfortunately, this has so far not necessarily been the case and in some countries, medicinals are taken off the market without justification. Although there certainly is a potential for Chinese medicines to be toxic, it should be considered that modern clinical experiences clearly demonstrate that the correct application of Chinese medicinals, with a few exceptions, is safe, and largely side-effect-free.

Traditional Safety Precautions

Following traditional guidelines concerning toxicity is a critical first step in the safe use of Chinese medicine. As was discussed earlier, all constituents of the Chinese materia medica have traditional evaluations of their relative toxicity and suitability for long-term use.

A second precaution is the correct application of medicinals and formulas. Each medicinal has traditional contraindications. Hot and acrid medicinals are contraindicated in *yin* vacuity with heat; bitter and cold medicinals are contraindicated in patients with cold in the middle burner. If these traditional contraindications are followed, the toxic potential of Chinese medicinals is strongly reduced.

An example is ephedra. Chinese medicine does not consider ephedra to be a toxic medicinal. It belongs to the exterior-resolving category and is acrid, bitter and very warm. It is used during acute exterior wind evil diseases for only short intervals. Further, like all dispersing and sweat-promoting medicinals, it is contraindicated in vacuity of *qi*, blood, and *yin*. As an acrid and very warm medicinal, it is further contraindicated in *yin* vacuity and heat conditions.

Ephedra contains alkaloids that stimulate the sympathetic nervous system, cause heart palpitations, and raise the blood pressure and is therefore contraindicated in such conditions. Interestingly, these are exactly the conditions that correspond to the Chinese medical patterns for which ephedra is traditionally contraindicated. Many more such examples could be added here. Hence, using the correct medicinals and formula according to the logic of Chinese medicine provides another very important safety barrier. The danger begins when Chinese medicinals are used outside of their context and according to single, pharmacologically proven functions by practitioners not thoroughly trained in their use.

A third traditional precaution is the traditional detoxification procedure. If medicinals are harvested and prepared according to traditional guidelines, their toxicity is often greatly reduced. An example is aconite, which was discussed earlier.

Regardless of all the methods of reducing toxicity, some medicinals still included in many modern materia medica are simply too toxic for any kind of modern application and should be considered "outdated relics." An example that still finds plenty of application in China is cinnabar. Cinnabar is mercuric sulfide and was used in Chinese medicine to clear heart fire and quiet the spirit. It is still prescribed today by arguing that the bound mercury would not be absorbed in the body. However, several studies have proven this to be wrong (Yeoh, Lee, & Lee 1989) and cinnabar simply should no longer be used. Other toxic medicinals that should no longer be used for internal administration in clinical practice are realgar, datura flower (*yang jin hua*), croton seed (*ba dou*), and calomelas (*qing fen*).

Safe Use of Herbs in Pregnancy

Another aspect of the safety of Chinese medicines is their use during pregnancy. Generally, it is advocated to take as little medicine as possible during pregnancy. With Chinese medicine, this is not always the case. Some Chinese herbs can have a very beneficial effect in treating pregnancy-related problems such as threatened abortion, bleeding, extreme fatigue, hypertension, migraine headaches, and so on. Chinese herbs may, when appropriate, be used during pregnancy. Still, there are some medicinals that are contraindicated during pregnancy. Just as with substances that are traditionally considered toxic, the fact that they are contraindicated during pregnancy has been recorded in different materia medica for hundreds of years. Generally, the principle holds true that most, if not all, downward-draining and downward-moving as well as most blood-quickening medicinals are contraindicated during pregnancy. Such medicinals disturb the quiet *yin* period the fetus requires to grow and develop. On the other hand, birth is considered an active *yang* expulsion phase, which requires a powerful downward movement of *qi*. Hence, to induce labor, such downward-moving medicinals as areca seed and husk (*bing lang* and *da fu pi*), talcum (*hua shi*), and poria are administered.

Drug–Herb Interactions

Drug–herb interactions must be considered given the fact that most patients visiting a Chinese medicine practitioner in the West take at least one if not several pharmaceutical drugs. The potential for interaction of Chinese medicinal formulas with modern pharmaceuticals is inexhaustible. There exists an almost limitless amount of Chinese medicinal combinations and an even greater amount of potential interactions with modern drugs. Hence, a systematic study is nearly impossible. However, there are ways of calculating possible interactions and thus minimizing the risk of causing them. For example, certain medicinal categories may have a greater potential to interact in the form of potentiation with a certain category of Western drugs. This seems to be true for the dampness-expelling, urine-disinhibiting medicinals with diuretic drugs; or for spirit-quieting or internal wind-extinguishing medicinals with sedative drugs. This is also true for blood-quickening medicinals with blood-thinning drugs. In this last category, research has actually confirmed two interactions: *tang kuei* and salvia root both interact with the clearance of warfarin and therefore lead over time to its build up in the blood and increase its strength. Potentially, this can lead to acute internal bleeding (Chan & Cheung 2003).

Another way of assessing interactions is to look at medicinal components and theoretically or in vitro study their interactions with the active ingredients of Western drugs. Most common here is the potential for precipitation of medicinal components such as tannic acids or minerals with Western drugs. However, these interactions can be avoided by simply not taking the Chinese and Western medicines in combination.

Besides these and very few other interactions, there have not been definite reports of problems. In China, herbal medicine is routinely prescribed in combination with modern pharmaceuticals. Although interactions are not being systematically studied, there are no indications that the Chinese medicines have a large potential to interact with pharmaceuticals. However, as with the issue of toxicity, further research must be conducted. Thereafter, considering the framework in which Chinese medicine works, further guidelines and rules to make interactions less likely and the combination of Chinese and Western medicine safety can be evaluated.

It is also interesting to consider that the Chinese long ago discussed drug–drug interactions. There are traditional lists of medicines that are considered incompatible with each other. These are called the 18 clashes (*shi ba fan*). Originally listing 18 herbs that should not be combined, the list has since been expanded. For example, according to this traditional list, the various aconite roots should not be combined with such herbs as fritillaria bulb, pinellia, trichosanthis fruit (*gua lou*), and so on. Or, licorice root should not be combined with sargassum (*hai zao*) or the overly strong purgatives euphorbia, knoxia roots or genkwa flower (*gan sui, da ji*, and *yuan hua*).

Furthermore, over the centuries, Chinese practitioners collected a list of 19 herbs that combine to 10 pairs that are said to antagonize each other. Today, most of these herbs are rarely used or toxic. Notable are the antago- nizing effect between ginseng and fly- ing squirrel droppings and between cinnamon bark (*rou gui*) and hallosite (*chi shi zhi*). Although these two lists are interesting, not every practitioner follows them and many consider them a relic of the past.

7

Chinese Dietetics

Mary Garvey

Introduction

As an agricultural nation, food has always been at the forefront of the Chinese mind. Many ideas about food and diet can be found in the *Yellow Emperor's Classic of Medicine*, and for much of the history of the development of Chinese medicine there was little distinction between diet and therapeutic herbal practices. The same substances that were used to improve the taste of foods were the substances that were known to have medicinal properties. To this day, the crossover between food preparation and medicinal therapy continues, and in most Chinese households there is a basic understanding of the nature of foods and the importance of eating in moderation.

The tradition of Chinese dietary therapy, as distinct from herbal therapy, began in the Tang dynasty (618–907 CE, see also p. 3 and pp. 50–51), with a chapter in Sun Si Miao's *Qian Jin Yao Fang (Thousand Gold Pieces Prescriptions)* devoted to dietary treatment. A Daoist scholar, Sun Si Miao (581–682 CE) was famous as a physician and a philosopher. His works include recommendations for daily living, implying diet, exercise, and work (either physical or mental work). Sun quotes lengthy sections from the *Classic*, emphasizing the necessity of moderation in eating and drinking, and he gives warnings and prohibitions concerning various foods and eating habits (see also pp. 36 and 226).

One of Sun Si Miao's most important suggestions is that dietary therapy should be applied first, prior to the use of herbal therapeutics for the simple reason that it is safer. He recognized that Chinese medicinal substances are therapeutically more potent than foods, but they can also be dangerous, a concept that was first made clear in *The Divine Husbandman's Materia Medica*. Sun and those who followed him assembled information from earlier texts concerning foods, created simple prescriptions, and discussed food preparation and cooking techniques. Sun Si Miao understood that one of the basic precepts of Chinese medicine, the prevention of disease, could be reinforced through diet and attention to the foods one ate and how they were cooked.

As discussed in Chapter 2, all of the viscera and bowels of the body need to function well for efficient production of the basic substances (*qi*, blood, essence, and fluids). However, Chinese medicine places a great deal of emphasis on the middle burner, the spleen, and the stomach, because this is where post-heaven *qi* production begins, and food and fluids are the fundamental substances required to produce the post-heaven *qi*. The quality of the food and fluids is very important in determining the quality of the post-heaven *qi* (see also **A** and **B**).

This chapter discusses some of the most important principles of diet according to Chinese medicine and presents recipes for improving diet and treating simple conditions.

A–B Ingredients and finished dish of a Korean soup of chicken (or Cornish hens) stuffed with sweet rice, red dates, ginseng, and garlic. Traditionally eaten in the height of summer on hot days, the soup has medical properties. Eating this dish makes you sweat and release toxins and cools you down, showing that truly food is medicine.

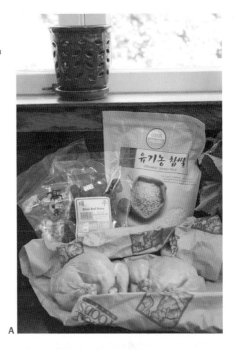

A

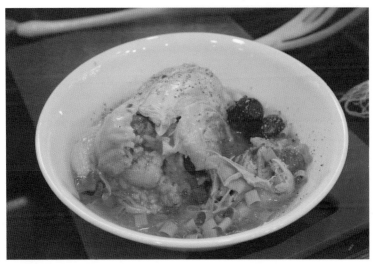

B

The Middle Burner
(Zhong Jiao 中焦)

The functions of the middle burner are fundamental to daily life. The internal–external relationship and complementary functions of the spleen and stomach are extremely closely connected. As the organs associated with the earth phase of the five phases, they constitute the center of the body and the place from which all other functions emanate. Although the pre-heaven essence that is stored in the kidneys determines our basic constitution, ultimately it is the grain *qi (gu qi)* from the middle burner that forms the post-heaven substances and maintains the overall health of the body. The quality of the *qi* of the middle burner is affected by our dietary habits, and a good, healthy, and balanced diet is essential to health.

The stomach receives the food and drink we ingest and begins its transformation into a form of *qi* that can be used. To accomplish this, the stomach requires a warm and wet environment. The stomach's "rotting and ripening" function is compared to a fermenting or cooking process, a process that requires a constant, low-level heat and sufficient moisture to keep the food from sticking. In the stomach, the digestate undergoes the first stage of separation, the initial separating of the clear *qi* and fluids for absorption from the turbid, which the stomach *qi* is responsible for downbearing to the intestines.

The spleen, on the other hand, requires a cool and dry environment for its role in transforming and transporting food *qi*. A cool, dry environment promotes the condensation of *qi*, and the elevation and separation of the five flavors. Spleen *qi* upbears the pure *qi* and fluids to the upper burner and distributes the five flavors to the five viscera. When we say that earth (the spleen and stomach) feeds the four sides, we mean that it transforms and transports water and food, nourishes the other four viscera, and sends the flavors to each of the viscera. (**A, B**)

Ideally, dietary habits and the foods ingested should conform to seasonal and other changes. According to the diurnal cycle, *qi* circulates through the 12 regular channels at specific times each day (see p. 169). The time when the stomach and spleen (the middle burner *qi*) is at its peak is from 7:00 a.m. to 11:00 a.m., explaining why the morning is the most important time to eat a good meal; 7:00 p.m. to 11:00 p.m. is possibly the worst time to eat a large meal because at this time the middle burner *qi* is at its lowest ebb (**C**) (see p. 168).

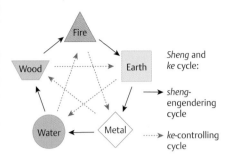

A The five phases with the engendering and controlling cycles. The spleen is the mother of the lung and together they instigate the formation and circulation of the vital substances *qi*, blood, and fluids.

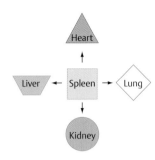

B The five phases organized with the spleen in the center. Earth at the center "feeds the four sides." The spleen and stomach transform and transport food and water to "feed the four sides," that is, the other organ systems and the whole body.

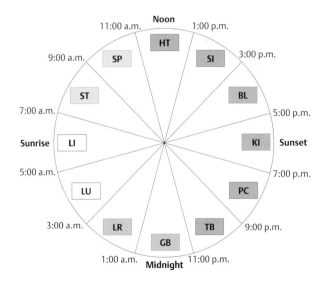

C Chinese organ clock. The *qi* of the middle burner is most abundant between 7:00 a.m. and 11:00 a.m. in the morning.

Diet and Disorder

As mentioned previously, moderation in diet is essential to health. Over-eating, under-eating, eating on an irregular schedule or without sufficient time, and eating inappropriate foods can all cause disharmony in the middle burner, resulting in digestive problems, and ultimately, problems with the production of *qi*.

Over-eating, eating on an irregular schedule or without sufficient time, and eating rich, greasy, or difficult-to-digest foods can obstruct the *qi* mechanism of the middle burner, causing food to accumulate in the stomach, possibly resulting in depressive heat, toxic heat, or stomach fire patterns. Eating food when it is too hot, or eating too much hot-natured or spicy food may overheat the middle burner and damage the *yin* fluids.

Under-eating, skipping meals, dieting, and eating excessively cold-natured or uncooked foods may injure the middle burner *qi* and damage the spleen *yang*, which is needed to cook and digest food. Frequently this results in *qi* and blood vacuity patterns. Furthermore, when the middle burner *yang qi* is depleted, fluid transformation does not occur as it should and dampness or phlegm accumulates. A diet heavy in sweet or fatty foods, or alcohol, will add to the creation of dampness, phlegm, and heat.

When the middle burner *qi* is depleted or obstructed, damp patterns are common. The spleen dislikes dampness, and as it accumulates in the middle burner, the function of the spleen weakens. Because the spleen governs the flesh, dampness may settle in the muscles and flesh, causing poor muscle tone and heaviness of the limbs. Additionally, according to the five phases, the spleen (earth) controls the kidney (water), and if dampness accumulates in the middle burner spleen earth may overwhelm kidney (water). This weakens the kidney so that over time the bones weaken and begin to ache. Accumulated dampness in the middle burner may also obstruct the upper burner, leading to difficulty breathing or palpitations. As the functions of the spleen weaken, the formation and transformation of *qi* blood, essence, and fluids are compromised.

Clinical manifestations of disorders of the middle burner include abdominal or epigastric discomfort, lack of appetite, gastrointestinal problems, lethargy, weakness, fluid retention, weight gain or weight loss, lack of concentration, and muddled thinking. Because spleen *qi* holds the blood in the vessels, spleen *qi* vacuity may also result in the extravasation of blood (bruising or bleeding problems).

To protect or restore the middle burner physiology, nourishing, easy-to-digest foods are recommended. Chinese medicine recommends regular meals, and cooked, warm, and soft diets rather than raw, hard-to-digest, cold foods. Mild foods (staples like grains, pulses, and vegetables) should form the bulk of our food intake. Eating foods that may be grown locally and are normally available during the current season also makes sense, because foods should be fresh, and they should look, smell, and taste good (**A–C**).

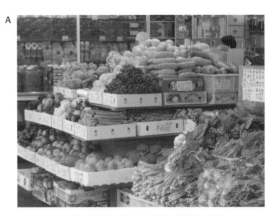

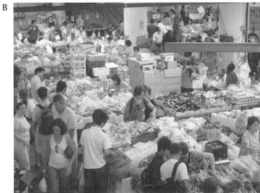

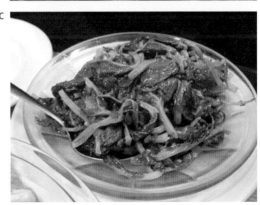

A–C Select foods that are fresh and in season.
Dishes should not only balance the five flavors but they should look, smell, and taste good.

From the Chinese medical viewpoint, the therapeutic value of foods and medicinal substances is described in terms of their *qi* or nature and their flavor. Further specificity is achieved when we take into consideration the channel that particular foods are said to enter. As discussed in Chapter 6, all substances, food included, enter specific channels and thus have greater influence on the organ associated with that channel. A good diet will be balanced in nature (neither too hot nor too cold), and will include a balanced proportion of all five flavors (see p. 232).

The Nature of Foods

The *qi* or nature of foods refers to the "temperature." This does not mean the actual temperature of foods, but rather it refers to the interaction between the food or substance and the body. If an ingested food is observed to increase body warmth and physiological activity, it has a warm nature. If the food cools or slows the body and its activities, it is a cool food. A food or substance may be hot, warm, neutral, cool, or cold. For example, pepper is hot, garlic is warm, eggs are neutral, tofu is cool, and pears are cold. See **A** for further examples.

The nature of foods helps to guide dietary intake in relation to individual constitution or, if illness is present, the characteristics of the disorder. For example, hot and warm foods are taken for cold disorders, and cool foods are recommended for heat patterns. A constitutionally hot person or an individual with a heat condition will feel worse after eating pepper, ginger, mutton, or other hot foods. Similarly, someone with a cold constitution or suffering from an illness of a cold nature, should avoid eating pears, watermelon, chilled foods and drinks, or other cold-natured foods.

Cooking affects a food's nature. For example, heating properties increase when foods are fried or roasted in oil. Baking without oil will have a heating and drying effect. Steaming and blanching can make foods more easily digestible, and will moderate warm/hot foods a little because of the watery cooking conditions. Prolonged steaming or boiling can slightly warm a cool-natured food. Appropriate processing, preparation, cooking, and blending of foods improves their palatability, aids digestion, and the availability of nutrients.

The Five Flavors

When the spleen distributes the five flavors, acrid goes to the lung, salty to the kidney, sour to the liver, bitter to the heart, and sweet to the spleen itself (see p. 232). Moderate amounts of all of the flavors are necessary to strengthen the viscera, but over-consumption of any flavor will damage organ functions. As we see in **B**, each of the five flavors acts on a particular organ. The dietetic qualities of foods explain their therapeutic benefits, and account for the problems resulting from over-consumption of any given flavor. The patterns and constitutional types that would benefit from particular foods and those to avoid or use with caution are noted.

Hot	Chili, dry ginger, pepper
Warm	Almonds, carrots, chicken, garlic, olives
Neutral	Chicken egg, grapes, potatoes, red beans, rice, sesame
Cool	Celery, green tea, peppermint, tofu, wheat
Cold	Banana, eggplant, pears, watermelon

A The nature of foods with examples.

Sour Contracts, astringes, gathers, stabilizes the *qi*, and can reduce swelling	**Sour benefits** fluids by stopping leakage; sour relieves stagnation, tones and tightens tissues; is used to treat loss of body fluids, incontinence, slack muscles, an erratic, changeable personality
Excess slows the *qi*, toughens the flesh, tightens the tendons	**Caution** with dampness and other lingering pathogenic factors, with muscle tension or diseases involving tendons and ligaments
Bitter Drains, dries, tightens, has a strengthening effect, leads the *qi* downwards	**Bitter benefits** the heart and spleen, drains downwards and improves the appetite; bitter + warm dries dampness, while bitter + cool clears heat, and reduces fever; used to treat slowness, lethargy, obesity, overheated-aggressive types
Excess weakens the spleen, withers the skin, dries and tightens the flesh	**Caution** with *yin*-blood vacuity, dry skin diseases; vacuity dryness or cold; dense, dry or congested stomach problems
Sweet Supplements, strengthens, harmonizes, relaxes, slows	**Sweet benefits** *qi* and blood vacuity patterns, is good for a thin, depleted constitution, nervous, weak scattered types, aggressive, impatient liverish types; used to strengthen weakness, relieve pain and relax tension; sweet and cool-natured foods engender fluids and moisten dryness
Excess slackens the muscles and flesh, causes dampness, aching bones	**Caution** with damp or phlegm patterns, spleen *qi* vacuity, people with excess weight, chronic fatigue, heart disease, or diabetes
Acrid Dissipates, moves, disperses, has an expanding-ascending direction	**Acrid benefits** the lung, promotes *qi* circulation, and benefits sluggish, dull, lethargic types; used to disperse stagnation (including evil *qi* lodged in the exterior), to dissipate and mobilize damp-cold and phlegm-damp
Excess knots the muscles, dissipates *qi* (→ *qi* vacuity), consumes *yin* (→ dryness)	**Caution** with hot, dry, wind problems, with *qi* and *yin* vacuity patterns, with thin, nervous types
Salty Softens hard masses, moistens, cleans, leads the *qi* inwards and downwards	**Salty benefits** the kidney and softens hard masses; used to treat muscle cramping, phlegm accumulation, phlegm-fire nodules and lumps, constipation, chronic inflammation, poor appetite, nervous types
Excess damages the arteries, the blood, and the bones	**Caution** with cardiovascular diseases, circulatory system problems, depression; can worsen damp patterns

B The five flavors.

Additionally, each flavor has a directional aspect (see also p.233): acrid is ascending, sour is contracting, bitter is draining, salty is inward and downward. Sweet is not directional because it enters the center. Bland, a sixth, neutral flavor (essentially the absence of the five flavors), disinhibits water and has a downward direction. It can drain or percolate excess fluids by benefiting urination. Many foods have more than one flavor, thus having an effect of multiple organ systems.

Because the spleen is the organ that sends the five flavors out to the four sides, it is essential that an appropriate amount of sweet food is consumed. However, nourishing sweet foods are not foods sweetened with refined sugars. Many natural foods are sweet, so sweet-flavored foods form the bulk of a healthy diet and are fundamentally nourishing for the middle qi. In Chinese medicine, sweet often refers to foods that are high in complex carbohydrates, and are mildly sweet in flavor. Most grains (for example, rice) and starchy vegetables (for example, sweet potato) fall into this category. Interestingly, these are also staple foods of the Chinese diet because they are readily available, inexpensive, and filling. Foods that are sweetened with refined sugars are overly sweet and can damage the spleen qi, resulting in digestive disorders.

Entering the Channels

The five flavors provide a guide for associating foods with the five viscera. The channel that a food enters gives additional, more specific information for treatment. Entering channels have been determined by observing the actions of foods on the body. That a particular food has a propensity to enter a given channel means that the qi of the food has been observed to affect particular organ systems. In other words, the food's nutritional benefits tend to have a more pronounced effect on those organs and their physiological activities.

For example, potatoes are sweet and so enter the spleen and stomach. They are used therapeutically to benefit the middle and strengthen the qi. Honey is sweet and neutral and enters the spleen, lung, and large intestine. The sweet flavor entering the spleen explains why honey supplements the middle. Sweet and neutral flavors together tend to engender fluids, so honey also moistens dryness, especially of the lung and large intestine. Its dietetic features explain why honey is used for tiredness, stomach ache, dry cough, and intestinal dryness constipation (**A**).

Chinese dietetics considers chicken flesh and chicken eggs to be very beneficial foods. Chicken eggs are sweet and neutral and enter the five zang and stomach. They are especially good to nourish blood, enrich the yin, and moisten dryness. Chicken is warm and sweet and enters the stomach, spleen, and kidney, so it supplements the qi and blood, invigorates the kidney, and nourishes the jing essence.

Sweet and neutral	Almonds, beef, beetroot, carrots, corn, eggs, green beans, lentils, oats, parsnips, peas, potatoes, rice, sesame, sweet potatoes
Sweet and warm	Carrots, cauliflower, chicken, coconut, fennel, lamb, miso, peaches, pinenuts, pumpkin, tempeh, trout, walnuts
Sweet and cool	Apples, barley, buckwheat, eggplant, mushrooms, radishes, spinach, squash, tofu, water chestnuts
Sweet and acrid	Basil, chives, cinnamon, coriander, garlic, ginger, mustard, nutmeg, onion, peppermint, rosemary, shallot, watercress
Sweet and sour	Aduki beans, olives, tomatoes, vinegar, yogurt, and most fruits (for example, apples, apricots, blackberries, grapes, grapefruit, mangoes, oranges, pears, pineapple, raspberries)
Bitter foods	Alfalfa, coffee, lettuce, oats, rye, turmeric, watercress
Bitter and sweet	Asparagus, broccoli, cabbage, celery, green tea, lettuce, paw-paw, wines and spirits
Bitter and sour	Vinegar
Bitter and acrid	Shallots, turnips, wines and spirits
Sour foods	Hawthorn berries (*shan zha*), lemon, lime, pickles, rosehips, sauerkraut, sour plum
Sour and acrid	Leeks, onions
Acrid and warm	Basil, coriander, fennel, garlic, ginger, horseradish, nutmeg, onions, shallots; chilies and peppers are acrid and hot
Acrid and cool	Elderflowers, kumquats, marjoram, peppermint, radishes
Acrid and neutral	Taro, turnips, kohlrabi
Salty and sweet	Seaweeds (kelp, nori, kombu, wakame), seafood (anchovies, lobster, oysters, prawns, salmon, squid), barley, millet, miso, pork, soy sauce
Salty and cool-cold	Clams, crab, kelp, salt

A Dietetic qualities and foods (Garvey 2008).

Tea enters the heart, lung, and stomach, and is sweet, bitter, and cool. Tea relieves thirst and restlessness, promotes urination, and benefits digestion. There is a good deal of research that appears to support tea's reputed anti-aging, anti-senility, and anti-hypertensive effects. Alcoholic wines and spirits are usually bitter, acrid, and sweet in flavor, and warm–hot in nature. Moderate consumption will promote *qi* and blood circulation, resolve dampness, relieve tiredness, and warm the middle *jiao* and the body to keep out the cold.

Lemon's warm nature and sour flavor enter the lung, spleen, and stomach. Lemon transforms phlegm and stops coughing, helps indigestion, supplements the spleen, moistens a dry throat and relieves thirst. Onion enters the lung, spleen, liver, and large intestine. Its warm-acrid qualities warm the interior and scatter cold pathogenic factors. Such features may be employed in the treatment of *qi*-blood stagnation patterns, the common cold, diarrhea, and worms.

A few slices of fresh ginger and a little raw sugar steeped in boiling water for a few minutes and sipped as tea, can be taken to relieve headache from cold, or cold-type period pains. For a wind–heat attack with dry sore throat, we can recommend peppermint tea with honey. Peppermint enters the lung and liver, so it can also help clear liver heat.

Oysters are salty and slightly cool. Oyster flesh strengthens *qi*, supplements *yin*-blood, and can benefit weak, nervous clients. Salt is salty and cold and can help cool the blood and clear pathogenic fire. For sunstroke with thirst and sweating, drink warm water that has a little salt and sugar dissolved in it (Garvey 2008).

Dietary Advice

The foods one chooses to eat and eating habits are often very personal, and can be quite difficult to change. Many clients, however, will want to adopt more appropriate dietary habits, and others may be able to gradually incorporate a few changes. General advice about regular mealtimes, cooked foods, and so on, can make a big difference therapeutically. Simple changes such as sitting down in a relaxed environment to eat a meal, can immediately benefit the stomach *qi*, and focus the person's attention towards lifestyle factors that might be contributing to their condition.

The Chinese medicine practitioner can also offer concrete suggestions about foods to avoid or include in the diet. The table on the previous page shows some effective combinations and examples. Regional and seasonal variations, preparation and cooking, and the other ingredients in a recipe can modify a food's dietetic qualities (**A–C**). The following recipes illustrate a few combinations and preparations, and may be used to illustrate the therapeutic application of Chinese dietetic principles for the treatment of *qi*, blood, and fluid disorders.

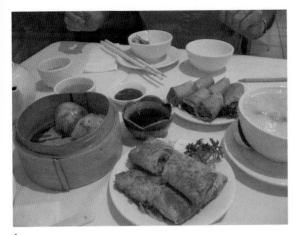

A

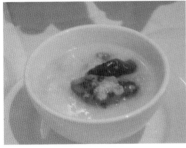

B

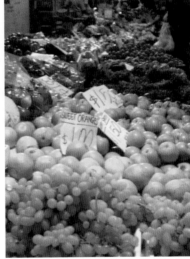

A–C Regional and seasonal variations,
preparation and cooking, and the
other ingredients can modify a food's
dietetic qualities.

C

Qi Stagnation in the Middle Burner: Mild Vegetable Curry

- 2 tablespoons ghee or vegetable oil
- 1 onion, diced
- Fresh ginger and garlic, minced, 2–3 teaspoons of each
- 1 teaspoon each of white mustard seeds, cumin seeds, coriander seeds, and fenugreek—dry fry till aromatic, then grind
- Ground cinnamon and turmeric, 1 teaspoon each
- 350 g of red lentils
- 1 l chicken or vegetable stock
- 1 diced potato
- 1 diced eggplant
- 1 diced carrot
- 2 diced tomatoes
- 1 bunch fresh coriander, roughly chopped
- Juice of 2 lemons

Melt the ghee or heat the oil in a large saucepan, add the onions, ginger, garlic, spices and lentils, stir to combine. Cook until the onion has softened. Add stock and cook for 20–30 minutes or until the lentils are soft. Add the potato, eggplant, carrots, and tomatoes to the lentils and stock, and cook for an-

other 20–25 minutes. Before serving, add the coriander and the lemon juice. Stir through the curry. Serve with rice, pappadam, or bread and your favorite condiments (**A–C**).

Discussion

- Ginger, garlic, and the spices used above are acrid, and very warm. They mobilize *qi*, dissipate stagnation, warm the middle burner, and aid digestion. Aromatic herbs and spices awaken the spleen to promote transformation and transportation, and their warm nature benefits spleen upbearing.
- Turmeric and fenugreek are bitter in flavor, dry dampness, and encourage the downbearing action of the stomach *qi*.

☒ Counsel the middle burner *qi* stagnation client against overeating, eating junk foods, and heavy, congesting foods (for example, cheese, eggs, dairy, red meats).

☑ Recommend eating less, eating slowly, eating light foods: a diet high in vegetables, low in carbohydrates, and with moderate to low meat intake.

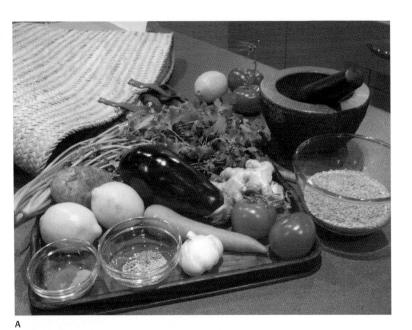

A

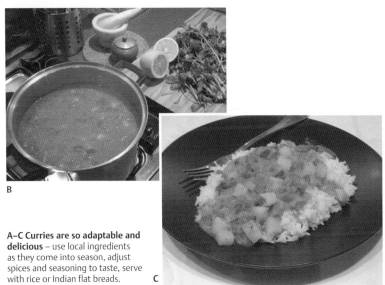

B

A–C Curries are so adaptable and delicious – use local ingredients as they come into season, adjust spices and seasoning to taste, serve with rice or Indian flat breads.

C

Liver Blood Vacuity:
Beetroot Risotto

- 2–3 tablespoons of extra virgin olive oil
- 1 red onion, diced
- 1 clove of garlic, minced (optional)
- 350g of Arborio rice
- 2 red beetroots, peeled and diced
- 125 ml of red wine (optional)
- 900 ml hot chicken/vegetable stock
- Bunch of baby spinach
- Grated parmesan cheese (optional)

Heat the oil in a large heavy-based saucepan. Add the onion and cook for 1–2 minutes until softened. Add the rice and beetroot, stir, and cook for 2 minutes until they are well coated with oil. Pour in the wine and stir until all liquid is absorbed. Add the stock a ladle at a time, stirring frequently and gently. Allow all the liquid to be absorbed before adding the next ladleful. Continue until the rice is creamy and al dente, about 25 minutes. Add roughly chopped spinach and stir through. Remove from heat, season with pepper and salt to taste, cover, and allow to stand for 2–3 minutes. Serve with grated Parmesan cheese (**A–C**).

Discussion

- Rice and beetroot are both sweet and neutral. Rice harmonizes the stomach, strengthens the spleen, and supplements *qi* and blood. Beetroot supplements the blood, soothes the liver, and benefits the heart.

- Cooking with alcohol warms the middle and upper burners and promotes *qi* and blood circulation. To avoid stagnation, enriching and supplementing dishes should include acrid foods to mobilize circulation. The acridity of the wine, onion, and garlic will help achieve this. Note: alcohol is generally contraindicated for clients with liver disease. The garlic may also be omitted if liver-heat is a problem.
- Cheese is neutral-cool, sweet and sour, and enters the stomach, spleen, lung, and liver. It supplements and moves the *qi*, nourishes *yin*, and moistens. Note: excessive cheese and other dairy products will aggravate damp-phlegm disorders.

☒ Counsel the blood vacuity client against over-eating, skipping meals, cold and uncooked foods.
☑ Recommend cooked, warm, simple meals with some quality protein (for example, organic chicken), and plenty of fresh, green, leafy vegetables, legumes, and root vegetables.

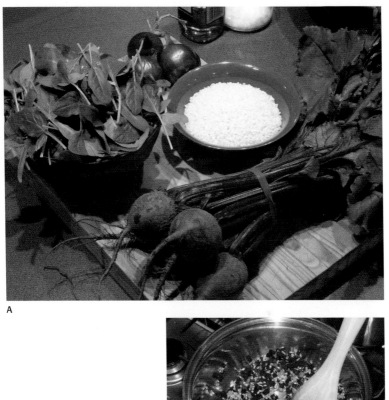

A

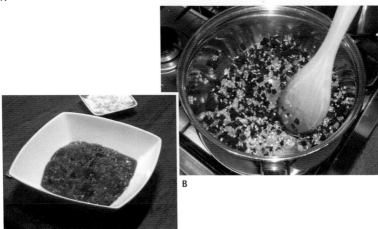

B

C

A–C Risotto is also an incredibly varied and adaptable dish. Slow cooking and gentle stirring release the starches from this plump Italian rice. The rice amounts can be varied depending on whether a more "soupy" risotto is preferred.

Lung *Yin* Vacuity Causing Dryness: Steamed Pears

- 4 or 5 pears
- Rock sugar
- Plain yogurt

Peel, core, and slice pears as desired. To prevent the flesh turning brown, toss with a little lemon juice. Place in an ovenproof dish and add a few pieces of rock sugar. Cover and steam for between 1 and 2 hours. Eat warm or when cooled, with yogurt (**A–C**).

Discussion

- Pears enter the lungs and stomach. Their cool nature, and sweet, slightly sour flavor clears heat and engenders fluids to moisten dryness. They are especially good when evil heat and dryness injure the lungs and throat.
- Rock sugar is neutral and sweet, enters the spleen and lungs, engenders fluids, and benefits digestion. White rock sugar is especially good for the lungs.
- Yogurt is cool-cold, with a sweet and sour flavor, qualities that nourish *yin*-fluids and clear heat. It relaxes the liver, moistens the lung, and quenches thirst.

☒ The *yin*-fluids vacuity client should avoid heating, acrid, and bitter foods (including chili, coffee, tobacco).

☑ Recommend sweet cool foods to moisten dryness (such as fruits, dairy, soy milk, barley).

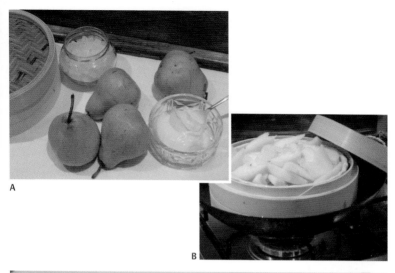

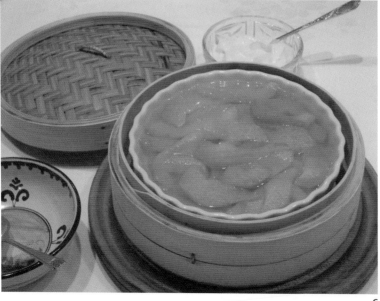

A–C Steamed pears, as shown here with rock sugar, are extremely helpful for the treatment of chronic dry coughs.

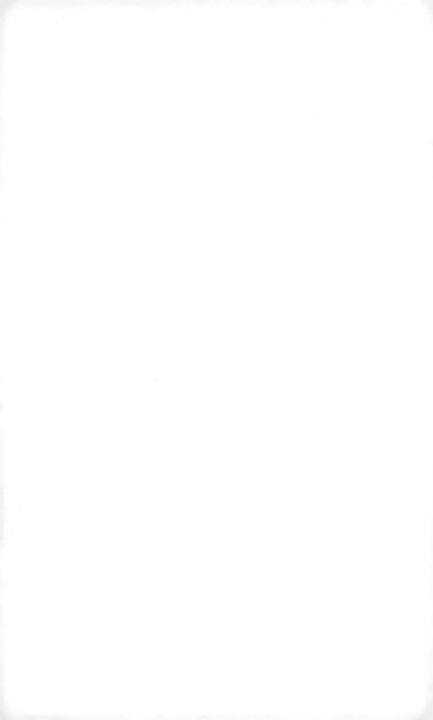

8

Qi Gong

Anne Reinard and Yves Réquéna

Historical Origins

The roots of *qi gong* date back to the time of Chinese shamanism, preceding the era of written records. As an agrarian civilization, the ancient Chinese were essentially dependent on the energy of the earth and the sky, and their survival and well-being were closely correlated to understanding and respecting the laws of nature. Through this direct connection to the earth and through their observation of the natural cycles of sowing and harvesting, of life and death, they learned the balancing principle of *yin* and *yang* and deduced the dynamics of *qi gong.*

The Yellow Emperor's Classic of Medicine, written during the Han Dynasty (206 BC–220 CE), explains that the ancient Chinese lived according to the "way of nature" (the Dao). They modulated their way of being according to *yin–yang*, numerology, and seasonal rhythms. The demands of their habitat generated a balanced lifestyle, which taught them "to avoid the 'perversions of exhaustion and the pirate winds' and, through calm and concentration, to maintain their natural breath in harmony, so as to be able to contain their spirit inside so that illness cannot strike" (translated from Réquéna 1998, p. 12).

Among the earliest recorded *qi gong* exercises are the shaman dances, which emulate the animals of the Chinese zodiac, and were practiced as a New Year's ritual during the Zhou dynasty (ca. 1100–256 BCE). The shaman would appear clad in a bear's fur and bejeweled with four golden eyes so as to see in all directions. He would be accompanied in his dance by all the villagers wearing animal masks (ibid.)

The *Book of Changes (Yi Jing* or *I Ching)*, the fundamental philosophical work that structured Chinese thought and culture, constitutes "the foundation of the reasonable and the basic tool for the intelligibility of the universe" (Réquéna 2003, p. 2) (**A**). According to the *Yi Jing* "Life engendering life, that is change" (Javary & Faure 2002, p. 1). The *Yi Jing* is a system of rules and patterns that elucidates the correlation between human, earth, and sky by incorporating the variable of change as the basic motive force of life. *Qi* is both the fuel and the agent of change. It is the connecting thread that holds everything together.

In around 300 BCE the Daoist poet-philosopher, Chuang Zi, claimed "that the ancients breathed down to their heels" suggesting that breath, in the form of *qi*, is projected and circulated throughout the body. A series of figurines painted on silk (from 168 BCE) was found during an archaeological tomb excavation (Ma Wang tombs) in Hunan Province in 1973. Partially damaged, this painted silk scroll constitutes a chart known as "Daoyin Tu," literally the map of the guiding thread of *qi*, and bears inscriptions relating to the therapeutic practice of *dao yin*, the term used to describe the practices that later provided the foundational concepts for *qi gong, tai ji quan*, and *tui na* self massage. **B** describes the eight basic *qi gong* movements, called the Eight Pieces of Brocade, used today.

A The *ba gua* (or eight trigrams) represents the transformation embodied in the concept of *yin* and *yang*. It forms the conceptual basis of several *qi gong* exercises. Shown here is Fu Xi's sequence (see also pp. 4–5) of the eight trigrams. Each of the eight trigrams is paired with all of the others to creat 8 x 8 or 64 hexagrams, the basis of the *Yi Jing*.

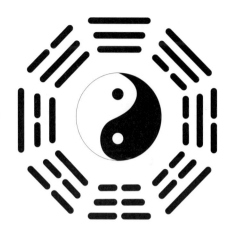

Movement	Therapeutic indication
1. "Hold the Sky"	By stimulating the triple burner, it strengthens the digestive system and balances energy in the internal organs.
2. "Draw the Bow to Shoot the Hawk"	Benefits the immune systems and strengthens heart and lung. Realigns the back muscles and spine.
3. "Separating Heaven and Earth"	By invigorating the torso with energy from the heavens and from the earth, it stimulates the stomach and spleen.
4. "Look Behind to Release Fatigue and Stress"	Strengthens the neck and eye muscles. Releases tension and benefits the nervous system.
5. "Sway the Head and Wag the Tail" (see p. 338–339)	Releases heart fire by regulating the function of heart and lungs.
6. "Two Hands Hold the Feet"	Stretches the spinal column. Strengthens the kidneys and the waist.
7. "Punch with Powerful Gaze"	By expelling tense and angry feelings, it increases general vitality and muscular strength.
8. "Bouncing on the Toes"	Generating waves of energy, it chases away 100 illnesses. Stimulates the kidneys and increases flow of blood to internal organs.

B The eight basic movements of *qi gong*, the *ba duan jin*, also called "Eight Pieces of Brocade" or "Eight Silken Movements," are a form of medical *qi gong*. In contrast to other religious or martial forms of *qi gong*, the eight basic movements have primarily been designated to improve health.

In the Zhou dynasty, Bian Que is said to have taught the practice of breathing to increase *qi* circulation. During the Han dynasty, Hua Tuo developed the "Frolics of the Five Animals" (*Wu Qin Xi*), a series of exercises that is mimetic of the movements of the tiger, bear, stag, monkey, and bird. The combination of breath (*nei gong*) and movement merges internal and external work. *Qi gong* works on the unfolding of the three treasures: essence (*jing*), *qi*, and spirit (*shen*) (**A**), which are regarded as key to vibrant health.

In the late fifth or early sixth century CE, Da Mo, a Mahayana Buddhist monk known as Bodhidharma, arrived in Shaolin, China from India and found the Shaolin monks feeble and lacking in discipline. His introduction of a practice based on a combination of movement with meditation invigorated the monks and strengthened their power. This was the beginning of the tradition of the superior martial artists of the Shaolin Temple, emblematic of the school of internal alchemy (*wai dan*). Martial *qi gong* develops the strength, endurance, and spirit of the warrior. *Wai dan* practice aims to fortify muscles and bones to develop physical invulnerability.

Daoist *qi gong* is aimed at alchemical transmutation, merging with nature, longevity, and immortality. It focuses on the three elixir fields (*dan tian*) and the transformation of the three treasures. First, essence (*shen*) is transformed into *qi* in the lower elixir field, then, thought-mind (*yi*, the mind of the spleen) conducts the *qi* into the central elixir field, at the level of the heart, where in turn it is transmuted and refined into spirit-mind (*shen*) in the upper elixir field. These original Daoist techniques are the jewels of contemporary *qi gong* practices.

Confucian *qi gong* focuses on the development of the spirit as the "commander of *qi*." It aspires to ethical development and refinement of personal temperament. It incorporates the ideas of the virtue of balance or the middle path, and of the perseverance or discipline required to generate effective results. See **B** for a table of the four different types of *qi gong*.

Buddhist *qi gong* seeks the refinement of the mind, the transcendence of illusory duality in order to liberate all sentient beings from suffering. Its prime focus is meditation to generate a transmutation of *qi* into compassion at the heart level, which is guided to the third eye with the intention of awakening benevolent wisdom in order to realize the state of non-duality, the ultimate goal of all Buddhist practices.

Medical *qi gong* augments the healing capabilities. It works on the three treasures and harmonizes energy on the physical, psychological, and emotional levels. Ideally, one draws from the pool of ancestral methods to choose the exercises that best fit the health and well-being of the student.

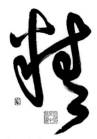 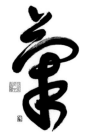 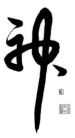

A *Jing, qi, shen.*

Daoist *qi gong*	Aimed at alchemical transmutation of the body, merging with nature and the macrocosm, and at longevity, and immortality in transcendence of the limitations of the human body
	Focuses on the three elixir fields *(dan tian)* in the human body and on the transformation and strengthening of the three treasures *(jing, qi,* and *shen)*
	Original Daoist techniques of self-cultivation in the context of longevity practices are the jewels of contemporary *qi gong* practices
Confucian *qi gong*	Focuses on the development of the spirit as the "commander of *qi*"
	Aspires to ethical development and refinement of personal temperament for the improvement of social relations and the individual's performance of duties to the community and family
	Strives to improve mental discipline, concentration, respect, moderation, and balance
Buddhist *qi gong*	Seeks the refinement of the mind and transcendence of the illusory duality in the mental world, in order to liberate all sentient beings from the suffering associated with life in the body
	Prime focus is meditation
	Buddhist monasteries famous for the development of martial arts for self defense and spiritual discipline
Medical *qi gong*	Practiced by both therapists and patients to improve health and cure disease
	Complements the other medical skills and techniques of the therapist in treating patients' bodies by applying his or her own *qi* to strengthen that of the patients and expel disease
	Is the root of the patients' ability to heal themselves by the power of *qi* cultivation
	Works on the three treasures and harmonizes energy on the physical, psychological, and emotional levels
	Incorporates all of the techniques invoked in the *dao yin*, (breathing, movement, posture, meditation, etc.), possibly adding other methods, such as the practice of therapeutic sounds, to enhance healing

B Different types of *qi gong.*

The patient becomes a responsible agent aware of the power he or she exercises on his or her own healing ability and healing process. The practice of *qi gong* entails the management of well-being, the reinforcement of health and vitality through one's own means. Medical *qi gong* incorporates all of the techniques invoked in the *dao yin*, possibly adding other methods, such as the practice of therapeutic sounds, to enhance healing.

The multiple lineages that have developed over the centuries all share common points. All forms of *qi gong* link work on the three treasures with channel-stimulating techniques associated with breathing. All schools cultivate a calm mind and value a virtuous spirit. These assorted techniques are variations on a basic scale whose adaptability resonates effectively in areas as varied as martial arts, medicine, and spiritual research.

Principles

Qi, literally breath, also implies the essential functions of life (see also pp. 22–23). The Chinese character for *qi* is made up of two elements, rice grains and breath, both of which are essential for life. The rice grain is a prime symbol for life. It is *yin* in its most concentrated, nourishing, and sustainable form. It holds the promise of future harvests. Breath, essentially *yang*, is evoked in its most mobile, invisible, and exciting guise, the vapor of rising steam. The composite meaning emerges through correlating these two elements.

The pictogram representative of *gong* associates a tool, a flat shovel used in wall construction, with the force that manipulates it. It implies the regular practice crucial to any fulfillment. "*Qi gong*" means exercising to cultivate vital energy. The objective of the practice is to promote the flow of *qi* and circulate *qi* through the channels. In Chinese medicine, *qi*, or that which animates all living organisms, maintains the body in good health. *Qi gong* practice stimulates the circulation of *qi* to convey it through the body and stimulate its self-healing abilities (**A**).

Concentration, Breath, and Posture: Indivisible Triad of the Dance of *Qi Gong*

Concentration, breath, and posture are the three ingredients whose combination embodies the essence of *qi gong*. The various lineages differentiate themselves through their particular focus. Some favor mental training, others focus on the breath or give preference to postures. Though each *qi gong* form has its specific function, stimulation through movement and breath is the distinctive hallmark of all forms. Forms vary to adjust to the needs of all, young or old, hyperactive or narcoleptic, remaining true in their essence to the *dao yin*. Movement, breath, and concentration mutually complete each other and work as components in the practice of *qi gong* to establish a profound sense of well-being.

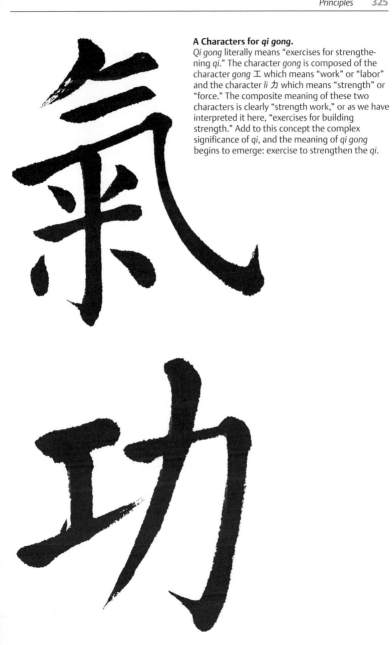

A Characters for *qi gong*.
Qi gong literally means "exercises for strengthening *qi*." The character *gong* is composed of the character *gong* 工 which means "work" or "labor" and the character *li* 力 which means "strength" or "force." The composite meaning of these two characters is clearly "strength work," or as we have interpreted it here, "exercises for building strength." Add to this concept the complex significance of *qi*, and the meaning of *qi gong* begins to emerge: exercise to strengthen the *qi*.

Posture is practiced in a frame of mind characterized by serenity and openness. Focusing on the body, the practitioner becomes aware of the four directions of his or her body and its dimension in space. Posture is both dynamic and relaxed; muscular tension is exercised through breathing and relaxation. Movement, relaxation, and tension in the muscles increase *qi* and its circulation along the channel network, which stimulates and influences the essential body functions. Generally speaking, body *qi* flows in the four cardinal directions (up, down, left, right).

Breathing is a distinctive feature of *qi gong* practice. More precisely translated as synchronous movement and breathing (*tu na*), *tu* (to dissipate, disperse, dispel, scatter) and *na* (to absorb) set the rhythm; exhalation and inhalation stimulate the flow of *qi*. The practitioner breathes naturally, deeply, slowly, and regularly through the nostrils. Inhalation is in accord with ascending *qi* movements, is *yin* in nature and energizing. Exhalation accompanies descending *qi* movements, is *yang* in nature and releases used *qi*. Although the various breathing techniques used in *qi gong* have their own characteristics, they all include regulating breath and calming the mind, allowing *qi* to descend and assemble in the lower elixir field, which plays a fundamental role in the distribution and transmutation of *qi* (**A**).

Concentration, intention, and visualization are the attributes of the mind that complete *qi gong* practice (**B**). The power of the mind moves matter by directing the flow of *qi*. Directing the mind is thus a key element in the practice of any *qi gong* movement. Conscious of his or her movement, the practitioner directs it mentally, the breath is guided by the mind, and visualization is added to reinforce the flow of *qi*. Typically, exhalation serves to eliminate used black or gray energy, whereas inhalation harnesses pure, white, and luminous energies. Visualization allows for a direct connection to the natural energies, which reinforces practice potential and lays the foundation for tackling internal *qi gong*, a subtle but powerful practice in which the spirit-mind is the commander.

Practiced regularly this synchronous handling of movement, breathing, and mind generates profound effects. The dynamic of *qi gong* is essentially harmonizing and contributes to a modification of body functions through the regular and extraordinary channels and the nervous system. According to Roger Jahnke, "the practice of *qi gong* triggers a wide array of physiological mechanisms which have profound healing benefits. It increases the delivery of oxygen to the tissues. It enhances the elimination of waste products as well as the transportation of immune cells through the lymph system. And it shifts the chemistry of the brain and the nervous system." (Jahnke Qigong).

A Ancient drawing representing the elixir fields within the body.

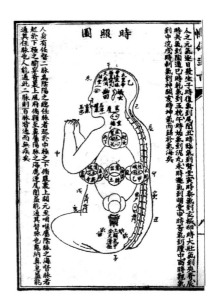

B Posture, Breathing, Concentration
(© by Thomas Langer,
reprinted with kind permission).

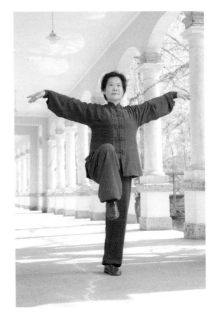

The Three Treasures and *Qi Gong*

Medical and Daoist *qi gong* is based on the transformative and connective power of *qi* that regulates the movement of the three treasures. Daoist practice consists in refining and transmuting essence into *qi* to nourish and unify the spirit-mind. In an advanced practice with a spiritual focus, spirit is transformed into emptiness.

Essence is the source of life and development. It is the substance that will be converted into *qi*. *Qi gong* as exercise for strengthening vital energy aims at reinforcing the transformation of the original essence of the practitioner into *qi*. Breathing harmonized with thought-mind is the key to *qi* movement. It gives the impetus to transform *qi* into spirit. Essence, *qi*, and spirit are merged into unity through Daoist *qi gong* practice.

Qi gong includes static postures, exercises in motion, and sitting practices. *Qi gong* movements and postures can also be differentiated according to the four types of *qi* movement: rising, descending, opening, and closing. *Qi* flows optimally through the channels when relaxation is at its highest. Insufficient relaxation hinders or blocks *qi* flow.

Research and Application Areas of *Qi Gong*

Qi gong represents one of the many therapeutic branches of Chinese medicine. It has been practiced for over 3000 years, both as a unique therapy and within the paradigm of traditional Chinese therapies. Acupuncture, Chinese herbal therapy, a custom-made diet, and an assortment of selected *qi gong* movements are the basic elements of a holistic, proactive, and efficient therapy that stimulates and refines *qi* quality and *qi* distribution, a therapy that incorporates all levels necessary to healing: physical, emotional, and spiritual.

During the Cultural Revolution *qi gong* was forbidden in China, due to its association with spiritual traditions like Daoism and Buddhism. Freed from its Chinese enclave in the liberal current of the 1980s, *qi gong* rapidly conquered the Western world. Less invasive than acupuncture, "the aspect of oriental medicine that has the potential to truly rock the Western world is *Qigong*" (Jahnke History). Indeed, the interest that *qi gong* has triggered as a therapeutic tool has led to an impressive number of scientific experiences and studies. Following the Chinese example, Western hospitals have begun using *qi gong* as a complementary therapy in treatments for hypertension, rheumatism, cancer, drug addiction/substance abuse, cardiopathy, psychological imbalance, shock, and so on. The efficiency presumption is such that it has given rise to substantial investments both in China and in the United States where the National Institute for Health has funded several clinical trials to assess the therapeutic potential of *qi gong*[*] (**A–D**).

---

[*]   For more details on the type and number of scientific studies on *qi gong* consult the website of the National Library of Medicine: http://www.ncbi.nlm.nih.gov/pubmed.

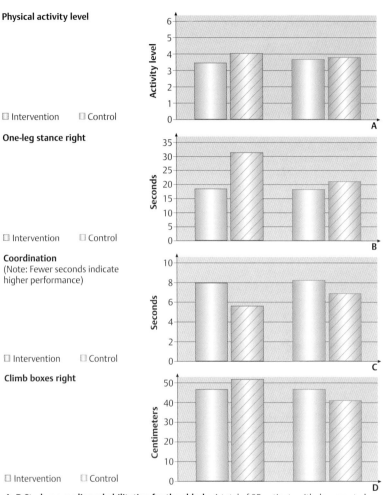

Physical activity level

☐ Intervention   ☐ Control

One-leg stance right

☐ Intervention   ☐ Control

Coordination
(Note: Fewer seconds indicate
higher performance)

☐ Intervention   ☐ Control

Climb boxes right

☐ Intervention   ☐ Control

A–D Study on cardiac rehabilitation for the elderly. A total of 95 patients with documented coronary artery disease were randomized to an intervention group (*n* = 48) or to a control group (*n* = 47). The intervention group met weekly over 3 months. The control group received usual care.
The striped bars describe the situation after the intervention and control respectively. A combination of *qi gong* and group discussions appear to be a promising rehabilitation for elderly cardiac patients in terms of improving self-reported physical activity, balance, and coordination. (Cardiac rehabilitation for the elderly: *qi gong* and group discussions. *Eur J Cardiovasc Prev Rehabil, 12.* 2005;1:5–11)

Qi gong practice strengthens the practitioner's sense of physical balance and contributes to the prevention of falls among the elderly. The regenerative effects induced by *qi gong* practice stimulate the mind and strengthen concentration capacity; they are particularly beneficial in the prevention of degenerative diseases. An additional advantage of *qi gong* is that it constitutes an accessible and wholesome practice for subjects of all ages, irrespective of their intellectual matrix or physical fitness.

In his studies relating to the use of *qi gong* in education, Heinrich Bölts quotes the experience of Rohrmoser who introduced *qi gong* to a group of adolescents with learning disabilities (Bölts 2003). Rohrmoser records a reinforcement of the adolescents' awareness of their individual value as well as an increase in self-esteem. Rohrmoser insists on the significance of *qi gong* practice in her work with adolescents who suffer from dyslexia, coordination problems, or feeble concentration, all of which are symptomatic of a lack of confidence and fear of failure. *Qi gong* practice entails the realization and experience of individual action potential, thus allowing us to experience an increase in regulation possibilities.

This dynamic breeds self-confidence and strengthens our awareness of our own competencies; it establishes a nurturing foundation that generates constructive transformation through individual initiative. The results of Bölts' studies (**A**) clearly demonstrate that regular *qi gong* practice improves the ability to regenerate by means of establishing restoration phases experienced as pleasurable moments of enjoyment. This regeneration strengthens our confidence in our own abilities and increases our potential for action, as well as our ability to face life more freely, and to meet the challenges of daily life with more serenity. *Qi gong* develops our ability to harmonize body, breath, and mind, and to incorporate this awareness actively into the repertory of lived experiences.

Qi gong is used successfully among socially problematic groups such as juvenile delinquents, drug addicts, or prison populations. *Qi gong* bio-energetics is beginning to be understood through research such as an investigation into the effectiveness of *qi gong* therapy in the detoxification of heroin addicts in a clinical trial in China. In addition to their own *qi gong* practice the *qi gong* group also received daily *qi* adjustments from a *qi gong* master. Reduction of withdrawal symptoms in the *qi gong* group occurred more rapidly than in the other groups, along with significantly lower mean symptom scores from day 1, and considerably lower anxiety scores. The amount of morphine in urine samples decreased much more rapidly, with negative results from day 5 for the *qi gong* group, compared with day 9 for the group detoxifying with lofexidine-HCl, and day 11 for the control group. (Li, Chen, & Mo 2002).

Current developments and studies portend a promising role in the range of modern therapeutics for *qi gong*.

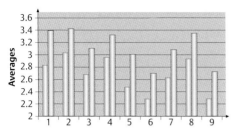

1) Mental and physical state
2) Body awareness
3) Awareness of body parts
4) Mental and physical perception
5) Mentally more dynamic
6) Able to concentrate better
7) Mental condition
8) Physical condition
9) Able to allow feelings

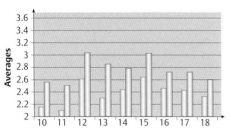

10) Able to express feelings
11) More secure
12) More powerful
13) Mentally more composed
14) More cheerful
15) More balanced
16) More optimistic
17) More thoughtful
18) More motivated

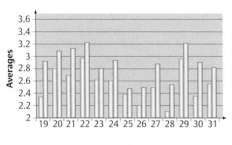

☐ First survey   ☐ Third survey

19) State of health
20) Awareness of bodily signals
21) Ability to regenerate
22) Awareness of physical disorders
23) Awareness of mental disorders
24) Self-acceptance
25) Reaction to environmental stimuli
26) Handling of harmful substances
27) Dealing with everyday problems
28) Everyday motivation
29) Everyday relaxation
30) Coping with hard times
31) Dealing with stressful times

A Comparison of the first and the third surveys of classes 8, 9, and 10 of the refresher course in *qi gong* according to the questionnaire QIE 2 (Qigong Evaluation 2) set up for this research (*n* = 58). The questionnaire for this research contained 31 items regarding health. Significant changes can be seen regarding health awareness, which are shown by improved physical perception (1–4, 7, 8) and awareness of mental state (6, 9, 10). The participants felt more secure, more balanced, and more active (11–15). A positive change is also recognized in the active handling of psychological imbalances. Responsiveness to physical and emotional states increased (19, 20, 22, 23) and everyday problems and stressful times are managed better (27, 30, 31) (Bölts 2003).

Qi gong opens the way for a paradigm shift in the Western therapist-patient dynamics as it helps to implement a most profound aspect of Asian medicine by establishing the root of self-care, thus turning the patient into an agent of his/her own healing. Indeed, the more one practices, the more *qi* circulates and the more *qi* there is to share, either to harmonize one's own energetic requirements, or as a therapist in relation to the available potential of *qi* that is transmitted via the hands. Every novice who practices the microcosmic orbit (see pp. 338–340) may experience the awakening of this energetic process. The practice of specific exercises increases the influx of energy; the tree posture (see pp. 334–336) charges the inferior elixir field with the vital energy that is connected to sexual energy. The respiratory dynamics causes the rise of *qi* inside the body, energy is distributed harmoniously, and practice generates a much stronger physical and intellectual resistance, a renewed vigor and greater sexual energy.

Furthermore, *qi gong* is naturally in line with the pursuit of a spiritual path. *Qi gong* exercises potentially grant access to meditative states that allow for the transmutation of the intrinsic quality of the energy that flows within us. The increase in vibratory rate causes a material purification with a purgatory effect on cellular memories, and as such sets a process in motion that is transformative on the transpersonal level that Dr. Alexander Lowen and Dr. Wilhelm Reich deal with in transpersonal psychotherapy. Engrams are memory traces left in the organism by the repetition of stimuli. These lasting, latent memories are engraved into the psyche, thus creating energy blocks and knots. The harmonizing combination of *qi gong* practice and breathing assists the energetic release of these blocks. The energetic unscrambling of these knots significantly frees the body of its engrams by enhancing *qi* quality and flow. *Qi gong* represents a truly multifunctional tool with major assets for any work dealing with personal development. The full array of *qi gong* methods not only endorses work on all aspects of personality that influence our daily communication, it also allows for the construction of an individualized practice that brings about energetic harmonization for a *better*-being on the physical, psychological, and emotional levels.

Qi gong is closely interwoven with dance: "the dance of life" (**A**). In this *pas de deux*, *gong* is conducted by *qi*, its guide and thread, certainly also a dance to live, to experience, play and grow with *qi*. Dance and *qi gong* activate and conduct *qi*, the "origin of both the form and substance of the whole universe" (Rose & Zhang 2001, p. 120). As such, *qi gong* is not merely creative in essence, and a remarkable tool to fuel creative potential, but an art in itself, which contains the seed for art therapy.

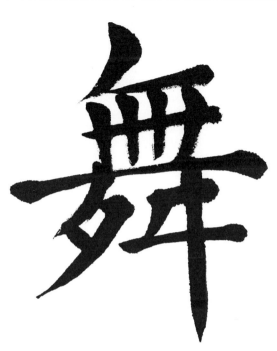

A The character depicted here, pronounced *wu*, is the character for dance. It encompasses the concept of dance, of moving about as if in a dance, of dancing with something in your hands, and of flourishing movement. Dance movement can conduct the flow of *qi* and can be a form of *qi gong*, just as *qi gong* is a form of dance and creativity.

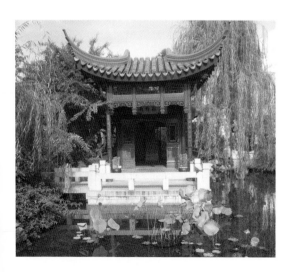

Qi Gong *Practice*

Dancers appreciate *qi gong* as an efficient method to prepare, strengthen, and protect their bodies. The development of *qi* gives rise to more spontaneous creativity, and *qi* distribution to the body periphery allows dancers to inhabit their choreography fully and harmoniously. *Qi gong* practice deepens self-confidence and helps to clear personal inhibitions; consequently it presents great potential as a tool for dance therapy and other art therapies.

The application of *qi gong* extends into all artistic realms. The interest aroused by *qi gong* practice and breathing techniques has led to the use of *qi gong* in many Western music conservatories as a means for improving body awareness to perfect body posture for optimal breath and voice. Singers and actors benefit from specific exercises that help to restore quality and strength of voice. Musicians find that regular *qi gong* practice brings about an interior transformation, which fuses the musician, the instrument, and the musical interpretation into a finely tuned unity.

Specific exercises prevent physical and psychological tension as well as stage fright. All creative artists know the importance of an empty mind to trigger and sustain the creative process, ultimately a transformational process of lived personal experience. *Qi gong* practice of empty mind activates the brain, which intensifies sensory perception and experience, and produces a feeling of alertness and vigilance that roots the practitioner within the present moment. This greater availability allows individual consciousness

spontaneous and powerful expression: "Poetry is the expression of the will or aspiration. Song is the recitation of sounds. Dance emotes and mobilizes form. These three originate in the heart, aroused by music. Thus deep feelings enlighten writing. It is the flourishing of *qi* that thus transforms the spirit. Its accumulation and harmonization in the center will draw out the excellence of the spirit" (*Book of Rites*, "Records of Music," cited in Rose & Zhang 2001, p. 62).

Static *Qi Gong*

Static *qi gong* teaches a variety of exercise types such as the postures associated with the eight trigrams, or the static animal postures. All *qi gong* begins with establishing a sound root, to ground the practitioner. The tree posture is most emblematic of static *qi gong*. It symbolizes both our roots with in the earth and growth and development in the direction of the sky.

The static tree posture (**A**) known as "embracing a tree" or "standing like a tree" is a simple form that combines body and mind. It stimulates essence, cultivates *qi*, and reinforces spirit. Essence stimulation enhances creativity, attention, and sleep quality. Immunity is boosted, vitality increased, and aging slowed down. The tree posture calms the mind, regulates blood circulation, digestion, and the bowels. It strengthens the sinews and joints while fortifying our sense of balance. Consequently, it reinforces tonus, physical performance, and endurance. The most notable effect of tree practice is the reinforcement of the immune system.

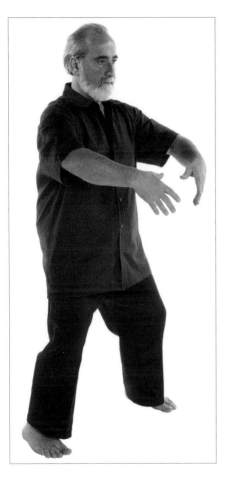

A The tree posture *song jing zhan li shi* (standing up relaxed and quiet).

- Position feet parallel to one another at shoulder width. Point toes slightly inward.
  Knees stay slightly bent, so that the body is in a comfortable seated posture.

- Slightly draw in the chin, slightly pull in the chest.

- Relax the shoulders, open the armpits.

- Bend the elbows, suspend them in the air with the elbows stretched to the exterior to empty the armpit hollows.

- The palms of your hands are facing the body, wrists are relaxed, fingers supple.

- The hands should be between the lower elixir field (navel level) and the middle elixir field (heart level). There should be a distance of about 30 cm between the hands and the front of the body.

- The eyes are downcast, focused on a fixed object 1–2 m ahead.

- Breathe in and out through your nose, using supple abdominal breathing to keep the muscles of the shoulders, back and chest free from tension.

This posture helps to ground the practitioner in terms of the body, by putting her/him in contact energetically with the earth. It establishes root by connecting with earth energy through the intention-breathing dynamics. This connection is made through the soles of the feet (*yong quan*, KI-1). Rooting is accomplished by focusing your mind beneath the connection point; visualize it spreading out underneath the earth. Practice of the tree posture consists of holding the posture, apparently motionless. Proper posture of the spine needs to be maintained and all of the joints must be slightly bent but extended to allow for *qi* to flow and be circulated efficiently. Posture time is gradually lengthened by a minute or two a week if practiced on a daily basis.

Qi Gong in Motion

Qi gong in motion resembles a dance (**A**). Fluidity of movement unfurls from the practitioner's roots within the earth to his or her connection with the sky; movement unfolds within the practitioner's awareness of the perfect vertical axis.

In practice, posture and *qi* motion are either in harmony, or they act through the association of opposing forces that simultaneously maintain and restrain each other. Raising the arms elevates *qi*; if the trunk is also in upward motion the ascending *qi* force increases through reciprocal reinforcement. Conversely, when lifting the arms while bringing the trunk down through lowering the buttocks and

bending the knees, *qi* ascension is more moderate. Here ascending and descending *qi* motions operate through opposing forces; they resonate at counterpoint, effecting a mutual restriction that harmonizes *qi* flow.

The dynamics of opening and closing movements is similar: during the opening, *qi*, guided by the mind, floods the body. Upon closure, *qi* converges from the extremities and superficial body areas. Movement and posture always begin with an opening to prime and spur *qi* flow. They conclude with an energetic closure to collect the energy generated in the practice and infuse the body with this energy.

The Head of the Turtle

The Head of the Turtle in forward motion: Stand upright, feet separated at shoulders' width, hands on the hips, head in vertebral alignment suspended by a thread above the *bai hui* acupuncture point (GV-20; Hundred Convergences), chin slightly drawn in. Inhale while lifting the chin vertically and stretch the cervical vertebrae, then exhale drawing a large circle towards the front with the chin. When the chin touches the sternum, inhale, and with the chin brushing against the breastbone realign the head within its axis. Continue the movement taking care to develop a supple fluidity tuned through synchronicity of breathing and movement. After a series of repetitions continue with the Head of the Turtle in backward motion: When the head has reached departure position exhale while lowering the chin and inhale upon raising the chin (**B**).

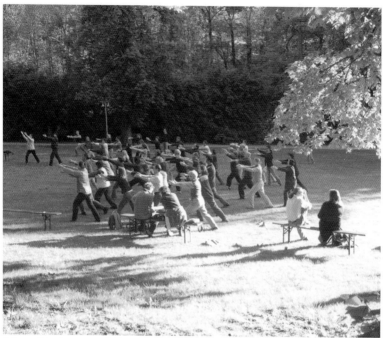

A Dance-like *qi gong* practitioners.

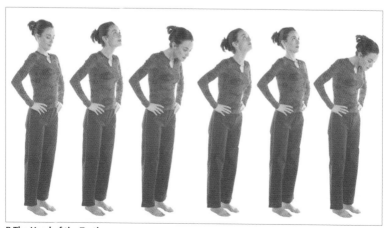

B The Head of the Turtle.

Therapeutic Indications

This exercise relieves the neck through an unblocking of vertebral joints, it activates the cranio-sacral pump, which nourishes the brain and stimulates essence. It releases the flow of energy along the neck channels, including GB, BL, SI, and GV.

Sway the Head and Wag the Tail

Open the feet widely, beyond shoulder width, place the palms on the inguinal creases. Tilt the chest forward 45°. Upon inhalation, bend the right knee and shift the body weight to the right leg. With the right hand, push hard on the bent leg. With the body, draw a circular arch and slant laterally in an oblique line. Align the head within the spinal axis, keeping the hips and shoulders facing front. Direct the eyes to the left and look at the left big toe. After 1–3 seconds exhale, draw your chest back to center. Repeat the movement on the opposite side. During inspiration concentrate on the *yong quan* acupuncture point (KI-1; Gushing Springm located on the side of the foot). When inhaling, the lung on the bent side absorbs and cools down heart fire, which is expelled from the body upon exhalation (**A**).

Therapeutic Indications

This movement contributes to massaging the heart. It calms agitation, anxiety, and distress, boosts sleep quality and is recommended practice to help and prevent palpitations and tachycardia.

Sitting *Qi Gong*

Some of the static poses, like the Head of the Turtle, can also be practiced sitting on the edge of a chair with the feet flat on the ground. There is an array of sitting practices that all associate visualization and breathing to generate *qi* flow within the channel system.

The Microcosmic Orbit

Settle comfortably on the edge of a chair with feet flat on the ground or sit on a cushion on the floor, legs folded, spinal column upright, chin slightly drawn in to align the head with the spinal axis. The head is suspended from a thread above *bai hui* (GV-20, located on the top of the heel). Free the shoulders from any tension, place the palms on the knees. Close the eyes and touch the tongue tip to the upper palate.

Relax into natural, abdominal breathing to calm the mind and grow conscious of the body's interior space. Upon inhalation, visualize the ascension of energy from the coccyx; make it rise along the governing vessel up the spine to the top of the head. Upon exhalation, concentrate on descending the energy from the top of the head through the nose and mouth, and then along the controlling vessel to the perineum. Continue to circulate the energy in this fashion: up via the spine during inhalation, down via the *ren* channel with exhalation. Breathing gives the tempo (**B**).

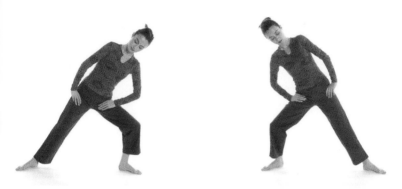

A Sway the Head and Wag the Tail (see p. 321).

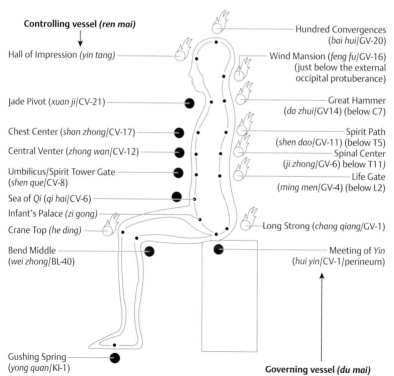

Controlling vessel *(ren mai)*

Hall of Impression *(yin tang)*

Jade Pivot *(xuan ji*/CV-21)

Chest Center *(shan zhong*/CV-17)

Central Venter *(zhong wan*/CV-12)

Umbilicus/Spirit Tower Gate
(shen que/CV-8)

Sea of *Qi (qi hai*/CV-6)

Infant's Palace *(zi gong)*

Crane Top *(he ding)*

Bend Middle
(wei zhong/BL-40)

Gushing Spring
(yong quan/KI-1)

Hundred Convergences
(bai hui/GV-20)

Wind Mansion *(feng fu*/GV-16)
(just below the external
occipital protuberance)

Great Hammer
(da zhui/GV14) (below C7)

Spirit Path
(shen dao/GV-11) (below T5)

Spinal Center
(ji zhong/GV-6) below T11)

Life Gate
(ming men/GV-4) (below L2)

Long Strong *(chang qiang*/GV-1)

Meeting of *Yin*
(hui yin/CV-1/perineum)

Governing vessel *(du mai)*

B The microcosmic orbit. The microcosmic orbit showing the *yin* (descending, in black),
and *yang* (ascending, flame) points.

After 5–10 minutes, cease the circulatory energy stimulation and let the energy collect in the inferior elixir field. Then cease concentration and return to natural breathing. After a moment, open the eyes on a deep inhalation. This exercise can be practiced using abdominal breathing, but inverted abdominal breathing is more conducive to initiating the energy wave.

Therapeutic Indications

This Daoist visualization eases the penetration of *jing* energy into the spinal cord/bone marrow, the brain, the nervous system, and the trunk organs. The microcosmic orbit regenerates the bone marrow and the brain; it contributes to a higher cerebral alertness and facilitates the development of further sensorial abilities.

Interior Smile for the Liver

Settle comfortably on the edge of a chair with feet flat on the ground or sit on a cushion on the floor, legs folded, spinal column upright, chin slightly drawn in to align the head with the spinal axis. The head is suspended from a thread above *bai hui* (GV-20). Free the shoulders from any tension, place the palms on the knees. Close the eyes and touch the tongue tip to the upper palate.

Breathe calmly. Lengthen inspiration and expiration progressively to make it totally fluid. Visualize your face in front of you. Visualize your face smiling, radiant, and illuminated or visualize the sun. Inhale capturing the energy and heat of the smile. Exhale still smiling inwardly toward the liver. Send this luminous, peaceful smile into the liver. Feel how it nourishes and fills itself with this appeasing and invigorating energy. Continue the practice until you feel the liver is full and content (5 minutes or more). Return to natural breathing. Open the eyes during an inspiration (**A**).

Therapeutic Indications

This exercise calms, relaxes, and nourishes the liver. It has an appeasing and balancing effect on the physical as well as the emotional level.

A The Interior Smile for the Liver.

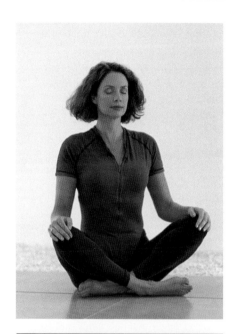

B The practice of the interior smile
is one that is found in Hindu, Buddhist, and Daoist traditions.

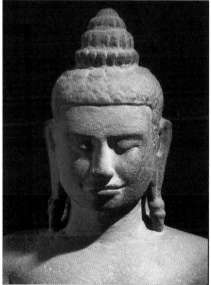

Qi Gong Self-massage

The sustained practice of moving and sending *qi* through the power of concentration opens the arm channels more widely and *qi gong* practice develops the ability to heal with your hands. This aspect is capitalized on and developed in different types of self-massage. *Qi gong* massage follows the channels through light brushing, caressing, tapping, or acupressure to release any tension induced by stress.

Nose Massage

Vigorously massage the nose with the index finger, from the ala nasi up the middle of the eyebrows and back. This simple massage is an efficient treatment to counteract acute head-cold symptoms or rhinitis. It stimulates the sense of smell and the lungs and it strengthens the mucous membranes of the nose (**A**).

Massage of *Ming Men* and *Dan Tian*

Ming men massage: With clenched fists, thumbs inside, vigorously massage the renal area in a circular motion (30–50 times one way, then the same number in the opposite motion). One should feel the heat infuse the area with energy. Then lightly tap the entire area with clenched fists, or with the interior sides of flat hands (30–50 times, **B**).

Dan tian massage: Place the palms flat on the belly and alternatively rub from the lower belly up to the navel area. Continue until the heat infuses the entire area and fills it with energy. Then lightly tap the entire area with clenched fists (about 50 times)

These two forms stimulate essence and constitute a general, preventive treatment. They stimulate the activity of the suprarenal and genital glands and the production of sexual hormones, while activating blood circulation in the kidney and genital spheres.

Eye Massage

With the thumbs and index fingers, massage the acupressure points around the eyes. Push on the point, maintaining the pressure for 3–5 seconds, then move on to the next point. Massage in order and on both sides simultaneously (see also pp. 216–217).

Points and Technique

Massage medial extremity of eyebrow, interior eye corner and suborbital hollow, then brush three times from the head to the tail of eyebrows. Then, massage the lateral extremity of eyebrow, and the hollow in the lateral extremity of the eye. Practiced in complement to the seventh movement of the *ba duan jin* (see p. 321), this massage stimulates the liver and is a thorough treatment to improve eyesight. An excellent preventive treatment to counteract overstress of the eyes (computer work, nocturnal driving, watching television). This technique also prevents failing liver energy (**C**).

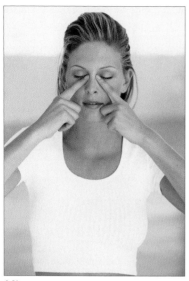

A Nose massage.

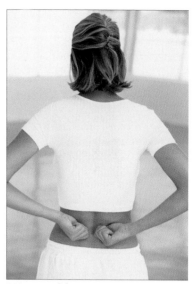

B Massage of the *ming men.*

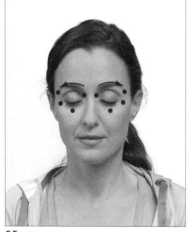

C Eye massage.

9

Tai Ji Quan

Douglas Wile

Introduction

In a little over a century, *tai ji quan*, whose name means "great ultimate martial art," has become the most popular health practice in China and just behind yoga and karate as an Asian cultural export. However, while yoga and karate have little public exposure in the lands of their origin, in China, every morning finds the parks teeming with practitioners performing the slow and flowing movements of *tai ji quan*'s hand and weapons forms and self-defense applications (**A, B**). Taipei holds the record for the largest simultaneous demonstration in one place with almost 15000 people. If yoga evolved as a spiritual philosophy that recruited somatic practices, *tai ji quan* and karate began as practical fighting arts that acquired philosophical trappings. Yoga in its modern incarnation has largely shed its links with Samkhya school of Indian philosophy, while *tai ji quan* has sought to wrap itself in Daoist robes. Yoga attempts to make a warrior of the philosopher; karate and *tai ji quan* attempt to make a philosopher of the warrior. In this sense, *tai ji quan* is more like the Olympics of ancient Greece, which began as martial training to become sport, religious ritual, and finally a reservoir of the culture's esthetic and philosophical ideals. If yoga is Venus and Karate Mars, *tai ji quan* falls neatly in between—the thinking person's martial art!

Often a gateway to Chinese culture, it is perhaps no exaggeration to say that more people in the West have come into contact with things Chinese through *tai ji quan* than all the language, history, art, philosophy, and religion courses combined. Few Westerners will attempt, much less attain, even a mediocre level of accomplishment in Chinese calligraphy or poetry, but millions have embraced *tai ji quan* and made it a part of their daily lives. Westerners are likely to have encountered it through travel to China or the countless schools, classes, tournaments, and demonstrations proliferating in the West. At first glance, the slow movements, vaguely suggestive of self-defense techniques, are unlike boxing, wrestling, sport, or dance. *Tai ji quan*'s plasticity has allowed it to be all things to all people, both in China and the West: the ultimate fighting art, preventative and restorative medicine, and a moving meditation. Thus, the meaning of a given posture may be explained as delivering a kick to the crotch, improving balance, or a standing meditation.

There is a cultural penchant in China to medicalize all human activities. The culinary arts, calligraphy, and sexology have all been pervaded by health concerns, so it is not surprising that the martial arts have acquired *qi gong* content or even been turned into *qi gongs*. Perhaps no art more than *tai ji quan* better embodies the ethos of an agrarian/bureaucratic empire: stability, moderation, and softness.

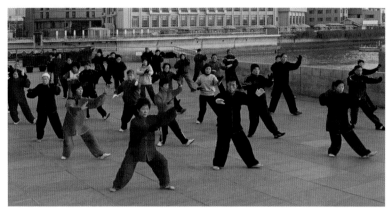

A *Tai ji quan* in the Bund area of modern Shanghai.

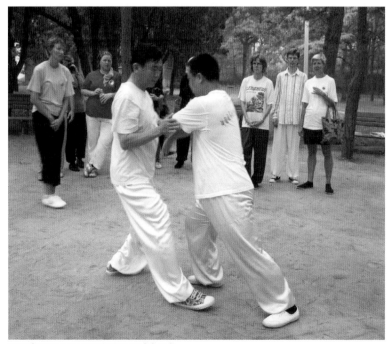

B Modern practitioners using push-hands.

Origins and Evolution

In China, the telling of *tai ji quan*'s history has been a major site of controversy between traditionalists and modernizers. Fundamentally, the various approaches to *tai ji quan*'s origins may be reduced to materialist and idealist. Among materialists there are those who emphasize the history of practice and those who emphasize the history of ideas; among idealists some trace its origins through myth and some through philosophical principles (Wile 1996).

If we tell *tai ji quan*'s story from the point of view of the development of a distinctive repertoire of named postures, then its history can be said to begin with Ming general Qi Ji Guang (1528–1587), who synthesized 16 styles into a 32-posture routine for troop training in his *Classic of Pugilism.* Twenty-nine of these postures appear in the Chen family art of Chen Village in Henan, possibly as early as Chen Wang Ting in the 17th century and certainly no later than Chen Chang Xing (1771–1853) and Chen Qing Ping (1795–1868) in the early 19th (Wile 2000). Family manuscripts examined by martial arts historian, Tang Hao, in the 1930 s listed seven forms, only two of which were still practiced (Tang 1935). The Chen style family lineage continued unbroken, but the transmission also passed to Yang Lu Chan (1799–1872) of Yongnian, Hebei, who developed the Yang style and taught the art to Wu Yu Xiang. Wu also journeyed to Chen village, and based on his study with Chen Qing Ping and Yang, created the Wu/Hao style, so named because it was perpetuated by Hao Wei Zhen (1842–1920), who learned the art from Wu's nephew Li Yi Yu (1832–1892). Yang's son Ban Hou transmitted the art to Wu Quan You (1834–1902), whose son Wu Jian Quan (1870–1942) standardized the Wu style, while Hao Wei Zhen transmitted it to Sun Lu Tang, who blended it with sister internal styles *xing yi* and *ba gua* to create the Sun style. These are the five most commonly practiced styles, with Yang being the most widely disseminated, followed by Chen and Wu, and then Sun and Wu/Hao. Each of these has many branches, and Zhao Bao and Wu Dang styles are also making strong bids for recognition (**A**).

If we ignore the external forms and focus on the development of a distinctive theory of internal training and defensive strategy, soft-style principles can be seen as early as Zhuang Zi's *On Swordsmanship* (Warring States period) and the story of the woman warrior, Yue Nü, in the *Annals of Wu and Yue* (Han dynasty). The first documented style based on these principles is Cotton Zhang's Close Boxing, described by Qi Ji Guang, followed by 17th-century philosopher Huang Zong Xi's "Epitaph for Wang Zhengnan" and his son Baijia's "Art of the Internal School" references to "stillness overcoming movement" and "reversing the principles of Shaolin."

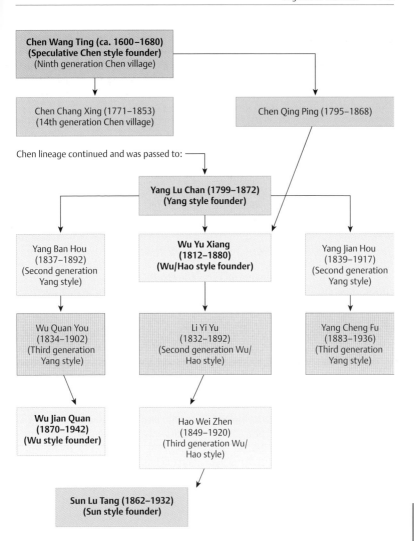

A *Tai ji quan* style founders and lineage chart.

The next stage is the addition of internal training to soft-style strategy, which we find in the writings of Chang Nai Zhou of the 18th century. Chang left us a detailed manual, describing a form completely unlike *tai ji quan* in its outer movements but sharing similar principles and even language with the *tai ji quan* "classics," whose first received texts date from the late 1800s. The body and soul of the art, its practices, and principles, finally come together, then, in a form recognizable today as the distinct style called *tai ji quan*, around the mid-19th century (Wile 2000).

Mythic accounts of *tai ji quan*'s genesis have fastened on the Huangs' allegorical tale of the Internal School, beginning with the God of War's revelation to the immortal Zhang San Feng or Zhang's inspiration from observing a fight between a stork and a snake. Many 19th- and 20th-century authors elided historical and stylistic discontinuities between the Internal School and *tai ji quan* and adopted the immortal Zhang for their own paternity. Not content with a medieval progenitor, some have traced the lineage all the way back to Lao Zi in the Zhou dynasty and through a series of legendary figures, including the immortal Zhang San Feng and quasi-historical figures Wang Zong Yue and Jiang Fa, finally entering the realm of recorded history with Chen Wang Ting in Chen village (Gu & Tang 1982) (**A**). Creationist ideologues have refused to give credit to the obscure and undistinguished Chen family, believing that only the likes of gods and immortals could have created the sublime art of *tai ji quan*. Sixty years of Marxist materialism, the belief in the production of knowledge through praxis, has not been able to eradicate this view, and today a subset of postmodern practitioners have revived the cult of Zhang San Feng and practice *tai ji quan* as a religious ritual (Wile 2007).

A closely allied group of idealists focus not so much on mythological lineages of supernatural and legendary figures but on the intellectual antecedents of the art. Believing that principle precedes practice and essence existence, they hold that *tai ji quan* is based on the cosmology of the *Book of Changes (Yi Jing* or *I Ching)*, the philosophy of Lao Zi, and the health prescriptions of *The Yellow Emperor's Classic of Medicine (Huang Di Nei Jing)*, as if the practical art sprang full blown from the heads of theoreticians. They deny the constant interplay of theory and practice, preferring to believe that principles exist in a perfect and transcendent realm, which geniuses tap into to create the practical arts. This tendency is particularly conspicuous in the writings of Sun Lu Tang, Wu Tu Nan, and Yang family disciples, Chen Wei Ming, Dong Ying Jie, and Zheng Man Qing (**A**, **B**).

Modern historians dismiss invented traditions, focusing instead on the evolution of *tai ji quan* as a construct combining body mechanics, military strategy, cosmology, Daoist philosophy, and *qi gong* in the context of changing social conditions.

A This building is in Chen Village.
The sign reads "Yang Luchan's *tai ji* learning place."

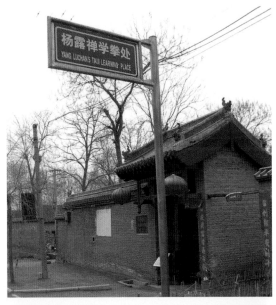

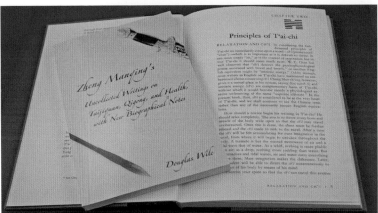

B Zheng Man Qing (1902-1975), his approach to teaching *tai ji quan*, and his writings captured the imaginations and practice styles of many American martial artists. Collections of his writings remain popular. The open page above, from an exposition of "T'ai-Chi" uses *Yi Jing* hexagrams throughout to illustrate the relationships between *tai ji quan* forms and the emerging from the permutations of the *ba gua* (eight trigrams) as the 64 hexagrams. Each of the hexagrams illustrate a moment in the dynamic interplay of *yin* and *yang*.

Chronology and Characteristics of Styles

Chen Style

Chen family accounts and most independent researchers credit Chen Wang Ting (ca. 1600–1680) with standardizing the family art into seven routines. Chen Fake (1887–1957) introduced the family art to the wider Chinese public, and in the 1980s his grandson Chen Xiao Wang brought it to the world. Although the other styles are all derived from the Chen family art, they lack the overtly martial quality preserved in the original (**A**).

Yang Style

Yang Lu Chan studied in Chen village and gained fame as a martial artist in the capital Beijing. His sons, Jian Hou and Ban Hou, were famous fighters, and his grandson, Yang Cheng Fu (1883–1936), spread the art nationally with the help of wealthy patrons and educated disciples. As Cheng Fu brought *tai ji quan* to a wider audience, he gradually eliminated the tempo changes, high kicks, and explosive punches to create a standard 108-posture form that could be practiced using high, medium, or low stances (**B**).

Wu/Hao Style

Wu Yu Xiang was a scholar from a wealthy and influential Hebei family, who along with his two brothers studied with Yang Lu Chan. Wu "discovered" and/or edited a number of short essays later canonized as the *Tai Ji Quan Classic*. He passed the transmission to nephew Li Yi Yu (1832–1892), who also authored a number of seminal works, and taught townsman Hao Wei Zhen (1842–1920), whose sons reduced the jumps and snap kicks in order to popularize the form in the 1920s. Wu/Hao style is the third in chronological order, but lacks family lineage, and is the last in worldwide dissemination (**C**).

Wu Style

Wu Quan You (1834–1902), a Manchu Yellow Bannerman and officer of the Imperial Guard, studied *tai ji quan* with Yang Ban Hou, oldest son of Lu Chan. Quan You's son Wu Jian Quan (1870–1942) modified and standardized the form for popularization and distinguished it from the parent Yang style. The family lineage was continued by sons, Gong Zao and Gong Yi, and grandson, Guang Yu (**D**).

Sun Style

Sun Lu Tang (1861–1933) was from a humble background in Hebei and learned Shaolin *kung fu* and *xing yi* as a boy. He studied *ba gua* in his thirties and *tai ji quan* in his early fifties from Hao Wei Zhen. Synthesizing the three styles and calling them "internal martial arts," he created his own style of *tai ji quan* and published the first book-length treatment with photographs in 1921. His contributions include emphasizing *tai ji quan*'s consonance with the *Yi Jing*, Daoist philosophy, and spiritual cultivation, and offering classes for women in his school (**E**).

1. Low, double-weighted stances.
2. Varied tempo from nearly standstill to explosive.
3. Leaping, stomping, and full-speed punches.
4. Open hand shape featuring hyperextension of fingers, abduction of index finger, and adduction of thumb.
5. Hook hand shape featuring thumb adduction, with other fingers folded into palm.
6. Reverse breathing, especially when issuing energy.
7. Spiral silk reeling energy and *dan tian* rotation.
8. In push-hands, partners face each other in mirror image (right leg opposite partner's left leg).
9. Demonstrating "shaking or vibrating" energy.

A Distinctive features of Chen style.

1. Open, expansive, and rounded arm movements directed by the waist.
2. Bow stances avoiding double-weightedness.
3. Rear foot at 45–90°angle to forward foot.
4. Slight forward inclination of torso when weight forward or back.
5. Concave palm with ulnar aspect (hypothenar eminence) leading on push.
6. Even tempo throughout form.

B Distinctive features of Yang style.

1. Compact, subtle movements.
2. High stances.
3. Hands do not extend beyond toes or cross center line of body.
4. Non-weight-bearing foot follows weight-bearing foot moving forward and backward.

C Distinctive features of Wu/Hao style.

1. High and narrow stances.
2. Parallel footwork.
3. Dorsiflexion of front foot when sitting back into rear leg.
4. Small circular hand techniques.
5. Incline plane alignment of head and heel.

D Distinctive features of Wu style.

1. High stances.
2. Quick footwork.
3. Following step by empty foot with forward and backward motion.
4. Few kicks and punches.
5. No horse or bow stances.
6. "Open-close" hand gestures at transitions for *qi* harmonization.

E Distinctive features of Sun style.

Movement Principles and Body Mechanics

Although the goal of *tai ji quan* is a state of body–mind integration, for convenience, we may analyze its movement principles into four aspects: external, internal, kinetic, and mental.

Externally, the general structural requirements include: holding the head as if suspended from above, releasing the shoulders, elbows, and chest, keeping the waist and pelvis horizontal, tucking the coccyx, and avoiding overextension of knees or pronation and supination of the feet.

Internally, the muscles are relaxed but alive. "Sinking the *qi* to the *dan tian*" encourages deep diaphragmatic breathing, "rooting" lowers the center of gravity, pressing the tongue against the upper palate forms the "magpie bridge" connecting controlling and governing channels, and constricting the anal sphincter raises *qi* from the *hui yin* point (CV-1) at the perineum.

From the kinetic point of view, all movement is "initiated in the soles of the feet, mounts up through the legs, is directed by the waist, and issues out through the hands." This coordinates upper and lower body and establishes an open power path from ground to hand, allowing us to gain economy of motion and mechanical advantage. A clear distinction of full and empty is achieved by avoiding double-weightedness, with 70–100 percent of the weight on one foot. Movement is slow and continuous, like "reeling silk" or a "flowing river." Nose and navel alignment unifies the movement of head and body. The pelvis and waist rotate like a horizontal wheel, never tilting.

The mind plays different roles at different levels of attainment. Initially, the mind is occupied with movement memory, but after the sequence becomes automatic, the mind concentrates in the *dan tian*, from where it monitors tension everywhere in the body. One may choose to focus on the breath, causing it to fill the *dan tian* or coordinate with movement; one may focus on key acupoints, such as the Gushing Spring (KI-1) in the ball of the foot or the Palace of Toil (PC-8) in the palm; or mental images may be used to develop movement qualities, such as "swimming on dry land," or project imaginary opponents. The practitioner may meditate on abstract principles, such as "finding stillness in movement and movement in stillness," or practice "mindfulness" by simply being at one with the movement, without discursive thoughts or distractions. At the highest level, there is a state of "no mind," where the body–mind dichotomy is erased as is the distinction of self and other. See **A** and **B** for examples of *tai ji quan* in practice.

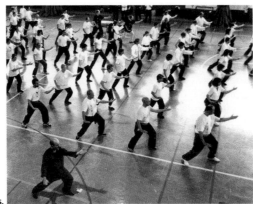

A *Tai ji quan* class.

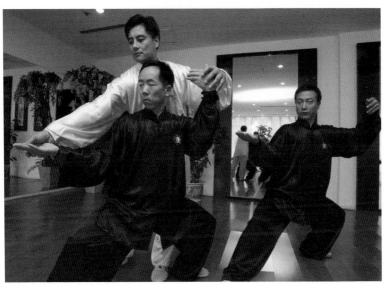

B Chinese *tai ji quan* master, Huang Zhongda, in white, teaches his students shadow boxing at his *tai ji quan* center in Shanghai July 2007.

Landmarks of Tai Ji Quan Literature

More than any other martial art, *tai ji quan* practitioners may be called "a people of the book." Although the provenance and date of the "classics" remain controversial, the *Tai Ji Quan Classic, Treatise on Tai Ji Quan*, and *Mental Elucidation of the Thirteen Postures in Tai Ji Quan*, together with the writings of Wu Yu Xiang and Li Yi Yu, have acquired scriptural authority (Davis 2004). On the practical level, they are normative prescriptions for developing skill, and on the literary level, they transport the reader to a realm of self-perfection: wholeness, power, and purity.

The first generation of writings dedicated to the distinctive art of *tai ji quan* and dated from the late 19th century, comprise short mnemonic verses and essays, as well as longer more systematic poems, redacted or composed by Wu Yu Xiang, his brothers, and nephew, Li Yi Yu. The second generation consists of transcriptions of the oral teachings of Yang Lu Chan, his sons and grandson, preserved as secret manuscripts and released by students in the third generation, mass market books, including history, theory, and practice, with photographs. The publication of these books coincides with China's humiliation by Japan and the West and represents an attempt, along with the founding of martial arts institutes, to promote native martial arts for health, pride, and a spirit of resistance.

Tai Ji Quan and Traditional Chinese Medicine

It is clear from the *tai ji quan* literature that many masters were conversant with traditional medicine. This is nowhere more apparent than in Chen Xin's *Introduction to Chen Family Tai Ji Quan* and Zheng Man Qing's *Master Zheng's Thirteen Chapters on Tai Ji Quan*. The tradition of therapeutic exercise traces back to the legendary Emperor Yu, who created a *qi gong* dance to drive out the dampness that afflicted his subjects, to the Han physician, Hua Tuo, who prescribed the "Frolics of the Five Animals" sequence for his patients, to Bodhidharma, who taught Shaolin boxing to his sedentary monks. The "Ma Wang Dui" manuscripts from the second century BCE contain illustrations of *qi gong* routines as part of a corpus of medical texts, and the great Yuan dynasty physician, Zhu Dan Xi, said, "Heaven has made all things to be in constant motion; man, too, must move to live."

Medicine and martial arts share a common language: *Yi Jing* cosmology. In *tai ji quan* theory, *yin* and *yang* are used to distinguish above and below, internal and external, mind and body, fast and slow, and hard and soft. *Tai ji quan*'s "13 postures" are analyzed according to five-phase theory (advance, withdraw, left, right, and central equilibrium) and the eight trigrams (ward-off, roll-back, press, push, pull-down, split, elbow-stroke, and shoulder-stroke). See **A** and **B** for examples of *tai ji quan* postures.

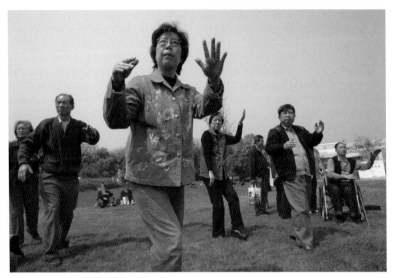

A Using *tai ji quan* for health and healing.

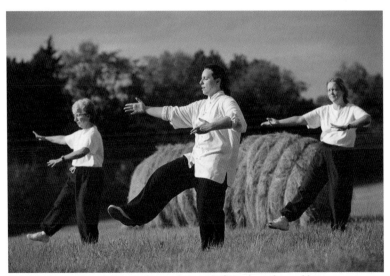

B Originating in China, *tai ji quan* has made inroads throughout the world. Here, a group of western students practice *tai ji quan* in a field.

The medical benefits and internal energetics of *tai ji quan* are often described in terms of channel theory. "Keeping the mind in the *dan tian*" and "sinking the *qi* to the *dan tian*" are the first steps in opening the "microcosmic orbit" (see p. 339) and circulating the *qi* in the controlling and governing vessels. By opening up the "macrocosmic orbit," a wave of *qi* can rise up from the Gushing Spring point, through the *yin* channels of the legs, up the governing channel in the spine, and out through the *yin* channels of the arms and hands. Most defensive techniques lead with the lateral aspect of the arm and hand, whose *yang* channels flow towards the body and are more resistant to attack. The complete curriculum of *tai ji quan* training includes grappling techniques that require an intimate knowledge of pressure points and can inflict instant paralysis or devastating delayed effects.

When it comes to organ theory, the most important connection for Chinese medicine, meditation, and martial arts is between the heart and kidney, or as expressed in five-phase theory, fire and water. "Maintaining the mind in the *dan tian*" places the heart's fire under the kidney's water, as in the auspicious hexagram "After Completion" (see **A**, **B**) and encourages *qi* and *jing* to rise up and eventually fill the brain and marrow (Zheng 1982). This also allows the prenatal "ministerial fire" of the "gate of life" between the kidneys to be enlivened but not overstimulated by the heart's "ruling fire." *Qi* circulating

in the liver keeps the liver fire calm, mind clear, eyes bright, and bones and sinews strong. Strong *qi* aids the spleen and stomach in transforming food and separating the clear and turbid elements. Deep breathing strengthens the lungs and delivers *qi* to the kidneys for storage and supply to all the other organs and encourages both lung and stomach *qi* to descend rather than become "rebellious." Since the *qi* and blood circulate in tandem, awakening the *qi* also stimulates the blood, and brings the nutritive *qi* traveling inside the blood vessels and defensive *qi* circulating outside the vessels into harmony (Qi 2005). The ideal of both medicine and meditation is stemming loss due to physical, mental, and sexual taxation, while avoiding the stagnation that results from inactivity. *Tai ji quan*, by cultivating "stillness in motion," seeks to store more than it spends and is ideal for conditions such as tuberculosis, where both bed rest and overexertion are contraindicated.

Tai ji quan form practice is also a kind of self-massage. There are 41 acupuncture points below the ankle and these receive deep massage as weight shifts from foot to foot. Bipedalism and erect posture in homo sapiens stacks the organs one on top of the other, causing them to be cramped and stagnate. Deep diaphragmatic breathing and slow, low impact movement massages the organs with the pumping of the diaphragm and turning of the waist (Zheng 1982).

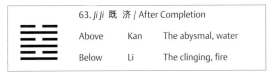

63. *Ji Ji* 既 济 / After Completion

| Above | Kan | The abysmal, water |
| Below | Li | The clinging, fire |

A The hexagram "After Completion" is a polyvalent symbol, consisting of the trigram *li* (fire) under *kan* (water). Metaphysically, this represents the union and fruitful interaction of fire, which tends to rise, and water, which tends to sink. In the political and social realm, because each of the six lines is in its numerologically correct position–unbroken *yang* lines in odd spaces and broken *yin* lines in even–it represents those in authority (*yang*) receiving compliant support by subordinates (*yin*) but not abusing their power. In Chinese sexual yoga, it is interpreted to symbolize the female superior position and the male strategy of playing the passive role in order to induce the female partner to release her *yang* energy. In self-cultivation and martial arts, "After Completion" represents body-mind integration through the process of holding the mind (fire) in the *dan tian* (watery region of the body), thus transforming water into steam, or *qi*, for health and strength.

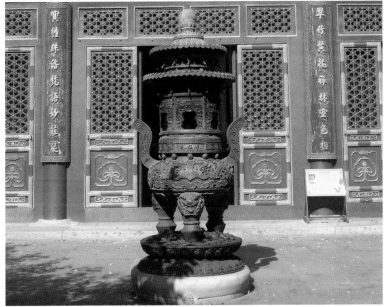

B The *ting* or tripod cauldron is an important ritual object in Chinese culture. This one stands in a temple courtyard in Hang Zhou. The *ting* was used to make sacrifices and is often used as an image of the interaction of fire and water described in the hexagram above. This relationship is seen in the life gate where the kidney water and kidney fire coexist. Additionally, the ting is an important vessel in Chinese alchemy (© Kevin Ergil).

Self-defense, Competition, and Weapons

Although today *tai ji quan* is practiced by many exclusively for its health benefits, the majority of teachers incorporate at least some self-defense applications in their instruction. The Chen family is credited with developing a unique form of self-defense training called "push-hands" (see p. 347), which allows partners to practice offensive and defensive techniques without protective gear and with minimal risk of injury. Through the principles of sticking to the partner, following, and listening, students gain tactile sensitivity and are able to cause incoming force to "land on emptiness" or "deflect a thousand pounds with four ounces." Stiffness or faulty alignment is immediately exploited by a skillful opponent's uprooting, locking, or throwing, while softness and yielding are rewarded by neutralizing the opponent's attacks. Students progress from one-hand to two-hand contact and from fixed stances to moving push-hands. There are many styles of push-hands, but one classic involves a continuous give and take exchange of push, press, ward-off, and roll-back. If no gaps or opportunities appear, more challenging techniques, such as pull-down, split, elbow-stroke, and shoulder-stroke may be introduced. For advanced students, there are choreographed self-defense duets called *da lü* and free sparring called *san shou* or *san da*.

In the 1950s, as Chinese martial arts were incorporated into a national system of physical education, simplified and standard routines were designed for popularization and competition (**A, B**). One of the most widely disseminated of these is the 24 Posture Simplified *tai ji quan*. There are now tournaments for all forms and push-hands competitions featuring synthetic and traditional family styles and for different weight divisions in push-hands. Full-contact matches attract athletes from different martial arts backgrounds, including *tai ji quan* practitioners.

As with other Asian martial arts, *tai ji quan* also has its arsenal of weapons. The most popular weapon in *tai ji quan* is the traditional choice of the Chinese literati, the two-edged sword, or *jian* (Chen, 2000) (**C**). This is followed by the broadsword, or *dao*, and then staff and spear. Again, the hallmark of *tai ji quan* weapon forms is slow tempo, continuity, and the extension of *qi* through the weapon. In fencing, as in push-hands, the key is sticking and following, waiting for gaps to appear, rather than forcing opportunities and exposing oneself.

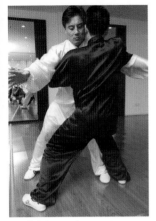 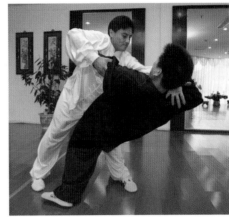

A Self-defense. Chinese *tai ji quan* master, Huang Zhongda, in white, teaches his students self-defense applications at his *tai ji quan* center in Shanghai July 2007.

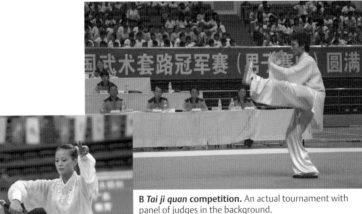

B *Tai ji quan* competition. An actual tournament with panel of judges in the background.

C *Tai ji* sword. Zhang Fang, the silver winner for female shadowboxing and *tai ji* sword from Guangdong Province in the 10th State Sports Meeting in October 2005.

Representative Postures

Across all styles, *tai ji quan* has a repertoire of around 30 postures, each embodying a generalized self-defense application. What follows are generic descriptions of three signature postures that are common to all styles, minus the fine points of hand shape, alignment, foot position, and weight distribution that distinguish one style from another.

Grasp Sparrow's Tail

The left foot is advanced, and as the weight is shifted to it, the left hand moves forward with the back of the hand facing out. Simultaneously the right hand moves down, with the palm leading, to a point lateral to the right hip. This is one hand ward-off. Now all the weight is concentrated on the left foot, as the right is elevated and steps out 90° to the right. Simultaneously, the right hand moves forward with the back of the hand leading and the left hand following closely behind, palm facing out. This is two hands ward-off. The waist continues to rotate another 45° to the right, and then as the weight is shifted back to the rear leg, the hands swing backward, with the right palm facing down and the left facing up. This is roll-back. The weight is now shifted to the forward foot as the hands move out with the back of the right hand facing out and the left palm lightly touching the right arm at the wrist or forearm. This is press. Now sit back into the rear leg, allowing the arms to separate and extend parallel in front of the body. Shift the weight forward again, pushing out with the two palms to form the posture push. This series is essentially a solo version of the two hands push-hands described above and illustrates two defensive and two offensive techniques. See **A**.

Single Whip

From the posture push, the weight is shifted back to the left foot, while simultaneously the waist rotates to the left and the empty right foot pivots left on the heel. Now the weight shifts to the right foot, while the right hand forms a hook suspended above the left hand held palm up. With the waist now facing 180° from the push direction, step out with left foot, while the two hands separate, the left moving out in front of the chest, palm rotating out, and the right hand, still holding the "hook," extending horizontally to the right. This foils an attack from the left rear, or alternatively represents a strike with the right hand or head twist with the left. See **B**.

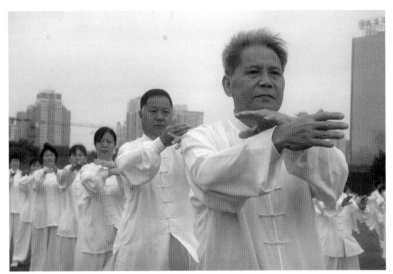

A Grasp Sparrow's Tail.

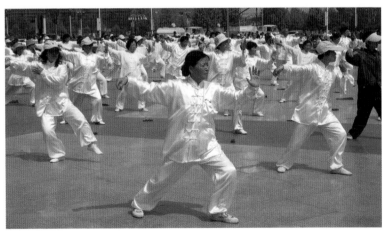

B Single Whip.

Golden Cock Stands on One Leg

From Single Whip lower posture, all the weight of the body is gathered in the left leg. As the body rises to an erect posture, the right knee thrusts upward, with the right elbow positioned just above it, fingers extended upward, and the left hand sweeping to the left, coming to rest, palm down, lateral to the left hip. Lowering the right foot to the ground and shifting all the weight to it, the left knee is elevated, the left elbow is suspended above it, and the right hand sweeps to the right, coming to rest palm down lateral to the hip. The rising knee and foot illustrate strikes to the abdomen and crotch, while the two hands illustrate sweeping and elevating blocks. See **A**.

Tai Ji Quan *and Western Medicine*

Tai ji quan's therapeutic potential has not escaped the attention of Western medicine, and hundreds of controlled, randomized, and observational clinical trials, together with cross-sectional and longitudinal studies attest to its preventative and restorative efficacy. The vast majority of research is in the area of geriatrics, but the range of conditions studied is stunning and may be grouped into primary, secondary, and holistic. Primary applications build skills by improving posture, balance, flexibility, agility, coordination, reaction time, and range of motion. Studies show consistent reduction in falls for the elderly after only short periods of training. Secondary applications improve digestive/bowel function, cardio-respiratory capacity, osteoporosis, arthritis, orthopedic injuries, insomnia, immune response, endocrine balance, pain management, and lymphatic circulation. Very specific diseases, such as Parkinson, shingles, Alzheimer, multiple sclerosis, and hypertension have also responded well to *tai ji quan* practice. Holistic benefits studied include stress reduction, social interaction, and mental calmness. *Tai ji quan* is also an attractive modality because of its safety and cost-effectiveness (Klein & Adams 2004) (**A**, **B**).

Tai ji quan, China's national treasure, has spread to every corner of the earth and continues to attract new practitioners for self-defense, health, and meditation. Its health benefits, having been promoted in China for more than a century and the subject of biomedical studies around the world for several decades, can be expected in the future to play a greater role in prevention, stress management, and geriatric medicine.

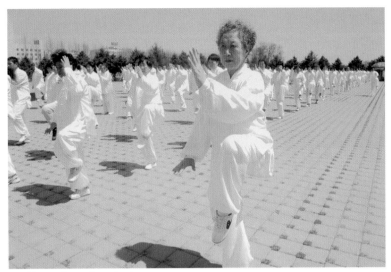

A Golden Cock Stands on One Leg.

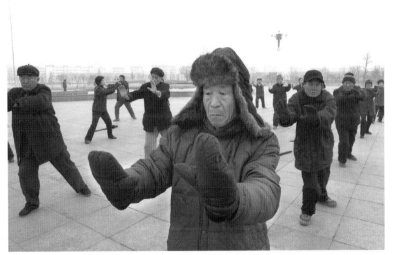

B Seniors undaunted by age or the elements practice outdoors in North China's bitter winter.

10

Acupuncture Research:
An Overview

Stephen Birch

This chapter discusses the types of research used to investigate acupuncture, and reviews the evidence from previous studies. It outlines where to find publications on acupuncture research and how to form judgements about that research. The chapter continues with a discussion of the limitations of previous research, major challenges for the future, and guidelines on how to pursue acupuncture research.

Types of Research

Research on acupuncture falls into two broad categories: studies that examine clinical practice and studies that examine mechanisms to explain how treatments work. There are two types of clinical practice studies: qualitative and quantitative. Qualitative approaches examine areas such as the nature of practice, who seeks treatment and why, who does the treatment, how people feel about their treatments, and so on (Cassidy 2000, 2002; Broom 2005; Richardson 2005). A qualitative study can capture data about feelings, beliefs, models, theories, and experiences. Quantitative approaches examine how effective a treatment is in comparison to something else. Quantitative approaches try to measure something specific, which requires that a specific thing, such as pain, be focused on, rather than the whole patient. Such studies try to measure objective changes using measurement technologies. Quantitative studies also try to measure subjective changes using validated questionnaires. In quantitative comparative studies, acupuncture treatment may be compared with usual medical intervention for the same condition, or treatment may be compared to a sham intervention.

Sham treatments are used to control for placebo effects. Studies attempt to control for placebo effects to know how effective the mechanism of the intervention is compared with the psychological impact of the intervention (Hyland 2003). In a properly designed placebo-controlled study, one can understand the relative effectiveness of treatment in comparison to placebo effects. A treatment is considered effective if it is shown to be significantly more effective then placebo.

There are more pragmatic clinical studies where acupuncture treatment is compared with the usual biomedical treatment for the same problem or where acupuncture is added to usual treatment in comparison to standard treatment (Thomas & Fitter, 1997, 2002; Sherman, Linde, & White 2007). Other clinical research approaches may examine questions such as the nature and accuracy of the diagnoses that a TCM practitioner makes (Birch 1997b; Schnyer, Birch, & MacPherson 2007; O'Brien, Abbas, Zhang, Wang, & Komesaroff in submission) (**A**).

An important way of consolidating and summarizing studies that fall into the same area of research is the meta-analysis or systematic review (Kane 2004; White & Schmidt 2005; Linde, Hammerschlag, & Lao 2007). Meta-analyses examine the quality of published studies and judge the level of evidence of the effectiveness of treatment for a particular problem.

Type of Question	Type of Research Design	Levels of External Collaboration Probably Necessary
Nature of practice (What do practitioners do in practice? How do they treat X?)	Literature reviews Expert panels	Often none Relevant experts
Demographics (Who does the treatments? Who goes for treatment?)	Surveys, interviews	Statistician and other relevant experts
Clinical practice results (How do patients describe the results of their treatments? How well do I do in my practice treating X?)	Clinical audit Targeted population audit Qualitative studies	Usually minimal Relevant medical expert and statistician and staff Relevant expert, e.g., medical anthropologist
Reliability of diagnosis and treatment (How much agreement do we have on the traditionally based diagnosis of patients?)	Controlled environment structured studies	Relevant expert, e.g., statistics, medical expert, staff
Development of assessment and outcome tools (How can I measure the results of my traditionally based treatments?)	Literature reviews, surveys, expert panels and controlled environment structured studies	Relevant expert, e.g., statistics, medical expert, biometrics expert, staff
Health services and economic studies "pragmatic trials" (How much does the treatment cost? Do patients use medical services less if they receive this treatment?)	Randomized controlled trial, e.g., acupuncture vs. standard therapy (e.g., drug) or standard therapy and acupuncture vs. standard therapy alone	Relevant experts— statistics, medical expert, staff
Comparative outcome research "pragmatic trial" (How effective is the treatment compared with standard medical treatment?)	Randomized controlled trial, e.g., acupuncture vs. standard therapy (e.g., drug) or standard therapy and acupuncture vs. standard therapy alone	Relevant experts— statistics, medical expert, staff
Placebo controlled studies to examine specific effects "explanatory trials" (How effective is acupuncture to treat X, i.e., are the specific mechanisms of action of acupuncture more effective than "placebo"?)	Randomized controlled trial, e.g., acupuncture vs. control acupuncture (sham)—sometimes also vs. standard therapy or no therapy	Relevant experts— statistics, medical expert, staff

A Clinical practice studies—questions and methods (based on Birch 2003).

Laboratory Research

Laboratory research can use various disciplines such as physics, engineering, biology, chemistry, pharmacology, or anatomy to answer questions such as how does the treatment work, or what physiological mechanisms does the therapy invoke? The laboratory may work with animal models, or use human volunteers, usually with some kind of technical measurement technique such as chemical analysis, electrical measurements, imaging methods such as X-ray, CAT scan, or functional magnetic resonance imaging (fMRI). For ethical and safety reasons, the research is usually done on ani- mals before it progresses to studies on human volunteers. Laboratory studies can also work in a more abstract manner. Instead of testing on the whole organism (animal or human), chemical derivatives or cells are tested to examine possible mechanisms of action.

Over the last century, especially the last three decades, considerable work has been done in all of these areas to investigate acupuncture. There are huge volumes of published studies in East Asia (Bensoussan 1991; Tang, Zhan, & Ernst 1999), with smaller (but quite significant) numbers of studies in the West (Han 1989; Pomeranz 1996, 1998).

While laboratory research of acupuncture has had its problems, the area is generally better received and reviewed than the clinical research, and more studies of East Asian origin are cited in Western reviews of the area. Bensoussan (1991) includes probably the best, but somewhat out-of-date summary of much of the Chinese acupuncture research. Pomeranz (1998) contains one of the best summaries of the studies examining the mechanisms of action of acupuncture. Researchers have concluded that acupuncture seems able to trigger various neurological pathways and neuropeptide mechanisms that are helpful for blocking pain, modulating pain, reducing inflammation, altering blood circulation, and so on (Han 1989; Pomeranz 1998; Hammerschlag, Langevin, Lao, & Lewith 2007). Among the mechanisms that have been uncovered, beta-endorphin is the best known and documented (Pomeranz 1998) (**A**).

FMRI has been applied to the investigation of acupuncture since the early 1990s (Cho et al. 1998). The emerging data suggests that acupuncture modulates neural activation and deactivation of specific areas of the brain in ways that are consistent with our understanding of the role that acupuncture has in releasing beta-endorphins and shows how acupuncture can be beneficial to patients with chronic pain (Hui 2000, 2005; Napadow 2007).

Recently, scientists have been discussing limitations of studies to date. Hammerschlag and colleagues (2007) identified that mechanism studies so far have been more of a "black-box" approach: apply a measured reproducible input and measure the output, but we don't really know what happens in between. As such, we have good models based on correlational data (when we do X, we measure Y), but no good documentation of the mechanisms of how X triggers Y.

Type of Question	Examples of Research Designs
How does acupuncture block acute pain?	Produce experimental pain in animals or humans, apply acupuncture to reduce the pain, then apply various methods to block the analgesic effects, such as injection of naloxone (which blocks endorphin)
How does acupuncture treat chronic pain?	Apply acupuncture to chronic pain patients. For those that have pain relief use PET scan imaging of the brain to explore neurological mechanisms that may be involved
What are the cardiovascular effects of acupuncture?	Measure heart rate, heart rate variability, vascular compliance, blood pressure, the electrocardiogram, and so on
What are the micro-circulatory effects of acupuncture?	Use the "rabbit ear chamber" method on rabbits to visualize the capillary bed and videotape changes in capillary flow
Do the acupuncture points have discrete electrical properties?	Using an electro-dermal measurement system, measure the electrical resistance of the skin at acupoints compared with surrounding skin
Do the acupuncture channels have discrete properties?	Inject radio-isotopes into the body near or into the channels and photograph the migration of the isotopes in the body
Does acupuncture have anti-inflammatory effects?	Measure, for example, blood cortisol levels
Does acupuncture have hormonal effects?	Measure the blood level of various hormones such as FSH, TSH, and so on

A Acupuncture mechanism studies—questions and methods.

Clinical Research

Unfortunately, the quality of the research conducted to test the clinical efficacy of acupuncture is variable. Problems such as inadequate treatment, inappropriate control intervention, inadequate numbers of patients, inadequate blinding or guarantees of blinding are common in Western acupuncture trials (Ezzo, Lao, & Berman 2000; White, Filshie, & Cummings 2001; Birch 2004). In Asia, problems with quality of research are more pervasive, including problems with outcome measurements, randomization, and inclusion/exclusion criteria. Since these are fundamental problems, most Asian research is not cited in Western publications. Further, much of the Asian research has not found its way into Indo-European languages, consequently most researchers in the West reviewing clinical studies have limited themselves to Western-origin, primarily English-language, publications. Birch, Keppel Hesselink, Jonkman, Hekker, & Bos (2004) published a broad summary of acupuncture clinical trial results by summarizing international reviews of the systematic reviews that had been conducted. They listed all the systematic reviews and meta-analyses of acupuncture that had been published. They then examined how review groups working for different health authorities or government agencies reviewed these reviews. By taking this meta-view of publications, analyses, and summaries, the authors were able to identify emerging international agreements concerning the levels of evidence of efficacy of acupuncture.

The various agency reviews themselves are also good summaries that should be examined (Acupuncture 1998; Filshie & White 1998; BMA 2000; Ezzo et al. 2000; Filshie & Linde et al. 2001; Tait, Brooks, & Harstall 2002; Vickers, Wilson, & Kleijnen 2002) (**A**).

One of the key issues for interpreting clinical acupuncture studies and their reviews is the role of placebo. Many studies and reviewers have assumed that when acupuncture is compared with some form of sham acupuncture, the sham acupuncture is inert, and the sham is thus equivalent to placebo. To date, however, no study has demonstrated that sham treatment is truly inert. The comparison in sham trials between the treatment and placebo effects becomes confused, and often impossible to interpret (Birch 2006). Additionally, what is labeled as incidental placebo effects are often specific parts of the treatment in acupuncture practice (Paterson & Dieppe 2005). This makes any attempt to simply control for those parts unfeasible and requires that acupuncture be approached as a "complex intervention" (ibid.), which necessarily has different research needs than a more simple intervention like a single drug therapy (Medical Research Council 2000).

Examination of the effectiveness of a therapy must be done hand in hand with examination of the safety of that therapy. A therapy that is highly effective but highly dangerous will be considered very differently than a therapy that shows some efficacy and has very little risk associated with it (**B**).

Conditions for which there is general agreement that acupuncture is effective (a) and where some reviews have claimed it to be effective (b)	(a) Nausea and vomiting from chemotherapy, following surgery; acute post-operative dental pain (b) Jaw pain (TMD); migraine; chronic low back pain
Conditions for which there is general agreement that acupuncture seems to be not very effective	Smoking cessation; losing weight; tinnitus
Conditions for which it is difficult to draw clear conclusions due to methodological problems, but where evidence is at least promising	Addictions; stroke rehabilitation; asthma; tension headache; neck pain; osteoarthritis; dysmenorrhea; post-operative pain; musculoskeletal pain; fibromyalgia
Conditions for which evidence is accumulating but has not yet been systematically reviewed	Angina pectoris; depression; breech version; increased success rate of success with IVF procedures; duration of labor; urological problems; xerostomia

A Summaries of acupuncture clinical trial research (based on Birch et al. 2004).

US National Institutes of Health Consensus Development Conference on Acupuncture (Acupuncture 1998)	"One of the advantages of acupuncture is that the incidence of adverse effects is substantially lower than that of many drugs or other accepted procedures for the same conditions"
British Medical Association Review (BMA 2000)	"In terms of safety, few major adverse reactions to acupuncture treatment are reported in comparison to adverse reactions to orthodox interventions"
UK National Health Service Review (Vickers 2001)	"Acupuncture appears a relatively safe treatment in the hands of suitably qualified practitioners, with serious adverse events being extremely rare"
Canadian/Alberta Health Authorities Review (Tait et al. 2002)	"The studies' conclusions are consistent in that they found that the rate or incidence of serious adverse events due to acupuncture treatment is low but that they do occur. MacPherson and colleagues stated that the adverse event rate, when compared with primary care drugs, suggests that acupuncture is a relatively safe treatment, and many researchers concur that it is a relatively safe technique"
Various surveys of adverse events in acupuncture (Birch 2004)	"No serious adverse events were found in four recent surveys in Japan, Sweden and the United Kingdom of 140,229 treatments (Yamashita, Tsukayama, Tanno, & Nishijo 1999; MacPherson, Thomas, Walters, & Fitter 2001; Oldsberg, Schill, & Haker 2001; White, Hayhoe, Hart, & Ernst 2001). Ernst and White reviewed these and five other surveys and found two cases of pneumothorax in nearly a quarter of a million treatments. From their review, they concluded: 'Serious adverse events are rare. Those responsible for establishing competence in acupuncture should consider how to reduce these risks' (Ernst & White 2001)"

B Conclusions of international studies and reviews of acupuncture safety.

Challenges Facing Acupuncture Research

Mechanism Studies

To date, mechanism studies have focused on uncovering the mechanisms of action of acupuncture with respect to observed effects of treatment rather than trying to understand the theoretical models behind those treatments. For example, acupuncture has been used as treatment for pain conditions, leading to the pursuit of analgesic mechanisms of action, such as endorphin, enkephalin, dynorphin, and serotonin changes (Stux & Hammerschlag 2000). Unfortunately, because these studies did not start with the theoretical assumptions of acupuncture (that treatment regulates the circulation of *qi*), but only tested hypotheses about the pathways of analgesia produced by acupuncture, they did not test hypotheses based on acupuncture theory (Birch & Lewith 2007). Nor did they attempt to understand what the traditional concepts and models of acupuncture refer to or how they might relate to known physiological mechanisms. Neurophysiological research has neither tested acupuncture as it is actually practiced, nor is it clear how the results help explain acupuncture practice.

Brain-imaging studies of acupuncture are gaining currency in acupuncture research (Cho, Na, Wang, Lee, & Hong 2000; Hui 2000, 2005; Napadow 2007), but it is not clear that they are able to investigate the traditional theoretical explanatory models behind the acupuncture treatments either (Scheid 2002; Kim 2006). Ultimately, such studies may be useful only to validate acupuncture as a therapy capable of doing something (as visualized via changes in the brain). Like the neurophysiological analgesia studies, brain imaging studies will most likely lead to replacement explanations of how acupuncture works *without actually having tested the explanations on which the treatment is based* (Kim 2006; Birch & Lewith 2007). This issue remains a considerable challenge for the acupuncture researcher if the research is to be meaningful to traditionally based practitioners.

Clinical Trials

Many clinical trials have focused on testing the effects of traditionally based acupuncture treatment on a known biomedical condition, such as asthma. When the traditionally based model of treatment offers a different basis for describing the nature of the symptom, and the descriptions do not make a clear correlation to a single biomedical condition (Kaptchuk 1983), this creates a problem not only for how to select an appropriate treatment for each patient, but also what the appropriate measures of change in the patients should be. One solution that has been offered is to recruit patients with condition X and then subdivide them into traditionally based diagnostic categories and administer treatment according to those categories (Lao, Ezzo, Berman, & Hammerschlag 2000). However, without evidence that these diagnoses are agreed upon by the community of practitioners (inter-rater agreement), then it becomes difficult to determine what the "correct" treatment should be. Few studies have used traditionally based diagnoses, and even fewer have investigated the reliability of the diagnoses (O'Brien & Birch in press; O'Brien et al. in submission).

Explanatory Models

Within TCM itself, and even more so in the broader field of Traditional East Asian Medicine (TEAM) there are multiple traditional explanations and models, both within a single country and its "tradition" (Birch & Sherman 1999; Scheid 2002) and between countries and traditions (MacPherson & Kaptchuk 1997; Birch & Felt 1999; Schnyer et al. 2007). This presents challenges for the researcher and may lead to difficulties with the selection of an appropriate treatment and sham treatment (Birch 1997a; Schnyer et al. 2007). Studies of a traditionally based system of practice need to document and work from a relatively clear model of that practice and not attempt to generalize from that system to the entire field (Birch 1997b; Schnyer et al. 2007). Studies of acupuncture often do not document the treatments they used, simply citing the texts upon which the treatments were based (Birch 1997b). Other studies state that they are "traditional" or "classical" acupuncture studies yet do not appear to be based at all on traditional theories (Birch 2002; Medici, Grebski, Wu, Hinz, & Wuthrich 2002).

Complex Intervention

Recent studies have demonstrated that acupuncture is a "complex interven-

tion" (Paterson & Dieppe 2005), which has different research needs than simple interventions (Medical Research Council 2000). Thus, it is critical that appropriate research methods be developed and approved if acupuncture is to be investigated in clinical trials.

Areas for Future Research

1. More exploratory studies are needed before large-scale studies are initiated (Aickin 2007). Many studies are undertaken with no or very few exploratory or pilot studies to establish the groundwork. Exploratory studies are small, do not have to be published as definitive studies, and can be undertaken for little cost by practitioners, schools, and practitioner organizations. They should be coordinated within a global agenda if they are to achieve the most useful outcomes (Birch 2003; Sherman & Cherkin 2003).

2. More survey and questionnaire qualitative studies are needed to investigate the nature of practice and what happens during treatment. Without data from these studies it is difficult to define precisely what to test in controlled clinical trials or laboratory studies. A few good published examples can be found (Cassidy 2000) and a large well-executed study from Germany will be published soon (Voigt 2008), but there is a general paucity of these studies.

3. More studies examining the nature and role of diagnosis in TCM acu-

puncture need to be conducted. Several studies using highly simplified diagnostic approaches have examined inter-rater agreement in TCM diagnosis (Zell, Hirata, Marcus, Ettinger, Pressman, & Ettinger 2000; Hogeboom, Sherman, & Cherkin 2001), but these do not reflect actual clinical practice (O'Brien & Birch in press; O'Brien et al. in press). A recent high-quality Australian study describes the reasons and methods for doing such studies and has some of the more significant inter-rater agreements on the basis of a more normal diagnostic assessment (O'Brien et al. in submission). More trials need to be performed using thoroughly applied traditionally based diagnostic categories such as those found in TCM or Japanese Meridian Therapy (Schnyer et al. 2007). Various models exist for doing this; among the most interesting is the use of the "manualized" diagnosis and treatment approach (Schnyer & Allen 2002; Schnyer et al. 2007).

Finding and Reading Publications on Acupuncture Research

Searching the Internet is becoming increasingly easier when one wants to track down information and data on a subject. A quick search on Google for "acupuncture research" on January 16, 2009 yielded 705 000 hits. Not only can it be very time-consuming sorting through these, but the quality of much that will come up is very poor or at least of questionable value. Thus, one needs to search in established databases if one wants a better quality yield. There are a number of electronic databases that are good sources for research publications. Many of these are peer-reviewed, meaning that the standards by which they are published should be better. Among the electronic databases one can search for studies of acupuncture are MEDLINE, EMBASE, AMED, and Cochrane controlled trials registry (Linde et al. 2007).

Probably the easiest place to start searching is through books that have focused on the topic of research on acupuncture. Here a number of high-quality publications can be found. One can then start tracking down more reliable information on the basis of the processes that the authors used to screen and include studies and databases for discussion.

A number of books and reviews have been published that summarize the literature. Some of these focus only on laboratory studies (Pomeranz 1998), some are more focused on clinical studies (BMA 2000; Birch et al. 2004), some include summaries of both areas (Ernst 1996; Acupuncture 1998; Filshie & White 1998; Stux & Hammerschlag 2000; MacPherson, Hammerschlag, Lewith, & Schnyer 2007). Reading these texts can give one a quick summary and overview of previous research and conclusions that can be drawn from it. However, sometimes the same data is analyzed differently, reflecting the different perspectives of the researchers performing each review (Ernst & White 1998; van Tulder, Cherkin, Berman,

Lao, & Koes 1999—see Linde et al. 2007).

In general if one wants to get a good overview of the research in acupuncture, start with reading the published books on that area and track the articles referenced in those books. But before reading any of the literature, if you have little or no experience of reading and *critically assessing* what you are reading, it is good to read up on how to do this too. There are a few publications that can give you some insights into this (Kane 2004; MacPherson et al. 2007).

If you are interested in clinical trials of acupuncture, many review papers have been published. It is a complex area that requires patient study if it is to be understood. In general, designing and conducting clinical trials can be a complex and expensive procedure (Meinert 1986). In a treatment like acupuncture there are additional issues that need to be thoroughly thought through and many problems that need to be addressed if the results of the trial are to be meaningful (Vincent & Lewith 1995; Lewith & Vincent 1996; Hammerschlag & Morris 1997; Hammerschlag 1998; Margolin, Avants, & Kleber 1998a, 1998b; White et al. 2001; Lewith, Jonas, & Walach 2002; Lewith, Walach, & Jonas 2002; Sherman & Cherkin 2003; Birch 2004; MacPherson, Hammerschlag, Lewith & Schnyer 2007). This is even more complicated when the study attempts to test a traditional form of treatment such as TCM acupuncture (Birch 1997b, 2004; MacPherson, Sherman, Hammerschlag, Birch, Lao, & Zaslawski 2002; Schnyer & Allen 2002). Even figuring out what constitutes an appropriate or adequate treatment in acupuncture trials has proven to be difficult (Birch 1997a; Stux & Birch 2000; White et al. 2001). In general, insufficient attention has been given to these issues. Recently the STRICTA (Standards for Reporting Interventions in Clinical Trials of Acupuncture) guidelines have been developed on how to report treatment in published trials of acupuncture; these guidelines thus inform what issues need to be attended to in clinical trials (MacPherson, White, Cummings, Jobst, Rose, & Niemtzow 2002). These are currently being updated so as to be incorporated with CONSORT (Consolidated Standards of Reporting Trials), the biomedical guidelines for reporting clinical trials.

For those interested in becoming involved in acupuncture research, an excellent discussion of how practitioners can become engaged has been written by Wayne, Sherman and Bovey (2007). The text by Hugh MacPherson, Richard Hammerschlag, George Lewith, and Rosa Schnyer is probably the most useful book concerning the status of and how to improve the condition of research in acupuncture (MacPherson et al. 2007).

References

History

DeBary W, Chan W, Watson B. *Sources of Chinese Tradition.* Vol 1. New York: Columbia University Press; 1960.

Ergil M. Chinese medicine in China: Education and learning strategies. Paper presented at Association for Asian Studies Annual Meeting: Boston, MA; 1994.

Ergil M, Ergil K. The translation of Chinese medical texts into English: Issues surrounding transparency, transmission, and clinical understanding. In: McCarthy M, Birch S, eds. *Thieme Almanac: Acupuncture and Chinese Medicine.* Stuttgart: Thieme; 2008:309–20.

Farquhar J. Problems of knowledge in contemporary Chinese medical discourse. *Soc Sci Med 24.* 1987;12:1013–21.

Hucker C. *China's Imperial Past: An Introduction to Chinese History and Culture.* Stanford, CA: Stanford University Press; 1975.

Needham J. *Clerks & Craftsmen in China & the West.* Cambridge: Cambridge University Press; 1970.

Reston J. Now, let me tell you about my appendectomy in Peking. *New York Times.* July 26, 1971. Available at: http://www.acupuncture.com/testimonials/restonexp.htm. Accessed 29 April, 2008.

Taylor K. *Chinese Medicine in Early Communist China: A Medicine of Revolution.* London: Routledge Curzon; 2005.

Unschuld P. *Medical Ethics in Imperial China: A Study in Historical Anthropology.* Berkeley, CA: University of California Press; 1979.

Unschuld P. *Medicine in China: A History of Ideas.* Berkeley, CA: University of California Press; 1985.

Unschuld P. *Nan-Ching: The Classic of Difficult Issues.* Berkeley, CA: University of California Press; 1986.

Unschuld P. *Huang Di Nei Jing Su Wen: Nature, Knowledge, Imagery in an Ancient Chinese Medical Text.* Berkeley, CA: University of California Press; 2003.

Wilhelm R, Byrnes C (translators). *The I Ching or Book of Changes.* Princeton, New Jersey: Princeton University Press; 1967.

Wiseman N, Ellis A. *Fundamentals of Chinese Medicine.* Brookline MA: Paradigm Publications; 1996.

Wiseman N, Ye F. *A Practical Dictionary of Chinese Medicine.* Brookline MA: Paradigm Publications; 1998.

Wiseman N. *Glossary of Chinese Medical Terms.* Brookline MA: Paradigm Publications; 1989.

Wiseman N. Approaches to Chinese medical term translation. Paper presented at American Association for Acupuncture & Oriental Medicine Annual Conference: Portland, OR; 2007.

Wong K., Wu T. *History of Chinese Medicine.* 2nd ed. Taipei, Taiwan: Southern Materials Center, Inc; 1985.

Fundamental Theory of Chinese Medicine

Ergil K. Chinese medicine. In: Micozzi M., ed. *Fundamentals of Complementary and Integrative Medicine.* St. Louis: Saunders Elsevier; 2006.

Larre C. *The Way of Heaven: Neijing Suwen Chapters 1 and 2.* Cambridge: Monkey Press; 1994.

Unschuld P. *Introductory Readings in Classical Chinese Medicine.* Boston: Kluwer Academic Publishers; 1988.

Unschuld P. *Medicine in China: A History of Ideas.* Berkeley, CA: University of California Press; 1985.

Veith I (translator). *The Yellow Emperor's Classic of Internal Medicine.* Berkeley: University of California Press; 1972.

Wiseman N, Ellis A. *Fundamentals of Chinese Medicine.* Brookline MA: Paradigm Publications; 1996.

Wiseman N, Ye F. *A Practical Dictionary of Chinese Medicine.* Brookline MA: Paradigm Publications; 1998.

Diagnosis in Chinese Medicine

Deng T. *Practical Diagnosis in Traditional Chinese Medicine.* Edited by Ergil K.

Translated by Ergil M. and Yi S. New York: Churchill Livingstone; 1999.

Huang B, Di F, Li X, et al. *Syndromes of Traditional Chinese Medicine.* Edited by Huang B. Translated by Ma D, Wang G, Sun S, Cao H. Heilongjiang: Heilongjiang Education Press; 1987.

Kaptchuk TJ. *The Web That Has No Weaver: Understanding Chinese Medicine.* Chicago: Contemporary (McGraw Hill); 2000.

Wiseman N, Ellis A. *Fundamentals of Chinese Medicine.* Brookline, MA: Paradigm Publications; 1996.

Acupuncture

Ellis A, Wiseman N, Boss K. *Fundamentals of Chinese Acupuncture.* Brooklyn, MA: Paradigm Publications; 1991.

Huang LC. *Auriculotherapy: Diagnosis & Treatment.* Texas: Longevity Press; 1996.

Low R. *The Secondary Vessels of Acupuncture.* New York: Thorsons Publishers Inc; 1983.

Ni YT. *Navigating the Channels of Traditional Chinese Medicine.* San Diego: Oriental Medicine Center; 1996.

Nogier PFM. *Handbook to Auriculotherapy.* France: Maisonneuve; 1981.

Nogier PFM. *From Auriculotherapy to Auriculomedicine.* France: Maisonneuve; 1983.

O'Connor J, Bensky D (translators). *Acupuncture: A Comprehensive Text.* Seattle, Shanghai College of Traditional Chinese Medicine: Eastland Press; 1981.

Unschuld P. *Medicine in China: A History of Ideas.* Berkeley, CA: University of California Press; 1985.

Wiseman N, Ye F. *A Practical Dictionary of Chinese Medicine.* Brookline, MA: Paradigm Publications; 1998.

Tui Na

Sun C, ed. *Chinese Massage Therapy.* Shangdong: Shandong Science and Technology Press; 1990.

Wang GC, Fan YL, Zheng G. 中国推拿/*Chinese Massage*, Vol 10 of *A Practical English-Chinese Library of Traditional Chinese Medicine.* Zhang Enqin, ed. Shanghai:

Publishing House of Shanghai College of Traditional Chinese Medicine; 1990.

Traditional Chinese Pharmacotherapy

Bensky D, Barolet R. *Chinese Herbal Medicine: Formulas and Strategies.* Seattle, WA: Eastland Press; 1990.

Chan K, Cheung L. *Interactions Between Chinese Herbal Medicinal Products and Orthodox Drugs.* London: Tayolr and Francis; 2003.

Merriam Webster's Collegiate Dictionary, 10th edition. Springfield, MA: Merriam Webster, Inc. 1997.

Unschuld P. *Medicine in China: A History of Pharmaceutics.* Berkeley, CA: University of California Press; 1986.

Yang SZo (translator). *The Divine Farmer's Materia Medica.* Boulder, CO: Blue Poppy Press; 1998.

Yeoh TS, Lee HS, Lee AS. Gastrointestinal absorption of mercury following oral administration of cinnabar in a traditional Chinese medicine. *Asia Pacific Journal of Pharmacology.* 1989;4(2):69–73.

Zhou YP. *Chinese Materia Medica: Chemistry, Pharmacology and Applications.* Amsterdam: Harwood Academic Publishers; 1998.

Chinese Dietetics

Garvey M. *Chinese Medicine Foundations 2: Course Notes.* Sydney: University of Technology; 2008.

Wiseman N, Ellis A. *Fundamentals of Chinese Medicine.* Brookline, MA: Paradigm Publications; 1996.

Qi Gong

Bölts J. *Lernziel: Gesundheitskompetenz; Der Beitrag des Qigong zur zukunftsfähigen Gesundheitsbildung in der Schule.* Oldenburg: BIS-Verlag; 2003. Extract can be downloaded from http://www.uni-oldenburg.de/ptch/.

Jahnke R. "History of Qi (Chi) Cultivation." 2007. Available at http://www.feeltheqi.com. Accessed: March 09, 2009.

Jahnke R. "Qi Gong (Chi Kung)." 2007. Available at http://www.feeltheqi.com. Accessed: March 09, 2009.

Javary C, Faure P (translators). *Yi Jing (The Book of Changes)*. Paris: Albin Michel; 2002.

Réquéna Y. *Le Guide du Bien-être Selon la Médecine Chinoise*, Paris: Guy Trédaniel; 2000.

Réquéna Y. Interview "Le qi gong—de corps et d'esprit." 2004. Available at: http://www.passeportsante.net/fr/Actualites/Entrevues/Fiche.aspx?doc=requena_y_20040105. Accessed: March 09, 2009.

Rose K, Zhang Y. *A Brief History of Qi*. Brookline: Paradigm Publications; 2001.

Vocca ML. Origini storiche del *qigong*. 2006. Available at: http://web.tiscali.it/qigong/italiano/origini%20storiche.htm. Accessed: March 09, 2009.

Yang JM. *Les Racines du Chi-Kung*. Noisy sur Ecole: Budo; 2003.

Tai Qi Juan

Davis B. *The Taijiquan Classics: An Annotated Translation*. Berkeley, CA: North Atlantic Books; 2004.

Gu L, Tang H. *Taijiquan Shu* (The Art of *Tai Ji Quan*). Shanghai: Jiaoyu chubanshe; 1982.

Klein P, Adams W. Comprehensive benefits of *taiji*: a critical review. *American Journal of Physical Medicine and Rehabilitation, 83*. 2004;9:735–45.

Qi H. *Taijiquan Yangsheng* (*Taijiquan* for Health). Beijing: Renmin tiyu chubanshe; 2005.

Tang H. *Neijiaquan de Yanjiu* (A Study of the Internal School of Martial Arts). Hong Kong: Unicorn Press (reprint); 1935.

Wile D. *Lost T'ai-chi Classics from the Late Ch'ing Dynasty*. Albany, NY: State University of New York Press; 1996.

Wile D. *T'ai-chi's Ancestors: The Making of an Internal Martial Art*. New City, NY: Sweet Ch'i Press; 2000.

Wile D. Taijiquan and Daoism: From Religion to Martial Art and Martial Art to Religion. *Journal of Asian Martial Arts, 16.* 2007;4:8–45.

Zheng M (translated by Wile). *Master Cheng's Thirteen Chapters on T'ai-chi Ch'üan*. Brooklyn, NY: Sweet Ch'i Press (original 1950); 1982.

Acupuncture Research: An Overview

Acupuncture. Acupuncture: NIH consensus development panel on acupuncture. *JAMA*. 1998;280(17):1518–24.

Aickin M. The importance of early phase research. *J Alt Complem Med*. 2007;13 (4):447–50.

Bensoussan A. *The Vital Meridian*. Edinburgh: Churchill Livingstone, 1991.

Birch S. Issues to consider in determining an adequate treatment in a clinical trial of acupuncture. *Complem Ther in Med*. 1997a;5:8–12.

Birch S. Testing the claims of traditionally based acupuncture. *Complem Ther Med*. 1997b;5:147–51.

Birch S. Letter to the editor: acupuncture and bronchial asthma, a long-term randomized study. *J Alt Complem Med*. 2002; 8(6):751–54.

Birch S. Developing a research strategy for the acupuncture profession: research questions, resources necessary to answer them and guidelines for matching resources to types of research. *Clin Acup Orient Med*. 2003;4(1):29–33.

Birch S. Clinical research of acupuncture. Part two—controlled clinical trials: an overview of their methods. *J Alt Complem Med*. 2004;10(3):481–98.

Birch S. A review and analysis of placebo treatments, placebo effects and placebo controls in trials of medical procedures when sham is not inert. *J Alt Complem Med*. 2006;12(3):303–10.

Birch S, Felt R. *Understanding Acupuncture*. Edinburgh: Churchill Livingstone; 1999.

Birch S, Keppel Hesselink J, Jonkman FAM, Hekker TAM, Bos A. Clinical research on acupuncture 1: what have reviews of the efficacy and safety of acupuncture told us so far? *J Alt Complem Med*. 2004; 10(3):468–80.

Birch S, Lewith G. Acupuncture research, the story so far. In: MacPherson H, Hammerschlag R, Lewith G, Schnyer R, eds. *Acupuncture Research: Strategies for Building an Evidence Base.* London: Elsevier; 2007:15–35.

Birch S, Sherman K. *Zhong Yi* acupuncture and low back pain: traditional Chinese medical acupuncture differential diagnoses and treatments for chronic lumbar pain. *J Alt Complem Med.* 1999;5(5):415–25.

BMA (British Medical Association). *Acupuncture: Efficacy, Safety and Practice.* London: Harwood Academic Publishers; 2000.

Broom A. Using qualitative interviews in CAM research: A guide to study design, data collection and data analysis. *Complem Ther in Med.* 2005;13(1):65–73.

Cassidy CM. Beyond numbers: qualitative research methods for Oriental medicine. In: Stux G, Hammerschlag R, eds. *Scientific Bases of Acupuncture in Basic and Clinical Research.* Berlin: Springer; 2000: 151–69.

Cassidy CM. *Methodological Issues in Investigations of Massage/Bodywork Therapy.* Evanston: American Massage Therapy Association Foundation; 2002.

Cho ZH, Chung SC, Jones JP, Park JB, Park HJ, Lee HJ, Wong EK, Min BI. New findings of the correlation between acupoints and corresponding brain cortices using functional MRI. *Proc Nat Acad Sci USA.* 1998;95:2670–73.

Cho ZH, Na CS, Wang EK, Lee SH, Hong IK. Functional magnetic resonance imaging of the brain in investigations of acupuncture. In: Stux G, Hammerschlag R, eds. *Scientific Bases of Acupuncture in Basic and Clinical Research.* Berlin: Springer; 2000:83–95.

Ernst E, ed. *Complementary Medicine: An Objective Appraisal.* Oxford: Butterworth Heinemann; 1996.

Ernst E, White AR. Acupuncture for back pain: a meta-analysis of randomized controlled trials. *Arch Int Med.* 1998;158: 2235–41.

Ernst E, White AR. Prospective studies of the safety of acupuncture: a systematic review. *Am J Med.* 2001;110(6):481–85.

Ezzo J, Lao LX, Berman B. Assessing clinical efficacy of acupuncture: what has been learned from systematic reviews of acupuncture? In: Stux G, Hammerschlag R, eds. *Clinical Acupuncture: Scientific Basis.* Berlin: Springer; 2000:113–30.

Filshie J, White A (eds.) *Medical Acupuncture.* Edinburgh: Churchill Livingstone; 1998.

Filshie J, White A. The clinical use of, and evidence for, acupuncture in the medical systems. In: Filshie J, White A, eds. *Medical Acupuncture.* Edinburgh: Churchill Livingstone; 1998:225–94.

Hammerschlag R. Methodological and ethical issues in clinical trials of acupuncture. *J Alt Complem Med.* 1998;4(2):159–71.

Hammerschlag R, Langevin HE, Lao LX, Lewith G. Physiological dynamics of acupuncture: correlations and mechanisms. In: MacPherson H, Hammerschlag R, Lewith G, Schnyer R, eds. *Acupuncture Research: Strategies for Building an Evidence Base.* London: Elsevier; 2007:181–97.

Hammerschlag R, Morris MM. Clinical trials comparing acupuncture with biomedical standard care: a criteria-based evaluation of research design and reporting. *Complem Ther Med.* 1997;5:133–40.

Han JS. Central neurotransmitters and acupuncture analgesia. In: Pomeranz B, Stux G, eds. *Scientific Bases of Acupuncture,* Berlin: Springer; 1989:7–33.

Hogeboom CJ, Sherman KJ, Cherkin DC. Variation in diagnosis and treatment of patients with chronic low back pain by traditional Chinese medical acupuncturists. *Complem Ther Med.* 2001;9:154–66.

Hui KK, Liu J, Makris N, Gollub RL, Chen AJ, Moore CI, Kennedy DN, Rosen BR,

Kwong KK. Acupuncture modulates the limbic system and subcortical gray structures of the human brain: evidence from fMRI studies in normal subjects. *Hum Brain Mapp.* 2000;9(1):13–25.

Hui KK, Liu J, Marina O, Napadow V, Haselgrove C, Kwong KK, Kennedy DN, Makris N. The integrated response of the human cerebro-cerebellar and limbic systems to acupuncture stimulation at ST 36 as evidenced by fMRI. *Neuroimage.* 2005 Sep;27(3):479–96.

Hyland ME. Methodology for the scientific evaluation of complementary and alternative medicine. *Complem Ther Med.* 2003;11:146–53.

Kane M. *Research Made Easy in Complementary and Alternative Medicine.* Edinburgh: Churchill Livingstone; 2004.

Kaptchuk TJ. *The Web That Has No Weaver.* New York: Congdon and Weed; 1983.

Kim JY. Beyond paradigm: Making transcultural connections in a scientific translation of acupuncture. *Soc Sci Med.* 2006;62(12):2960–72.

Lao L, Ezzo J, Berman BM, Hammerschlag R. Assessing clinical efficacy of acupuncture: considerations for designing future acupuncture trials. In: Stux G, Hammerschlag R, eds. *Scientific Bases of Acupuncture in Basic and Clinical Research.* Berlin: Springer; 2000:187–209.

Lewith G, Jonas WB, Walach H. *Clinical Research in Complementary Therapies.* Edinburgh: Churchill Livingstone; 2002.

Lewith G, Vincent C. On the evaluation of the clinical effects of acupuncture: a problem reassessed and a framework for future research. *J Alt Complem Med.* 1996;2(1):79–90.

Lewith G, Walach H, Jonas WB. Balanced research strategies for complementary and alternative medicine. In Lewith G, Jonas WB, Walach H, eds. *Clinical Research in Complementary Therapies.* Edinburgh: Churchill Livingstone; 2002:3–27.

Linde K, Hammerschlag R, Lao LX. Evidence overviews: the role of systematic reviews and meta-analyses. In: MacPherson H., Hammerschlag R., Lewith G., Schnyer R, eds. *Acupuncture Research: Strategies for Building an Evidence Base.* London: Elsevier; 2007:199–217.

Linde K, Vickers A, Hondras M, et al. Systematic reviews of complementary therapies—an annotated bibliography. Part 1: Acupuncture. *BMC Complem Alt Med.* 2001;1:3.

MacPherson H, Hammerschlag R, Lewith G, Schnyer R. *Acupuncture Research: Strategies for Building an Evidence Base.* London: Elsevier; 2007.

MacPherson H, Kaptchuk TJ. *Acupuncture in Practice.* New York: Churchill Livingstone; 1997.

MacPherson H, Sherman K, Hammerschlag R, Birch S, Lao L, Zaslawski C. The clinical evaluation of East Asian systems of medicine. *Clin Acup Orient Med.* 2002;3(1):16–19.

MacPherson H, Thomas K, Walters S, Fitter M. The York acupuncture safety study: a prospective survey of 34,000 treatments by traditional acupuncturists. *BMJ.* 2001; 323:486–87.

MacPherson H, White A, Cummings M, Jobst K, Rose K, Niemtzow R. Standards for reporting interventions in controlled trials of acupuncture: the STRICTA recommendations. *J Alt Complem Med* 2002;8(1):85–89.

Margolin A, Avants SK, Kleber HD. Rationale and design of the cocaine alternative treatments study (CATS): a randomized, controlled trial of acupuncture. *J Alt Complem Med.* 1998a;4(4):405–18.

Margolin A, Avants SK, Kleber HD. Investigating alternative medicine therapies in randomized controlled trials. *JAMA.* 1998b;280(18):1626–28.

McDowell I, Newell C. *Measuring Health: A Guide to Rating Scales and Questionnaires.* Oxford: Oxford University Press; 1987.

Medical Research Council. A framework for development and evaluation of RCTs for complex interventions to improve health; 2000. Available at: http://www.mrc.ac.uk/Utilities/Documentrecord/index.htm

?d=MRC003372. Accessed November 4, 2008.

Medici TC, Grebski E, Wu J, Hinz G, Wuthrich B. Acupuncture and bronchial asthma: a long-term randomized study of the effects of real versus sham acupuncture compared to controls in patients with bronchial asthma. *J Alt Complem Med.* 2002;8(6):737–50.

Meinert CL. *Clinical Trials: Design, Conduct and Analysis.* Oxford: Oxford University Press; 1986.

Melzack R. Short-form McGill pain questionnaire. *Pain.* 1987;30:191–97.

Napadow V, Kettner N, Liu J, Li M, Kwong KK, Vangel M, Makris N, Audette J, Hui KK. Hypothalamus and amygdala response to acupuncture stimuli in Carpal Tunnel Syndrome. *Pain.* 2007 Aug;130(3):254–66. Epub 2007 Jan 19.

O'Brien KA, Abbas E, Zhang J, Wang WC, Komesaroff P. Examining the reliability of a Chinese examination. In submission.

O'Brien KA, Birch S. A review of the reliability of traditional East Asian medicine diagnoses. In press. *Alt Complem Med.*

Oldsberg A, Schill U, Haker E. Acupuncture treatment: side effects and complications reported by Swedish physiotherapists. *Complem Ther Med.* 2001;9:17–20.

Paterson C, Dieppe P. Characteristic and incidental (placebo) effects in complex interventions such as acupuncture. *BMJ.* 2005;330:1202–05.

Pomeranz B. Scientific research into acupuncture for the relief of pain. *J Alt Complem Med.* 1996;2(1):53–60.

Pomeranz B. Scientific basis of acupuncture. In: Stux G, Pomeranz B. *Basics of Acupuncture.* 4th ed. Berlin: Springer; 1998: 6–72.

Richardson J. Design and conduct a survey. *Complem Ther in Med.* 2005;13(1):47–53.

Scheid V. *Chinese Medicine in Contemporary China. Plurality and Synthesis.* Durham, CA and London: Duke University Press; 2002.

Schnyer RN, Allen JJB. Bridging the gap in complementary and alternative medicine research: manualization as a means of promoting standardization and flexibility of treatment in clinical trials of acupuncture. *J Alt Complem Med.* 2002;8(5):623–34.

Schnyer R, Birch S, MacPherson H. Acupuncture practice as the foundation for clinical evaluation. In: MacPherson H, Hammerschlag R, Lewith G, Schnyer R, eds. *Acupuncture Research: Strategies for Building an Evidence Base.* London: Elsevier; 2007:153–79.

Sherman KJ, Cherkin DC. Challenges of acupuncture research: study design considerations. *Clin Acup Orient Med.* 2003; 3(4):200–06.

Sherman K, Linde K, White A. Comparing treatment effects of acupuncture and other types of healthcare. In: MacPherson H, Hammerschlag R, Lewith G, Schnyer R, eds. *Acupuncture Research: Strategies for Building an Evidence Base.* London: Elsevier; 2007:111–31.

Stux G, Birch S. Proposed standards of acupuncture treatments for clinical studies. In: Stux G, Hammerschlag R, eds. *Scientific Bases of Acupuncture in Basic and Clinical Research.* Berlin: Springer; 2000:171–85.

Stux G, Hammerschlag R, eds. *Scientific Bases of Acupuncture in Basic and Clinical Research.* Berlin: Springer; 2000.

Tait PL, Brooks L, Harstall C. *Acupuncture: Evidence from Systematic Reviews and Meta-analyses.* Alberta, Canada: Alberta Heritage Foundation for Medical Research; 2002.

Tang JL, Zhan SY, Ernst E. Review of randomised controlled trials of traditional Chinese medicine. *BMJ.* 1999;319(7203): 160–61.

Thomas KJ, Fitter MJ. Evaluating complementary therapies for use in the National Health Service: "Horses for courses." Part 2: alternative research strategies. *Complem Ther in Med.* 1997;5:94–98.

Thomas K, Fitter M. Possible research strategies for evaluating CAM therapies. In: Lewith G, Jonas WB, Walach H. *Clinical*

Research in Complementary Therapies. Edinburgh: Churchill Livingstone; 2002: 59–91.

van Tulder MW, Cherkin DC, Berman B, Lao L, Koes BW. The effectiveness of acupuncture in the management of acute and chronic low back pain. A systematic review within the framework of the Cochrane Collaboration Back Review Group. *Spine.* 1999;24(11):1113–23.

Vickers. Acupuncture. NHS Centre for Reviews and Dissemination. *Effective Health Care.* 2001;7(2):1–12.

Vickers A, Wilson P, Kleijnen J. Effectiveness bulletin: acupuncture. *Qual Saf Health Care.* 2002;11:92–97.

Vincent C, Lewith G. Placebo controls for acupuncture studies. *J Royal Soc Med.* 1995;88:199–202.

Voigt J. Qualitative acupuncture research in Germany. In: McCarthy M, Birch S, eds. *Thieme Almanac: Acupuncture and Chinese Medicine.* Stuttgart: Thieme; 2008: 30–35.

Ware JE, Sherbourne CD. The MOS 36-item short-form health survey (SF-36); 1. Conceptual framework and item selection. *Medical Care.* 1992;30(6):473–83.

Wayne P, Sherman K, Bovey M. Engaging acupuncturists in research—some practical guidelines. In: MacPherson H, Hammerschlag R, Lewith G, Schnyer R, eds. *Acupuncture Research: Strategies for Building an Evidence Base.* London: Elsevier; 2007:219–37.

White AR, Filshie J, Cummings TM. Clinical trials of acupuncture: consensus recommendations for optimal treatment, sham controls and blinding. *Complem Res Ther.* 2001;9:237–45.

White A, Hayhoe S, Hart A, Ernst E. Adverse events following acupuncture: prospective survey of 32,000 consultations with doctors and physical therapists. *BMJ.* 2001;323:485–6.

White A, Schmidt K. Systematic literature reviews. *Complem Ther in Med.* 2005;13 (1):54–60.

Yamashita H, Tsukayama H, Tanno Y, Nishijo K. Adverse events in acupuncture and moxibustion treatment: a six-year survey at a national clinic in Japan. *J Alt Complem Med.* 1999;5:229–36.

Zell B, Hirata J, Marcus A, Ettinger B, Pressman A, Ettinger KM. Diagnosis of symptomatic postmenopausal women by traditional Chinese medicine practitioners. *Menopause.* 2000;2:129–33.

Further Reading

History

Contemporary Traditional Chinese Medicine emerges as the cultural and intellectual product of over 2000 years of recorded Chinese history. While the definitive history of the development of Chinese medicine has yet to be written, and may never be, the texts below offer the reader authoritative and reliable points of entry to the historical development of Chinese medicine as well as its contemporary expression as a product of cultural and historical processes. The editors strongly recommend, as a starting point, Paul Unschuld's *Medicine in China: A History of Ideas* (1985) and *Medicine in China: A History of Pharmaceutics* (1986).

Furth C. *A Flourishing Yin: Gender in China's Medical History, 960–1665.* Berkeley, CA: University of California Press; 1999.

Lu GJ, Needham J. *Celestial Lancets: A History and Rationale of Acupuncture and Moxa.* London/New York: RoutledgeCurzon; 2002.

Scheid V. *Currents of Tradition in Chinese Medicine 1626–2006.* Seattle: Eastland Press; 2007.

Taylor K. *Chinese Medicine in Communist China, 1945–63: A Medicine of Revolution.* London/New York: RoutledgeCurzon; 2005.

Unschuld P. *Medicine in China: A History of Ideas.* Berkeley, CA: University of California Press; 1985.

Unschuld P. *Medicine in China: A History of Pharmaceutics.* Berkeley, CA: University of California Press; 1986.

Veith I (translator). *The Yellow Emperor's Classic of Internal Medicine.* Berkeley, CA: University of California Press; 1972.

Wong K, Wu T. *History of Chinese Medicine.* 2nd ed. Taipei, Taiwan: Southern Materials Center, Inc; 1985.

Fundamental Theory of Chinese Medicine

Fidelity to core concepts and principles developed over millennia remains fundamental to understanding the theory and practice of Traditional Chinese Medicine. Among the many textbooks available in the West that address the foundational concepts of Chinese medicine, very few retain a close linkage to traditional concepts. Ted Kaptchuk's recently revised *The Web That Has No Weaver* (2000) remains an important first step in learning about Chinese medicine. Manfred Porkert deserves tremendous credit for recognizing the criticality of linguistic rigor to understanding Chinese medicine concepts and his book, *The Theoretical Foundations of Chinese Medicine: Systems of Correspondence* (1982), remains a pioneering effort. Wiseman and Ellis's more accessible approach to linguistic fidelity and systematic term choice in *Fundamentals of Chinese Medicine* (1995) has however, emerged as the definitive standard for understanding Chinese medicine concepts.

Kaptchuk TJ. *The Web That Has No Weaver: Understanding Chinese Medicine.* Chicago: Contemporary (McGraw Hill); 2000.

Porkert M. *The Theoretical Foundations of Chinese Medicine: Systems of Correspondence.* Cambridge, MA/London: MIT Press; 1982.

Wiseman N, Ellis A. *Fundamentals of Chinese Medicine.* Revised ed. Brookline, MA: Paradigm Publications; 1996.

Diagnosis in Chinese Medicine

The concerns expressed above with regard to language and theory apply equivalently to Chinese medicine diagnostics. Tietao Deng's seminal *Practical Diagnosis in Chinese Medicine* (1999) offers a faithful portrait of Traditional Chinese Medicine diagnostics. The other works presented below are distinctive for the excellence of their organization, illustrations, and innovative approaches.

Deng, TT. *Practical Diagnosis in Traditional Chinese Medicine.* Ergil K (ed.). Ergil M, Yi SM (translators). New York: Churchill Livingstone; 1999.

Kirschbaum B. *Atlas of Chinese Tongue Diagnosis. Vols 1 and 2.* Seattle: Eastland Press; 2000.

Li Shi Zhen (translator Hoc Ku Huynh). *Pulse Diagnosis.* Brookline, MA: Paradigm Publications; 1981.

Lin ZH (translated by Li M). *Pocket Atlas of Pulse Diagnosis.* Stuttgart, New York: Thieme; 2008.

Porkert M. *The Essentials of Chinese Diagnostics.* Zurich: ACTA Medicinae Sinensis Chinese Medicine Publications Inc.; 1983.

Schnorrenberger CC, Schnorrenberger B. *Pocket Atlas of Tongue Diagnosis.* Thieme; 2005.

Wiseman N, Ellis A. *Fundamentals of Chinese Medicine.* Revised ed. Brookline, MA: Paradigm Publications; 1995.

Acupuncture

We have selected the following texts based on the choices we routinely make to train our students. These books represent what we consider to be the best currently available English language reference works to guide point location, point selection, and therapeutic application in Chinese acupuncture.

Deadman P, Al-Khafaji M. *A Manual of Acupuncture.* Hove, UK: Journal of Chinese Medicine Publications; 1998.

Ellis A, Wiseman N, Boss K. *Fundamentals of*

Chinese Acupuncture. Brooklyn, MA: Paradigm Publications; 1991.

Hempen C-H, Wortman Chow V. *Pocket Atlas of Acupuncture.* Stuttgart, New York: Thieme; 2006.

Low R. *The Secondary Vessels of Acupuncture.* New York: Thorsons Publishers Inc; 1983.

MacLean W, Lyttleton J. *Clinical Handbook of Internal Medicine Vols I and II.* Macarthur, Australia: University of Western Sydney Press; 1998.

Ni YT. *Navigating the Channels of Traditional Chinese Medicine.* San Diego: Oriental Medicine Center; 1996.

Nogier R. *Auriculotherapy.* Stuttgart/New York: Thieme; 2009.

Oleson T. *International Handbook of Ear Reflex Points.* Los Angeles: Health Care Alternatives; 1995.

Shanghai College of Traditional Medicine (John O'Connor and Dan Bensky translators). *Acupuncture: A Comprehensive Text.* Seattle: Eastland Press; 1981.

Wiseman N, Ellis A. *Fundamentals of Chinese Medicine.* Revised ed. Brookline, MA: Paradigm Publications; 1995.

Wu Y, Fischer W. *Practical Therapeutics of Traditional Chinese Medicine.* Brookline, MA: Paradigm Publications; 1997.

Tui Na

There are many titles about *tui na* (Chinese massage), representing different practice styles and individual clinical approaches. We have chosen a selection of books that we feel provide a useful and accessible introduction to *tui na*. Among these, Sun's *Chinese Massage Therapy* (1990) is considered to be an authoritative resource by many practitioners, and Tom Bisio's *A Tooth From the Tiger's Mouth* (2004) is a very accessible introduction to the application of *tui na* and bone-righting principles in patient care.

Bisio T. *A Tooth From the Tiger's Mouth: How to Treat your Injuries with Powerful Healing Secrets of the Great Chinese Warriors.* New York: Simon & Schuster; 2004.

Bisio T, Butler F. *Zheng Gu Tui Na.* New York: Zheng Gu Tui Na; 2007.

Cao XZ. *The Massotherapy of Traditional Chinese Medicine.* Hong Kong: Hai Feng Publishing Company; 1985.

Cline K. *Chinese Paediatric Massage.* Rochester, VT: Healing Arts Press; 2000.

Luan C. *Concise Tuina Therapy.* Shandong: Shandong Science and Technology Press; 1992.

Marcus A. *Musculoskeletal Disorders, Healing Methods from Chinese Medicine, Orthopaedic Medicine and Osteopathy.* Berkeley, CA: North Atlantic Books; 1998.

McCarthy M. Skin and touch as intermediates of body experience with reference to gender, culture and clinical experience. *J Bodywork Movement Ther 2.* 1998;3:175–83.

McCarthy M. Palpatory literacy and Chinese therapeutic bodywork (tui na) and the remediation of head, neck and shoulder pain. *J Bodywork Movement Ther 7.* 2003;4:262–77.

Sun CN, ed. *Chinese Massage Therapy.* Shangdong: Shandong Science and Technology Press; 1990.

Sun CN, ed. *Chinese Bodywork, A Complete Manual of Chinese Therapeutic Massage.* Berkeley, CA: Pacific View Press; 1993.

Xu MZ. *Manual Treatment for Traumatic Injuries.* Beijing: Foreign Languages Press; 1997.

Zhu JH (compiler), Ding XH (translator). *Chinese–English Illustrated Tuina Therapies for Common Diseases.* Shanghai: Shanghai Scientific and Technical Publishers; 2006.

Traditional Chinese Pharmacotherapy

We have selected the following texts based on the choices we routinely make to train our students. These books represent what we consider to be the best currently available English-language reference works to guide one's study of the materia medica, formulas, and the clinical application of Chinese herbs. These selections include standard references, terminologically correct textbooks such as Brand and Wiseman's *Concise Chinese Materia Medica* (2008), guides to clinical practice such as Yan Wu and Warren Fischer's *Practical Therapeutics of Traditional Chinese Medicine* (1997), and advanced texts based on the observations of senior practitioners such as the Jiao Shu De (2001–06) series.

Bensky D, Clavey S, Stöger E. *Chinese Herbal Medicine: Materia Medica*. Seattle, WA: Eastland Press; 2004.

Bisio T. *A Tooth From the Tiger's Mouth: How to Treat your Injuries with Powerful Healing Secrets of the Great Chinese Warriors*. New York: Simon & Schuster; 2004.

Brand E, Wiseman N. *Concise Chinese Materia Medica*. Brooklyn, MA: Paradigm Publications; 2008.

Chen J, Chen T. *Chinese Medical Herbology and Pharmacology*. City of Industry, CA: Art of Medicine Press; 2004.

Foster S, Yue Chongxi. *Herbal Emissaries: Bringing Chinese Herbs to the West*. Rochester, VT: Healing Arts Press; 1992.

Jiao SD. *Ten Lectures on the Use of Formulas from the Personal Experience of Jiao Shu De*. Brooklyn, MA: Paradigm Publications; 2005.

Jiao SD. *Ten Lectures on the Use of Medicinals from the Personal Experience of Jiao Shu De*. Brooklyn, MA: Paradigm Publications; 2001.

Jiao SD. *Case Studies on Pattern Identification*. Brooklyn, MA: Paradigm Publications; 2006.

MacLean W, Lyttleton J. *Clinical Handbook of Internal Medicine Vols I and II*. Macarthur, Australia: University of Western Sydney Press; 1998.

Scheid V et al. *Formulas and Strategies*. 2nd ed. Seattle: Eastland Press; 2009.

Wu Y, Fischer W. *Practical Therapeutics of Traditional Chinese Medicine*. Brookline, MA: Paradigm Publications; 1997.

Chinese Dietetics

There are few reliable books on Traditional Chinese Medicine dietetics. Many Western authors incorporate a limited discussion of traditional dietetic principles into substantially Western perspectives on health and diet, such as macrobiotics or whole foods nutrition. While these integrative efforts may be valuable, the texts we list below engage traditional Chinese dietetics on its own terms and represent its practices accurately. We particularly recommend Jeorg Kastner's *Chinese Nutrition Therapy* (2009) as probably the most useful comprehensive textbook on this subject available in English. *Chinese Medicated Diet* (Enqin Zhang 1990), while challenging to read, conveys a fully traditional perspective on Chinese dietetics. Bob Flaws' *Book of Jook* (2001) introduces the Western reader to a distinctive Chinese cuisine that is very important in the therapeutic application of Chinese dietetics.

Cai JF. *Eating Your Way to Health: Dietotherapy in Traditional Chinese Medicine*. Beijing: Foreign Languages Press; 1993.

Flaws B. *Book of Jook: Chinese Medicinal Porridges, A Healthy Alternative to the Typical Western Breakfast*. Boulder, CO: Blue Poppy Press; 2001.

Kastner J, MD, LAc. *Chinese Nutrition Therapy*. 2nd ed. Stuttgart: Thieme; 2009.

Liu J. *Chinese Dietary Therapy*. Edinburgh: Churchill Livingstone; 1995.

Maclean W, Lyttleton J. *Clinical Handbook of Internal Medicine. Vol. 2: Spleen and Stomach*. Penrith: University of Western Sydney; 2002.

Zhang E, ed. *Chinese Medicated Diet*. Shanghai: Publishing House of Shanghai College of Traditional Chinese Medicine; 1990.

Zhao Z, Ellis G. *The Healing Cuisine of China: 300 Recipes for Vibrant Health and Longevity*. Rochester, VT: Healing Arts Press; 1998.

Qi Gong

There are innumerable "how-to" titles about *qi gong*, representing many different styles and thousands of masters. Rather than inadvertently leave out one or more masters or traditions of practice, we have chosen a small selection of books that we feel provide a general point of access to the wide-ranging topic of *qi gong*. These books are written by experts in the field but are by no means exhaustive.

Cohen KS. *The Way of Qigong*. New York: Ballantine Books; 1997.

Ding L. *Transmitting the Qi along the Meridian: Meridian Qigong*. Beijing: Foreign Languages Press; 1988.

Jwing Ming Yang. *The Root of Chinese Chi Kung—The Secret of Chi Kung Training*. Wolfeboro, NH: Yang's Martial Arts Association; 1989.

Liang SY, Wu WC. *Qi Gong Empowerment*. East Providence: The Way of the Dragon Publishing; 1996.

MacRitchie J. *Chi Kung: Cultivating Personal Energy*. Rockport, MA: Element Books; 1993.

Réquéna Y. *Qi Gong Gymnastique Chinoise de Santé & de Longévité*. Paris: Guy Trédaniel; 1998.

Réquéna Y. *La Gymnastique des Gens Heureux: Qi Gong*. Paris: Guy Trédaniel; 2003.

Websites

http://www.feeltheqi.com.

Tai Ji Quan

Although how-to books on *tai ji quan's* ten or more schools abound, there are few scholarly studies of *tai ji's* history and seminal literature. The following titles cut through myth and parochialism to present *tai ji's* origins and development, primary sources, and role in Chinese culture in an objective and unbiased fashion. They also include ample bibliographies for further reading.

Davis B. *The Taijiquan Classics: An Annotated Translation*. Berkeley, CA: North Atlantic Books; 2004.

Wile D. *Lost T'ai-chi Classics from the Late Ch'ing Dynasty*. Albany, NY: State University of New York Press; 1996.

Acupuncture Research: An Overview

Staying abreast of research in Traditional Chinese Medicine requires a constant engagement with recently published journal articles. This topic is discussed in the chapter on Research, and guidance is provided to the reader. The books below provide useful perspectives on the conduct and understanding of research in Traditional Chinese Medicine, or summarize the results of research in specific areas up to the date of publication. *Clinical Acupuncture: Scientific Basis* edited by Stux and Hammerschlag (2001), although slightly dated, remains the most complete single text on developments in acupuncture research. *Acupuncture Research* by Hugh MacPherson (2007) offers the most up-to-date insights on issues confronting acupuncture research.

Bensoussan A. *The Vital Meridian*. Edinburgh: Churchill Livingstone, 1991.

Flaws B, Chace C. *Recent TCM Research from China: 1991–94*. Boulder, CO: Blue Poppy Press; 1994.

Lewith G, Jonas WB, Walach H. *Clinical Research in Complementary Therapies*. Edinburgh: Churchill Livingstone; 2002.

MacPherson H, Hammerschlag R, Lewith G, Schnyer R. *Acupuncture Research: Strategies for Building an Evidence Base*. London: Elsevier; 2007.

Stux G, Hammerschlag R, eds. *Clinical Acupuncture: Scientific Basis*. Berlin: Springer; 2001.

Photos and Illustrations

Front cover: Thomas Gefaell, Thomas Möller, Michael McCarthy, Kevin Ergil; pages 5A, 25C, 43B: Patrick Ryan; pages 5B, 13A, 167A, 173A, 175A, 181A-D, 327B: Bob Felt/ Paradigm Publications; pages 7A, 17B, 27B, 31B, 41A, 337A: Angelika-M. Findgott; page 9A: photolibrary; page 11A: David Sibai; pages 11B and C, 47A: Yuhuan Grant; page 23B: Velia Wortman Chow; page 25A: Julien Mohr; page 27A: Ahazan; page 31C: Alastair Clark; page 33B: Kate James; page 35B: Amrit MacIntyre; page 37A: China Purmed GmbH; page 43A: Ralph Harpuder; page 95A: Corbis; pages 107B, 161A, 163A, 169A, 175B, 185A, 359B: Marnae and Kevin Ergil; page 121: Markus Voll; pages 161B, 195C: 3B Scientific/Stefan Baudis; page 197A: Raphael Nogier; page 219A: Karl Wesker; pages 301A and B: Christine Zilka; page 327A: Thomas Langer; page 341A: imagesource; page 341B: Corel Stock; pages 343A and B: MEV; pages 347A and B, 355B, 357A, 361A-C, 363A and B, 365A and B: Imaginechina; page 351A: Sunya Dickman; page 355A: Asociaso Catalana Kun Fu; page 357B: Corbis.

Calligraphies on pages 9B, 13B, 19B, 23A, 325A, and 333A: Tan Sheng Yan; calligraphies on page 323B: Helmut Magel.

The publisher wishes to thank Kevin Ergil for taking more than 70 photos for chapters that he did not author.

Index

Page numbers in *italics* refer to illustrations or tables